FOOD SCIENCE AND TECHNOLOGY SERIES

This publishing programme provides an organised coverage on food science for professional technologists, research workers, and students in universities and polytechnics.

Series Editors:
Professor E. D. Morton, Head of Food Science,
Queen Elizabeth College, University of London;

Dr. R. Scott, formerly Reading University,

and **Dr. R. Osner**, Sheffield City Polytechnic

FUNDAMENTALS OF FOOD CHEMISTRY
W. HEIMANN, Director, Institute for Food Chemistry, University of Karlsruhe, Germany.

HYGIENIC DESIGN AND OPERATION OF FOOD PLANT
Edited by RONALD JOWITT, National College of Food Technology, University of Reading

HANDBOOK OF DOMESTIC ENGINEERING
D. KIRK and A. MILSON, Sheffield City Polytechnic.

DESIGN AND OPERATION OF CATERING EQUIPMENT
D. KIRK and A. MILSON, Sheffield City Polytechnic.

HYGIENIC DESIGN AND OPERATION OF FOOD PLANT

Editor:
RONALD JOWITT
National College of Food Technology,
University of Reading

Published for the
SOCIETY OF CHEMICAL
INDUSTRY, London

by
ELLIS HORWOOD LTD.,
Publishers, Chichester

First published in 1980 by

ELLIS HORWOOD LIMITED
Market Cross House, Cooper Street, Chichester, West Sussex, PO19 1EB, England

The publisher's colophon is reproduced from James Gillison's drawing of the ancient Market Cross, Chichester.

Distributors:

Australia, New Zealand, South-east Asia:
Jacaranda-Wiley Ltd., Jacaranda Press,
JOHN WILEY & SONS INC.,
G.P.O. Box 859, Brisbane, Queensland 40001, Australia.

Europe, Africa:
JOHN WILEY & SONS LIMITED
Baffins Lane, Chichester, West Sussex, England.

The Americas, Japan, The Phillipines:
AVI PUBLISHING COMPANY
250 Post Road East, Westport, Connecticut 06880, U.S.A.

British Library Cataloguing in Publication Data
Hygienic design and operation of food plant. –
(Ellis Horwood food science and technology series).
1. Food industry and trade – Hygienic aspects
I. Jowitt, R
613.6'2 RC965.F58 79–40990
ISBN 0-85312-133-8 (Ellis Horwood Ltd., Publishers, Library Edition)
ISBN 0-85312-153-2 (Ellis Horwood Ltd., Publishers, Student Edition)
ISBN 0-87055-345-3 (The AVI Publishing Co.)

Typeset in Press Roman by Ellis Horwood Ltd.
Printed in Great Britain by Fakenham Press Ltd.

Table of Contents

Preface

In 1966, the Joint Technical Committee of the Food Manufacturers' Federation and the Food Machinery Association set up a working party on the Hygienic Design of Food Plant under the Chairmanship of David Shore (see 'Introduction'). The 'guide to good practice'† which it produced was published in 1967 and has remained the only text of its kind in Britain, although it endorsed the principles proposed by the American 3A Sanitary Standards Committee and published in *Food Processing* for October 1964 and April 1965.

In 1971 the Food Machinery Association was subsumed by the Process Plant Association, which later formed a Food Machinery Division, and the joint technical committee of the FMF-FMA lapsed until late 1978 when it was succeeded by a joint technical committee of the FMF Food Engineering Committee and representative of the Food Machinery Division of the PPA.

During the discussions that preceded this latest regrouping it was early recognized that the work of the previous joint technical committee in the field of hygienic design of food plant had been valuable and widely appreciated, but that the *guide to good practice* was now in need of updating and expansion to take account of developments in the intervening decade, to cover wider scope than the original, and to include hygienic aspects of food process plant *operation,* as this is clearly inseparable from consideration of the hygienic design of such plant.

However, after much deliberation that committee decided that it could not undertake such a task, but instead agreed to the alternative suggestion of jointly sponsoring a symposium on the subject with the prime objective of subsequent publication of the proceedings as a successor to the original *guide*, The present book is the result. Each of the chapters is a version of the corresponding paper presented at the symposium, adapted for publication; and the discussion which

† 'Hygienic Design of Food Plant: a guide to good practice with particular reference to the design of tanks, pumps and pipework', Food Manufacturers' Federation and Food Machinery Association, reproduced in Appendix, pp. 241–273.

followed likewise follows each chapter, in near original form, as recorded magnetically and in manuscript. Only one of the papers‡ presented has not become available for publication in this way.

It was felt that for completeness it would be valuable if the original *Guide* could also be reproduced in this volume. The Food Manufacturers' Federation's agreement to this is gratefully acknowledged.

The symposium, held on 19 and 20 April 1978 at the National College of Food Technology, was organized by the Food Engineering Panel of the Society of Chemical Industry on behalf of the FMF, the FMA, and the Food Research Association, Leatherhead. The contributions of the representatives of these bodies and others on the planning committee are recorded with appreciation, in particular that of Dr Arthur Brown, Secretary of the Planning Committee and of the Food Engineering Panel at the time.

The Committee records its thanks to the Chairmen of the four sessions, Mr D. T. Shore, Dr E. H. T. Hoblyn, Dr J. G. Davis, and Mr R. Jowitt.

Last but not least, the invaluable assistance of Mrs A. Pearson with the manuscripts and the record of the discussions is warmly acknowledged.

Ronald Jowitt
Weybridge
December 1978

‡ 'Post-process sanitation in can and pouch handling' by R. H. Thorpe (Campden Food Preservation R. A.).

Introduction

D. T. Shore, APV Co. Ltd.

The Process Plant Association, and before it the Food Machinery Association, recognized the contribution that engineers could make to design aspects other than the containment of material, the strength of components, and energy transfer in food equipment.

The FMA/FMF joint technical committee, in 1966, recognising the lack of a code of practice in the UK, set up a working party which, after some two years' deliberation, produced a booklet entitled 'Hygienic Design of Food Plant'. This document dealt specifically with the design of tanks, pumps, and pipework, and it remained an objective of that committee to see the work continued. It was hoped that the industry would, in a quiet way, develop an equivalent of the American 3A Standards which, with some additional or alternative State requirements, are common throughout the USA. No food equipment supplier would dream of putting equipment on the market which would fail to meet the 3A Standards. I am somewhat disappointed that with the disbanding of the PPA/FMF joint technical committee there has been no further study of the subject.

I have frequent opportunities to compare the design aspects of food plants engineered by a variety of suppliers throughout Europe and North America, and I would like, by way of introduction to the subject, to draw from my own experience and make a few general remarks.

1. A well-designed plant is no safeguard against bacterial infection or other contamination unless it is accompanied by sound instructions for its installation, operation, cleaning, and maintenance.
2. Factory management must ensure good housekeeping and, what is more, be constantly vigilant against any bad housekeeping.
3. We should recognize that there is no such thing as a foolproof plant or process, and man shows an extraordinary ingenuity in finding ways around the operating instructions if, in his view, his own method of working makes life a little easier. Simplicity will always pay off.

4. For successful operation of the plant, consideration at the layout and general design stage should include the engineer, the food chemist, and the microbiologist. In this way the operating procedures can be coupled with the necessary quality controls. I would add to this that success also requires that the agreed procedures are properly communicated to all those who must operate the plant.
5. Where are we going to with the plants of today or tomorrow? Certainly plants are becoming bigger, they are of greater capacity, and we are pumping more materials through longer pipelines. There is less inspection of internal surfaces and a greater reliance on automatic in-place cleaning. There is also automatic start-up and shut-down. While this provides less opportunity for human error, it also gives less chance of spotting that a performance error, has occurred.
6. Food processes are operating for much longer running periods, and for non-aseptic plants (they are the majority) this means that there is more bacteriological build-up in the plant as the run proceeds. There must, for product quality reasons, be safe levels set for this build-up. Often this is not recognised in the same way as, for example, the fouling of a plate heat exchanger where, after a long running period, there may be either an increased pressure drop or 'saturation' of the temperature control system. Such events would trigger an automatic cleaning procedure. If the change is only a bacterial build-up it might be undetected, and those in charge of quality control must, with the process engineers, determine the timing of satisfactory cleaning and sterilising routines.
7. Hygienic design of a very high standard is essential in the modern plant to minimize down-time for cleaning and sterilizing. With more concern for pollution it must be recognized that the minimum effective cleaning for any process cycle means minimum trade effluent, and the fewer the cleaning periods the less product loss by dilution with rinse water.

CHAPTER 1

Hygienic Design of Food Plants and Equipment

S. Holm, Alfa-Laval A.B.

INTRODUCTION

Hygiene in food plant is necessary for the prevention of food poisoning and to reduce food spoilage. The main factors affecting this are biological, but others such as chemical and physical factors also contribute.

The ideal way of absorbing nutrients is used by a foetus in its mother. In spite of the closed system: production – transportation – consumption, a special check must be carried out to ensure that the unborn consumer will not be affected by toxins or the wrong nutrients in the product. However, these nutrients are not usually regarded as food. It is only after the baby has been born that one talks about the absorption of nutritious matter from food. Initially the only difference is that the product is 'packed' to enable it to be, consumed at intervals instead of continuously. Considering the extremely good packing system used in this case, we are probably as close to the ideal situation as is possible.

Later, we move further and further away from this ideal situation into a system which is not so closed and direct. The real responsibility for the necessary hygienic precautions is then transferred to those who handle food intended for others. 'Handling' includes processing and other operations such as storage and transportation, as well as catering and food service.

As the biological effects can be devastating so far as the suitability of food is concerned, it is very important to understand something about microbial development and to be able to understand the consequences if unrestrained growth is permitted. A micro-organism's development takes place rapidly, as the following examples illustrate.

One bacterium is very small – about 0.01 mm long. If it were enlarged to a length of 6 cm then a normal human being (enlarged to the same scale) would be about 8500 m tall. As the bacterium is so minute it can hide in pores, cracks, and crevices. Reproduction, by fission, takes place rapidly—in about 20 minutes. If there are 1000 bacteria at 7 o'clock in the morning, by breakfast time (about

9 15 am) there would be about 128 000, and by lunch time (12 noon) there would be approximately 33 million.

Bacteria, yeasts, and fungi are the most important micro-organisms where food is concerned. Many of them have a beneficial effect and have been used for a long time in the production and preservation of food. However, there are others which are pathogenic or can spoil food and thereby render it unfit for human consumption. With this background it is easy to understand how important correct design of food equipment is.

Before dealing with equipment, some other important factors will be discussed.

BUILDINGS, MATERIALS, LAYOUT

It is extremely important that when architects design buildings for food installations they should consult a hygiene specialist. When the building costs are estimated, allowance should be made for proper hygiene.

The value of a well-coordinated project organization cannot be overestimated. Hygiene plays a very important part in nearly all the problems which arise, and it frequently influences the choice of the solution to the problem as well as deciding the costs. However, it is also important not to overestimate this: demands are different for different ranges of application. Different types of rooms in an industrial building may require different standards. There should be a classification of rooms which have similar hygienic demands. Certain rooms require a modest standard of hygiene, whereas others demand a very high standard.

Examples of types of premises requiring increasing standards of hygiene are:

1. Dry rooms which do not become dirty and require only dry cleaning.
2. Dry rooms which become dirty (for example, reception of raw materials). These should be scrubbed once a week.
3. Wet rooms:
   a) Very wet rooms which become dirty from, for example, soil. These require frequent flushing and scrubbing.
   b) Very wet rooms of varying temperature, for example process rooms. These require frequent flushing and cleaning with strong detergents.
4. Other rooms such as staff rooms, especially wash rooms and toilets. Here a very high standard of hygiene is required.

These requirements are complicated nowadays by the increasing demand for lower noise levels.

Ventilation

Ventilation is of great importance where hygiene is concerned, especially in rooms where excess heat produced has to be removed. The ventilation must be suited to the different types of rooms, and it is important that, in processing rooms in particular, it has the flexibility to meet the needs of any alterations in production which might occur.

Both the air intake and discharge often need filtration, and steps to prevent draughts must also be taken.

The cost of an optimum ventilation system can be considerable but must be regarded as necessary in order to achieve a high standard of personal and production hygiene.

EQUIPMENT DESIGN

'Machines, equipment, containers, and other equipment used when handling food should not be of such a nature that the food is in danger of becoming unfit for human consumption.'

A legal paragraph can be worded in this manner, and one must work accordingly. It does not say anything concrete but requires that one lives up to the principle.

The designer is required to design both machines and plants in such a way that the results will be satisfactory. The planning of a plant is just as important as the design of a machine. A good machine can be dangerous if the planning is bad. The reverse is also possible, if less common.

Today, good hygiene is a necessity in all food industries. The consumer has the right to demand both good quality and good shelf life. Mechanization and automation have made great progress in the cleaning of equipment which was previously cleaned by hand. In earlier days all the machines were opened every day, and if certain parts were not specially hygienic they were given an extra cleaning. Then came CIP (Cleaning In Place). At first, control was by a single panel with push buttons. Now it is fully automatic, using a large automatic panel, and recently has become computer controlled. This will not affect the cleaning efficiency of individual components, but the computer helps to optimize the total cleaning result.

The designer is now burdened with the responsibility of ensuring that the equipment is properly cleaned by means of automatic cleaning – month after month. He has to reckon with the fact that the equipment will not be taken apart before it falls apart. Naturally there are periodic checks, but regular inspection of 1000 valves, for example, is so extensive that one cannot be sure of it, and one should design as if inspections did not exist – and then inspect anyway!

A CIP system often means that a cleaning solution flows through a system which is separated only by a valve from another system through which product flows. Cross-contamination of these two liquids – even if they both happen to be clean – must be regarded as unhygienic, so it is important to ensure that the liquids cannot mix. In addition, by having a higher pressure in the product line, one can make certain that any leakage that might occur is of product into the cleaning solution and not vice versa.

A safer solution to the problem is to use two valves, mounted and connected so that there is always an opening towards the atmosphere between the two liquids. Any leakage that might occur will flow to a leakage area where no pressure can build up – if the drain opening is large enough. The valves in such a system are interlocked in relation to each other, and the process cannot start until all the valves are in the correct position. This system is safer but more expensive than the former because it requires twice the number of valves at certain points and also more piping.

Choice of materials

One could say that it is easy to choose materials for machines used in the food industry; that is, for those parts in contact with the food product or which are used as protection for the machines. The other parts come into the category of normal machine construction.

Stainless steel is the only generally usable construction material in the food industry today, even if it does have its weaknesses. For example, sometimes it tolerates a solution such as brine, and sometimes it does not. This depends on many things – concentration, temperature, crevices, flow rate, cleaning etc. An alternative material is used when stainless steel cannot tolerate a certain liquid or when a cheaper material such as plastic can be used.

Normally only two grades of stainless steel are used: AISI 304 and AISI 316 – a molybdenum alloy stainless steel which is acid-proof. Both are weldable and can be machined by normal machine tools. As a bar stock AISI 316 is approximately 30% more expensive per kg than AISI 304 (1978 prices).

AISI 304 is nearly always used externally as it is needed only for protecting the machine from the atmosphere, water, and sometimes spilled liquids. One must choose between AISI 304 and AISI 316 for parts which are in contact with the product. AISI 304 tolerates most food products which do not contain acids. It also tolerates the most common cleaning solutions and is suitable for most purposes. AISI 316 is used for more aggressive liquids such as juices which contain fruit acids.

If a machine is designed for use with a variety of products some of which might be acid, it is often more economical to use AISI 316 for all the parts which come into contact with the product – especially if the machines are manufactured in large runs, particularly where lighter constructions are concerned. For example, only a few *tanks* are made at a time and usually to order, so one can choose the material for each individual case. It is not possible to specify the limit where one can standardize onthe use of one material, because it depends on how much stainless steel the construction contains, the production run, the stock, intracompany interest, etc.

There are also other types of stainless steel – some with a lower chromium or nickel content and some which have other alloying materials added, such as niobium, titanium, or tantalum alloyed with AISI 316, mostly for weldability. In addition to these, pure titanium and Hastelloy are obtainable. Generally speaking the low-alloy stainless steels tolerate only water and weaker chemicals, and the more 'exotic' metals such as titanium are so exclusive that those who work with liquids which require these materials are usually familiar with them. It is said 'Any food which requires machines made of titanium is not fit for human consumption', but certain liquids which contain chlorine may require titanium.

Bronze, including chrome-plated bronze, can be used for different external parts of the machines. On the other hand beware of copper or copper alloys if they may come into contact with oil or fat, as copper hastens oxidation. In such cases keep to stainless steel or possibly aluminium; but bear in mind that aluminium does not tolerate certain liquid detergents.

Rubber and plastics really need a chapter to themselves, but let a few general pieces of advice suffice. Some of the grades of rubber and certain plastics contain lead or other toxic components.

Before one decides upon a certain grade of rubber or plastic which will come into contact with food one must obviously make sure that it is suitable for the particular food. It is always best to consult the manufacturer or his agent. One should also check other properties such as whether nitrile rubber deteriorates, or whether it resists oil (EP rubber has good temperature qualities but does not tolerate oils) and if it may also have a relatively high compression set. Does the plastic I intend using tolerate detergents and sterilizing temperature?

One also has to exercise a little care where carbon seals are concerned, because different substances such as lead, are sometimes used for impregnating the carbon or for increasing its durability.

PRINCIPLES OF HYGIENIC DESIGN

The most important aim is to avoid pockets and crevices, the present author's definition being that a pocket is relatively large whereas a crevice is narrow and deep.

Normally, a pocket is nothing to be afraid of: it is more important to avoid crevices. For example, my company has studied a case where a plate heat exchanger is opened every six months. A pocket forms between each pair of plates. However, it is large enough to be cleaned. After all, a pump is only a very large pocket if it is assembled with the outlet upwards – and it does get cleaned.

It is the small crevices which can cause trouble, because the detergent solution is not able to rinse them clean.

Fixed packings

Some pipe fittings might create a crevice which is rather difficult to clean, or a crevice which is shallow but becomes clean. If the crevice has been eliminated, the packing may be easy to clean, but a disadvantage is that the packing can easily be sucked into the pipe if there is a vacuum in the pipe and if the fitting is not tightened properly. This disadvantage disappears when the ISO and screwed and clamp fittings are used. In these fittings the rubber is formed so that it remains in place even when there is a vacuum in the pipe.

Packings in places where flow velocities are high should not fit loosely or be glued, but should preferably be clamped firmly. Examples are valve seats and plugs where great forces affect the packing during the moment of opening and closing. A glued packing can easily come loose, resulting in a leak; but before this happens cracks may appear in the cement, and bacteria may grow.

Rotating seals

There are many available types of mechanical shaft seals, but the majority of them are unsuitable for food as they cannot be cleaned-in-place. When choosing such a seal one must be extremely careful and also consider any undesirable component in the material.

Radial shaft seals should not be used for food unless they are specially designed.

Seal-flushing liquids can be used with double shaft seals. Water is usually used for vacuum purposes, for example in evaporation plant, in order to avoid air being sucked into the product, and also to keep the seals clean when sticky liquids such as sugar solutions are pumped. Steam is used for aseptic seal purposes. During operation the steam pressure should not exceed atmospheric pressure as the seal can become dry and damaged.

Reciprocating movement

The observations made on fixed seals also apply to O rings.

Lip seals efficiently scrape away the liquid from the moving stem. A sealing lip should also be turned towards the atmospheric side in order to seal if there is vacuum on the machine.

For aseptic purposes one can seal with bellows or a diaphragm or use a barrier medium in order to avoid bacteria following the movement of the stem in any scratches which might occur. Where there is a barrier medium the barrier chamber must be longer than the stroke, if the mandrel does not move so slowly that it is sterilized during the stroke.

Liquids containing chlorine, such as common salt and hypochlorite, are particularly dangerous in small crevices because free chlorine can form and attack the material. In this case it is extremely important that crevices, if there are any, are large and that the equipment is rinsed immediately after use.

Undrained Pockets

Undrained pockets can often be avoided by mounting pumps and valves etc. correctly and, for example, by maintaining a level lower edge in pipes of varying bore. The pipelines should slope in the right direction, and it should be possible to blow them empty. When CIP cleaning the equipment, there must be no part where the flow pattern causes a 'shadow' which does not get cleaned.

SOLID PRODUCTS

Most of the foregoing observations refer mainly to liquid products, but quite a lot can be applied to solid products, such as the processing of meat and vegetables. Automatic cleaning has recently been introduced at more and more points where these products are handled. For example, a conveyor in the form of a wide chain passes through a box for a short distance. The conveyor can then be cleaned automatically after use with the help of cleaning nozzles. A great deal of manual work can be saved, as this type of conveyor is common in the food industry. It is very much more difficult when it comes to machines such as grinders and certain packaging machines. These often have to be completely dismantled for cleaning, but the dismantling could be made simpler in many cases and involve fewer parts. These parts should be easy to remove. The spaces which are then to be cleaned should be open and incline outwards so that all product material and cleaning liquids can easily drain from the machine. Much has already been done in this field, but I believe that the food industry could encourage the manufacturers of the machines to make their machines easier to clean – and eventually automatically cleanable – whether it is a filling machine for juices or mayonnaise or a meat-mincing machine. This could be achieved by built-in devices or with extra equipment. It might mean an increase in the price of the machine, but if manual labour is considerably reduced that should mean a reduction in cost overall.

CONCLUSION

Whatever the specialists might do to attain a satisfactory result, their work can be frustrated. A well-designed machine can be neglected, and because of insufficient service it can be in such a condition that it does not meet the necessary requirements.

It is necessary to understand that good maintenance and handling of the equipment is of the utmost importance. This can happen only if the staff are sufficiently well-trained and motivated. There is possibly a risk that, with more and more use of automatic processes, one can be led to believe that it is less important for the staff to be careful and particular.

DISCUSSION

Mr J. Brentnall (Mars Limited): Mine is more an endorsement of the remarks that were made that with the remote control plants we are moving, as other people are, to remote control rooms where the operating staff are based rather than being directly interfaced with the plant. We are finding just this problem that the cleaning of the plant is not so good as it was because the operators are remote from the actual equipment. I have no answer to this but it does endorse the point.

Mr D. T. Shore (Chairman): Would you like to comment, Mr Holm? Is the removal of the plant operators in the control room away from the plant influencing the effectiveness of the operation, particularly cleaning?

Mr Holm (Alfa-Laval A.B): Oh yes, I would agree to that, and I think you could say generally there is a similar debate going on on the automation side. Shall you have a central automation room or shall you automate locally? In computers should you have one computer for complete control or a minor computer for each of the processes? One should not take all the people away from the process room. It is funny that it has an influence but it has – you should keep some of the process operators in the room.

Mr R. Jowitt (NCFT): Could I ask Mr Holm, Mr Chairman, if he can put any figures to the amount of enlargement of crevices in order to make them into pockets? I think he gave a qualitative distinction between the two; could he give a quantitative distinction and how much does this depend upon individual circumstances such as the method of cleaning used, detergent systems, nature of the soil?

Mr Holm: I am sorry I don't have any figure to give you; that is of course dependent on different things, but I agree that if I say that a pocket is a large crevice, I should know what I am talking about, but it is depending on the state of the product passing the crevices and so on. But in the case I quoted it was very narrow initially and was opened to, I think, 1.5 mm or so. But it depends on the product which is deposited. The important thing is that it is almost always the case that you can open a crevice to a pocket.

CHAPTER 2

An "Emblem" to Denote Hygienic Standards of Food Plant Design

K. Cook, Henry Simon Ltd.

In the summer of 1976 the first executive meeting of the newly formed Food Process Plant Association was held at the Association's headquarters in London.

Discussion revealed that the executive was clearly concerned that unless it could publish a programme which offered some positive commercial benefit to food machinery companies then the section membership would be unlikely to grow, and would make of doubtful value the very existence of the section. All present were reluctant to include the Health and Safety at work Act or to make noise about noise. After all, those subjects were being debated ad nauseam in a multitude of committees, and it was considered that to publish an initial agenda containing these items would hardly set the world on fire.

Further discussions revealed that several members of the committee had experience of selling in North America, and all other factors being equal had found difficulty in establishing themselves until such time as they had a reference point within the United States. Offshore references were often not acceptable, and even when they were the recurrent problem seemed to be 'I would like the machine/plant but does it meet United States hygiene/health standards?' There was a general awareness among the members present that in most cases we did not know if our machinery/plant met American regulations. Indeed, we were only too conscious of the fact that with the advent of the Health and Safety at Work Act we may not even be complying with the UK regulations.

Here, then, seemed to be an area in which we could work to the benefit of PPA members in particular and the UK food industry in general. If an acceptable and recognized standard of hygiene could be established for a range of food manufacturing equipment within the UK, then possibly the standard could be submitted to the United States and Common Market authorities for consideration and possible acceptance.

You may recall that in 1976 'The Britain Has Had It Brigade' were holding considerable sway; nevertheless, we felt that British engineering institutions, standards institutes, and inspection bodies were still highly regarded worldwide, and their assistance and seal of approval properly used would undoubtedly benefit British industry.

To save ourselves from possible wasted effort an approach was made to the Department of Industry sponsoring branch to ensure that the proposed scheme would not contravene the Trade Descriptions or any other Act. Conditional clearance was given on the understanding that the scheme would not have Government backing, although it was recognized that the scheme would have a possible role to play in any future EEC policy-making on hygiene. The Department of Industry also suggested that the Environmental Health Officers' Association should be invited to participate in the development of the scheme.

It was quite clear that unless the scheme was acceptable to and recognized by the British food industry it had no chance of getting off the ground internationally, so to achieve acceptance and recognition we considered that a reasonable approach was to involve the food manufacturers as early as possible, ask for their opinion and if this was favourable to seek their active cooperation. A prospectus was prepared and presented to the Food Manufacturers' Federation with a request for a meeting with a representative committee. The prospectus contained a précis of the then situation:

At present in the UK there is a general requirement under the Food Hygiene (General) Regulations 1970 (S.I. 1970 No. 1172) regarding cleanliness of equipment as follows:

> 'Articles or equipment with which food comes into contact, or is liable to come into contact, in the course of a food business shall be kept clean and with the exception of non-returnable containers, shall be so constructed, be of such materials and be kept in such good order, repair and condition as to:
> a) enable them to be thoroughly cleaned;
> b) prevent, so far as is reasonably practicable, any matter being absorbed by them; and
> c) prevent, so far as is reasonably practicable, any risk of contamination of the food'.

This is, however, too general to be of direct help to designers, manufacturers, and users. To achieve the objective of the Regulations in relation to equipment, more specific guidance is needed, and we are strongly of the opinion that this would be best provided by a code of practice. It is suggested that such a code should be largely based on the principles outlined in the American document, 'Sanitary Design' (Printed in *Food Processing Catalog* 1964/5).

The principles, seven in all, were endorsed by the joint technical committee, Food Manufacturers' Federation/Food Machinery Association, responsible for the preparation of the publication in the late 1960s of *Hygienic Design of Food Plant – a guide to good practice.*

An outline of the code and the five principles on which a minimum standard could be established were given:

1. All surfaces in contact with food must be inert to the food under the conditions of use and must not migrate to or be absorbed by the food.
2. All surfaces in contact with food must be smooth and non-porous so that tiny particles of food, bacteria, or insect eggs are not caught in microscopic surface crevices and become difficult to dislodge, thus becoming a potential source of contamination.
3. The equipment should be so designed that all surfaces in contact with food can be readily disassembled for manual cleaning.
4. Equipment must be so designed as to protect the contents from external contamination.
5. The exterior or non-product contact surfaces should be so arranged to prevent harbouring of soils, bacteria, or pests in and on the equipment itself as well as in its contact with other equipment, and as far as possible with floors, walls, and hanging supports.

It is proposed that the compilation of the code of practice should be undertaken by a joint working party consisting of representatives from the Food Manufacturers' Federation (FMF), the Food Process Machinery Section of the Process Plant Association (PPA) and the Association of Public Health Inspectors.

Appropriate British Standards will be incorporated, and cooperation may be necessary with the BSI in certain aspects.

In drawing up the code due attention will also be paid to any relevant standards, codes, directives, regulations applying or in prospect in the EEC, USA (for example, regulations), or other countries.

After digesting our submission the Food Manufacturers' Federation agreed to a meeting which turned out to be the precusor to the establishment of the joint working party consisting of members from the Food Manufacturers' Federation, the Association of Public Health Inspectors, and the Process Plant Association.

For several months we had fought to have our ideas accepted, despite the many buckets of cold water which from time to time had been poured over them; and it was most heartening to find enthusiastic encouragement from members of the Food Manufacturers' Federation.

Help came in several forms: ideas, guidance, and offers of assistance in testing involving both people and premises.

The working party quickly knocked into shape the five principles which ultimately turned out to be six, which in their final form are:

1. All surfaces in contact with food should be inert to the food under the conditions of use, and constituents from their surfaces must not migrate into the food or be absorbed by the food in quantities which could endanger health.
2. All surfaces in contact with food should be smooth and non-porous so that particles of food, bacteria, or insect eggs are not caught in microscopic sur-

face discontinuities and become difficult to dislodge, thus becoming a potential source of contamination.
3. Equipment should be so designed internally to provide the minimum number of crevices and dead spaces where any particles could collect.
4. The equipment should be so designed that all surfaces in contact with food can be properly cleaned. In accordance with current practice clean-in-place techniques are preferred, but where this is not practicable the design must allow for the ready dismantling of the relevant parts for manual cleaning.
5. Equipment should be so designed as to protect the contents from external contamination including accidental ingress of foreign matter, for example bolts, nuts, washers, and gaskets etc.
6. The exterior or non-product contact surfaces should be arranged to prevent harbouring of soils, bacteria, or pests in and on the equipment.'

Having disposed of these six points attention was then focussed on what to test, and who should test it. On *who* should test, it was agreed that it had to be an independent body of stature, the actual choice being left to a small subcommittee. The subject of *what* to test, however, was not so simply resolved, in fact is still not completely so. There was considerable initial support for keeping things simple – for example consideration of surface finish, internal finish of pipework, the design of valves and pumps, etc., but the PPA members felt that unless complete machines were included at an early stage the scheme would lose its impact. Eventually an offer to provide a list of machines which were recurrently found to be unhygienic was accepted, and to date here the matter rests with a list in the course of preparation. When the list is finally established the action will be to approach manufacturers within the PPA to advise them of the situation and invite them to submit their revised designs for consideration.

For criticism and testing the Leatherhead Food Research Association has kindly agreed to cooperate. The detailed methods and costs have yet to be established. These will be determined when the first hygienic designs appear over the horizon.

Amongst all the serious committee work a more lighthearted exercise was the choosing of the actual emblem for the scheme. This was eventually achieved, and it is shown in Fig. 2.1.

In following our chosen course we accept that we are laying ourselves open to criticism from the 'purists', but our declared aim is to help the British food machinery manufacturer to sell his products by giving a guarantee of an acceptable hygienic design. Of course, many other considerations will affect the user's final choice of machinery, but all other considerations being equal we feel that the emblem scheme will carry some weight.

I had hoped to be able to announce at this conference that the scheme had really got off the ground and the first machinery examined and approved. Unfortunately this is not the case, and we expect that another 6 to 12 months will elapse before equipment bearing the emblem begins to make an appearance.

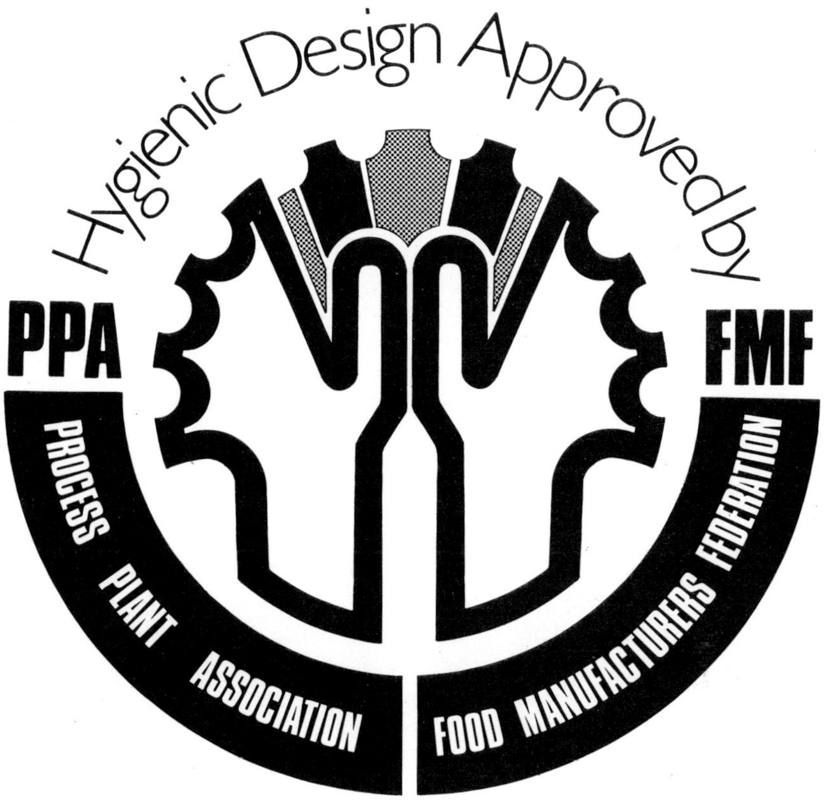

Fig. 2.1 – The Emblem.

DISCUSSION

Mr T. Cleather (APV Company): The scheme, as outlined, certainly seems highly laudable; I am sure we will all be grateful when it arrives, but I understand it is going to apply to unit items of equipment. Now, in a complete process plant, the items are interconnected by sections of pipework which can provide a serious hazard in themselves if they are not properly designed. How does the working party view this aspect, as far as approval is concerned?

Mr K. Cook: This really comes back to the long arguments and discussions that took place in committee of exactly where we should start and, of course, logically I suppose you would start with surface finish, but you are then going to spend, I think, a lifetime without making any progress. Obviously there is a commercial element to this from the food machinery manufacturers' side. In looking for somewhere to start, we felt that we could find unit pieces of equipment that the finger can be pointed at consistently. There are a number of pieces of equipment that are used in the food industry that were never designed for the food industry: for instance; sieving or dust-collecting equipment which is used in the food industry but never actually designed for it. Those are the areas that we want to try to look at first. I think it will give a bigger pay back, and we can then say 'yes we have achieved something'. How it will develop after that, time will tell, but I think to look at complete process plants and all the pipes and all the couplings and everything else to start with just wouldn't be practical.

Dr G. B. Lawson (Unilever Research Ltd): I would like to ask Mr Cook how the emblem scheme committee is going to deal with the difficult task of deciding when a piece of equipment is acceptable for one part of the food industry and not for another. For example, some of our products are very stable products, and hygiene with such products is less important than the other end of the spectrum – fish and meat, for example, where hygiene becomes a much more important consideration. A single piece of machinery bearing an emblem might be perfectly acceptable to one and might be a disaster for another.

Mr K. Cook: Yes I accept that. I was going to say I'll duck the question and say that it all depends on how we get on with the Leatherhead Food RA. We have to get the thing off the ground, and we are obviously not going to pick pieces of equipment initially that are used right across the food industry. I think to start with we are going to have to pick things which are simple; but, having said that, we are also looking for equipment which is used regularly. I don't think there is any point at all in picking a piece of equipment which is *very* highly specialized and which we can spend years on. So we are going to pick simple equipment which is probably not designed for the food industry but is universally used right throughout it. So I duck the question because I don't know what the answer will be.

Mr J. Priestly, (Associated Dairies Ltd.): Just a suggestion: would it be useful in your code of practice that you intend to produce, to insist that meaningful cleaning schedules should be provided with all approved machinery that you intend to market? At the moment we usually find that when machinery arrives in the factory or dairy, we have then to start to produce the cleaning schedule for the machinery at the factory.

Mr. K. Cook: Yes, I think that it is a very useful suggestion, and from the machinery manufacturers' side I think that all are very very conscious that this kind of thing has got to be done now, bearing in mind things like the Health and Safety at Work Act, because I think if you don't lay down how your plant should be maintained then you are leaving yourself wide open to criticism in the future.

Mr J. Milledge (NCFT): What sort of yardstick are you going to use to measure hygienic design? It may well be a very simple matter to regard certain pieces of equipment as being unhygienic, but the lack of quantitative criteria for measuring hygienic design could lose the emblem scheme some of its impact.

Mr K. Cook: What we are going to do is to work out with Leatherhead just what the code of practice and the six points that have been laid down mean in terms of the piece of equipment or the type of equipment we are looking at at the time; and, for instance, equipment that is used for handling powders will need assessing in a completely different way from something which, for instance, is handling fresh meat or fish. So I think it will be done from a practical point of view rather than from a theoretical or absolute point of view.

Mr R. Jowitt, (NCFT): Mr Chairman, if I could follow that up, I don't think it is a distinction so much between 'theoretical' and 'practical' but between 'quantitative' and 'qualitative'! in other words, if you can say that hold-up of this particular vessel is so many millilitres per square foot whereas the other is so much less, then the other is self-evidently more hygienic. I share Mr. Milledge's fears that unless you can quantify the criteria by which the alternative pieces of equipment are judged, you are putting somebody in an awfully hot seat who has to pronounce judgement on competitive equipment and say that subjectively one is more or less hygienic than the other. Is it intended that the basis of the award of the emblem will be quantitative rather than qualitative?

Mr K. Cook: It will, I hope, be quantitative. This is the whole purpose of going to the Leatherhead Food RA; and although we are rather like a sponsoring body, we certainly will not be the inspection body, and based on the code that we have laid down we will expect them to come up with the quantitative method of measuring the hygienic design of pieces of equipment.

Mr W. E. Whitman, (Leatherhead Food RA): A number of these points are of course of extreme interest to us because we are very much learning in this field and, until we have actually got some pieces of plant to cut our teeth on, it is very difficult to know precisely how we are going to be able to apply any set of criteria apart from a general adherence to the principles which have been laid down as fundamental. We will, wherever possible, move toward systems of quantitation. The problems of using microbiological standards of cleanliness are enormous because as soon as one has put sterilizing solutions through a piece of plant that even has been improperly cleaned, the chances are that the population of remaining micro-organisms are down to such a low level that it is very difficult to establish relative degrees of cleanliness; and, although I think I can fairly claim we have some of the best microbioligists in the country available to us they are not at all happy at the moment with the idea of applying microbiological techniques to assess cleanliness in a quantitative manner. So I think to some extent we are going to come back to physical measurement techniques, and to some extent also we are going to have to come back to questions of judgement, and there I hope we will not be dependent on judgements of individuals who may be prejudiced but of some form of jury system where three or four well reputed and independent people can each look at and pass views on the drawings and on the equipment itself. I am conscious that what I have said is not a complete solution to the problem. It is by no means as cut and dried and as hard and fast as I should very much like it to be, but I don't really at the moment think that there is any more positive answer that I can offer.

Mr P. C. Stauber, (British American Tobacco Co Ltd): I would suggest that a simple way of assessing whether the machine is hygienic or not is the effect on the product. I would suggest that if the machine in the first instance does not make an *uncontrolled* contribution to the outgoing portion of the product, then it is a reasonably sound machine, and it isn't a difficult matter in fact to quantify that, whereas it might be very difficult to quantify whether or not a cleaning procedure has removed the last few bugs from that machinery.

Mr D. Newman, (Urschel International Ltd.): Whilst I appreciate, and think very laudable, the concept of the emblem scheme in producing these high standards of food machinery, there is obviously the commercial aspect in that you state you are promoting a high standard of *British* made processing machinery. Does this place imported machinery such as made by my company at a disadvantage ultimately in not being able to fly the emblem? As I understand it, the PPA excludes companies not manufacturing in this country such as ourselves and thereby makes it impossible for us to fly this emblem.

Mr K. Cook: that is in fact not so. One of the conditions of getting Government permission is that any company can apply for the emblem.

Dr Lawson (Unilever Research): Does that mean the initiative will be from the manufacturer of a piece of equipment to make such equipment available for tests, or will the committee give some guidance calling for manufacturers of, say, dicing machinery or whatever to make their machinery available for testing?

Mr K. Cook: Well, initially, obviously what we will try to do is to select equipment which is being made currently by PPA members. Obviously there is an advantage in dealing with PPA because you have some idea of what machinery is going to be looked at. But in the longer term if, for instance, a particular type of machinery is obviously being tested and the emblem awarded, then there is nothing to stop anybody that manufactures that particular type of equipment putting it forward for testing.

Mr D. T. Shore: I'd like to say a few words from my privileged position in the Chair.

Reference was made in my opening remarks and also by Mr Cook to the American 3A standard. What we have to remember about any emblem system is that it cannot in itself constitute the entire design criteria any more than designing process equipment to the American ASME standard can. You can merely say that you have complied with it, but you may still have your own in-house rules of design to suit your own methods of manufacture, and indeed so that the plant will stand up. It could well be that if I design a vessel to emblem standards it would fall over the first time it was put on the floor. That's an absurd example just to illustrate.

The second point I would make is that there is a serious problem in trying to get quantitative answers. Reference was made earlier to 'the effect on the product'. Again in my opening remarks I carefully drew the distinction between the few plants that must operate *aseptically,* in which case you can have a very strict standard and make a measurement, and the more common type of plant which will have a bacterial build-up during periods of operation: *will.* The problems of producing products 'semi-sterile' are, as have been referred to before, like talking of being 'semi-pregnant'! You have really to be very careful in drawing standards for cleanliness. The booklet referred to, produced by the Food Machinery, now Process Plant Association, is still available, and this does cover a great number of the points which would be the starting point for any continuation of this work. The seven points quoted by Mr Cook from the American publications caused us untold problems when we were trying to decide to reproduce those or to produce our own. Several meetings were taken up in the slight language difference between the Americans and the English. We eventually reproduced them in identical form except for the changing of one word. We changed 'sanitary' to 'hygienic'.

Every meeting where we decided to look at putting together pumps, pipes, valves, produced a text which at the next meeting somebody could quarrel with. It is again, as I said in my opening remarks, a very subjective matter. The proof of the pudding is whether or not the equipment works well. How do we develop those yardsticks? Well, I do think that we *have* to try to develop them. It is only 50 years ago that the designers of heat exchangers talked about the 'water equivalent' of the apparatus because they were applied physicists. The question of a heat transfer coefficient had never been thought of. Now perhaps we could project our thinking forward into saying that we will develop some criteria for a quantitative measurement.

CHAPTER 3

Solving Hygiene Problems by Process Design

V. R. Charlish and **K. G. Warman**, Colman Foods

INTRODUCTION

This paper is about some specific hygiene problems encountered by one food company during the manufacture of its products, and the solving of them by process design.

The Company is the Food and Wine Division of a well-known, worldwide company with factories in many different countries. The Division is located in Norwich on an 80-acre site, and it employs some 1700 people. It manufactures a wide range of products including various mustards, soft drinks, baby foods, wet and dry sauces, sweet and savoury condiments, preserves, and wines. In addition it manufactures a significant proportion of all the different containers used for packaging the products, including tins of all shapes and sizes, PVC and HDPE bottles etc, cartons, caps, plugs, and labels, since the company aims to operate on as self-contained a basis as is economically justified.

In this company the responsibility for the technical development of products and processes rests with the Food Research Department. This department specifies formulations, processes, ingredient raw materials, packaging materials, and legal, quality control, and hygiene requirements. The responsibility for ensuring that the specified criteria are properly complied with, together with those for the development of cleaning methods to attain the specified hygiene standards and the monitoring of their effectiveness, is vested in the Factory Quality Control Department.

Before discussing specific problems associated with the process design, some general observations will be made by way of introduction.

First, the design and quality of a process adopted for the manufacture of a food product must be dictated by a knowledge of the way in which the product will behave so as to attain the appeal and shelf life expected of it. The main technologies for preserving food products are illustrated in Fig. 3.1.

Unless effective action as indicated in Fig. 3.1 is 'built into' the process design and operation, then hygiene hazards can exist which could lead to ineffective heat treatment, to recontamination *after* some vital stage of the process such as sterilization has occurred, or to a hygiene condition difficult in its own right to overcome, calling for some additional process stage later in the total sequence.

Particularly important are products which contain no natural or inherent preservative and where a UHT (ultra high temperature) treatment combined with aseptic filling would be the process selected. Such a process demands a very high standard of hygienic design to ensure that sterility is maintained after the heat treatment and while the product is sealed into its container.

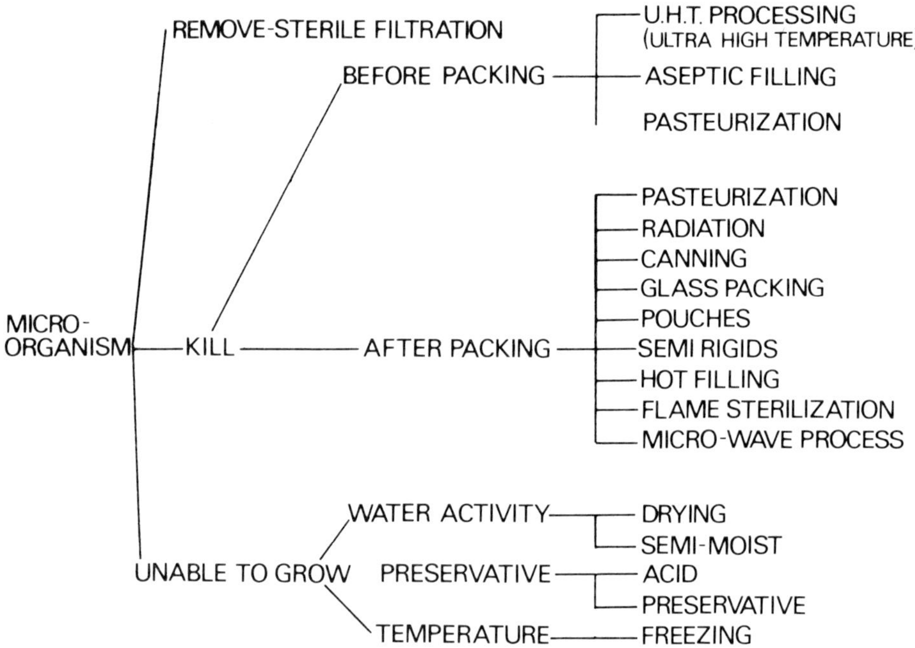

Fig. 3.1 – Food preservation technologies.

It is suggested that from a food manufacturer's point of view hygiene considerations in process plant fall into three main categories necessitating –

1. The selection of specialized equipment already available such as mixers, dicers, extruders, mincers, and pumps where alternatives exist and the user company is able to assess whether the available equipment will perform to the required specification, and will meet its hygiene standards in terms of materials of construction, design suitability, and cleanability.
2. The selection of other specialized equipment which by its nature leaves little choice such as certain pumps, reactor vessels, and certain mixers. If such equipment is *not* up to the required standards, then the user company modifies it as necessary to meet its own design and hygiene criteria, or even on occasions designs and produces its own.
3. The design and control of the process proper.

The evaluation of plant in categories 1 and 2 is the responsibility of this particular company's Food Research Department, who first establish the effectiveness of the equipment to perform the process duty required and then, in conjunction with Production and Quality Control, assess the hygiene and cleaning aspects of the design. Specific examples of problems arising from these evaluations and ways of overcoming them are referred to later, but before moving on to this some general points will be made on Item 3 which cover the linking together of items of equipment to form a complete process. This involves tanks, pipes, pumps, and valves, together with control equipment, flowmeters, temperature and level sensors, etc.

Fig. 3.2 illustrates a process flow sheet for the manufacture of a sweet condiment product, which will be used to indicate some of the more obvious hygiene points which had to be taken into account when designing the process. The product is sugar-based and will readily ferment under poor hygiene conditions. It is therefore vital that all contact areas of the plant should be smooth and free from crevices and dead spots.

Process vessels

The main process vessels, whether of open or closed design and whether operating under pressure or vacuum, have well-rounded corners with all welds properly dressed and capable of withstanding flexing under load which could create hollows or pockets in which product can become diluted or develop microbial growth. For this reason the vessels are capable of complete drainage of the product and of cleaning fluids, and the tank bottom and outlet are designed to permit this. Internal agitators are, where possible, of the top entry type and incorporate product spinners and mechanical seals to prevent product contamination. Fig. 3.3 illustrates some examples of bad practice which could result in dilution of the product and microbial growth.

Piping systems

Over the years the company has used a number of different product piping systems in our processes including glass, Durapipe, stainless steel, and occasionally various examples of flexible pipe. For this particular process crevice-free stainless steel piping was selected, which provides a completely smooth and continous bore which can easily be cleaned and is ideally suited for the CIP systems which will be referred to later. (See Fig. 3.4.)

Flowmeters

Most fall short of good sanitary design; for this application a smooth bore electromagnetic flowmeter which posed no hygiene problems was chosen.

Pumps

There are many types of pumps available with considerable differences in hygienic character. In this process it was possible to cover all the duties with a single design of pump, a stainless steel lobe type which is relatively easy to strip down for manual cleaning.

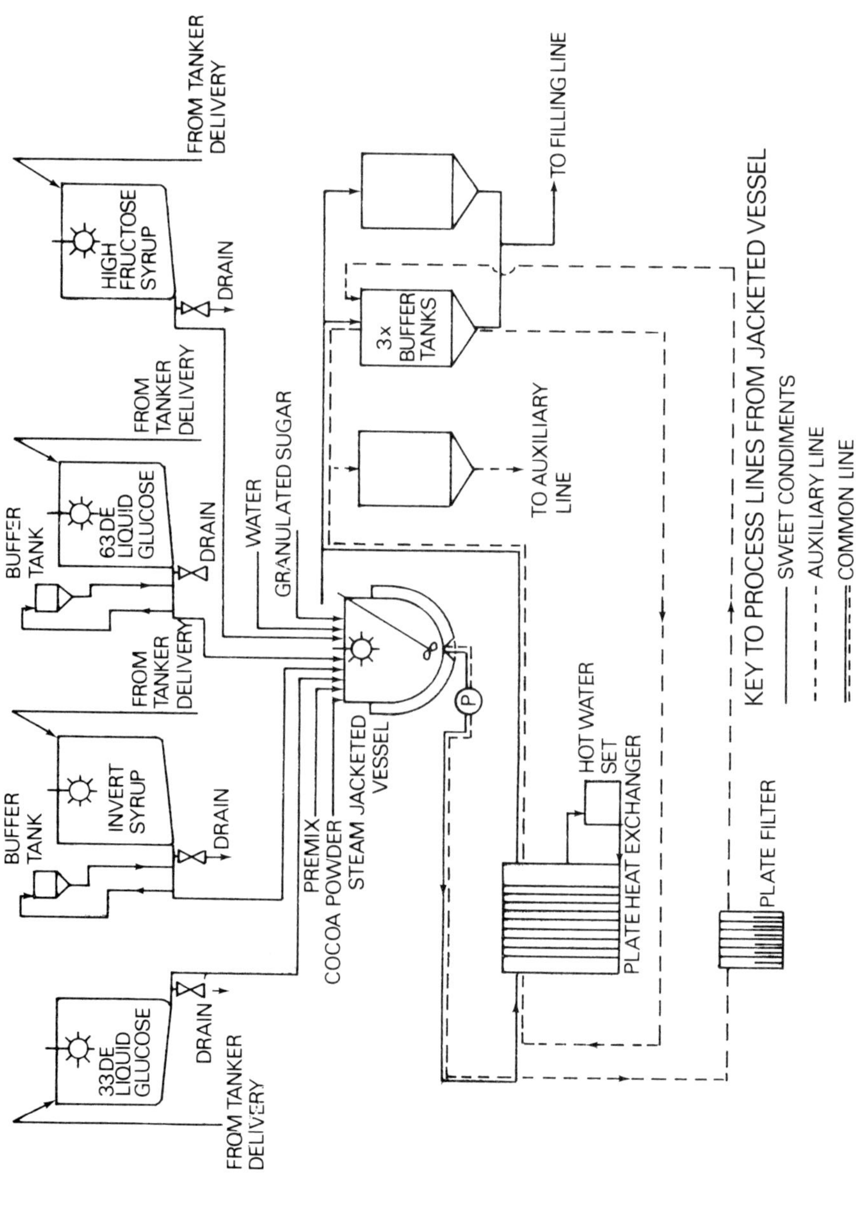

Fig. 3.2 – Flow sheet for production of sweet condiment.

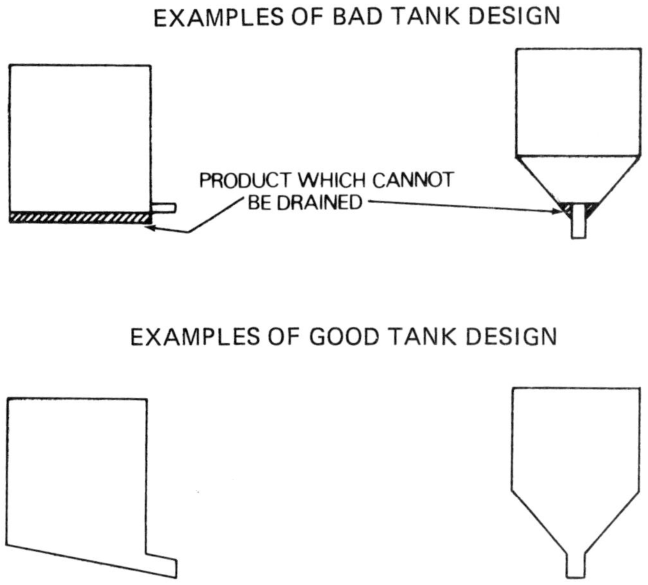

Fig. 3.3 – Tank designs.

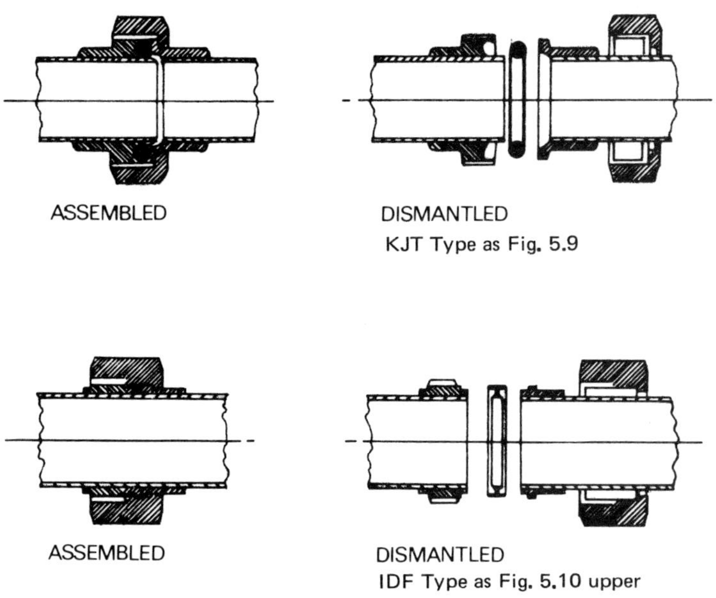

Fig. 3.4(a) – Piping systems.

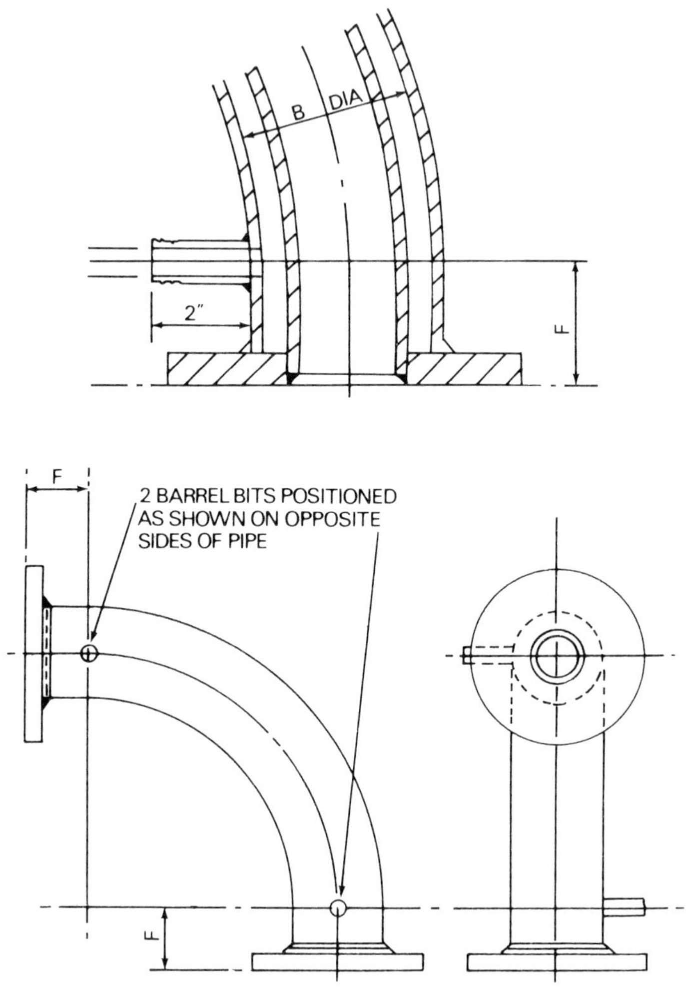

Fig. 3.4(b) – Piping systems (continued).

SERVICES

At this point it is necessary to make a few general points on services regarding the back-up necessary when providing facilities that are satisfactory from the product and hygiene point of view.

Water

Borehole water drawn from the site is used wherever possible, chlorinated and dechlorinated before general use as process water. Where there would be a hygiene hazard in its use, for example, if used to dilute a syrup after the syrup has been pasteurized or sterilized, the chlorination step is followed by local cartridge filters capable of removing bacteria from the water.

Steam

Where live steam is used as a direct heating medium as in direct steam injectors (see Fig. 3.5), a combined filtration system which is capable of removing entrainment down to 2 microns is used. This takes the form of a centrifugal spinning device and a sintered stainless steel cartridge filter, and it ensures that the steam delivered satisfies an approved hygiene standard. It is, of course, essential to exercise control of feed water additives used in the boiler plant.

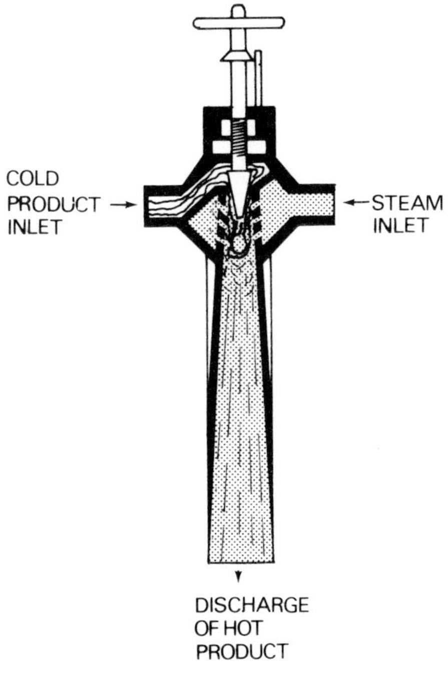

Fig. 3.5 – Steam injector.

Air

Where air is allowed into storage vessels, for example to prevent collapse under vacuum when the vessels are emptied, this air is carefully filtered to ensure sterility and no contamination of the vessel contents during storage. If compressed air is used and is likely to come into contact with product, it is filtered to ensure that it is oil and water-free; in certain cases the water removal is achieved by refrigeration.

PROCESS CONSIDERATIONS

Having dealt with the individual plant items and the special attention called for, some of the techniques adopted by this company to eliminate hygiene hazards within the process are now referred to in product groups.

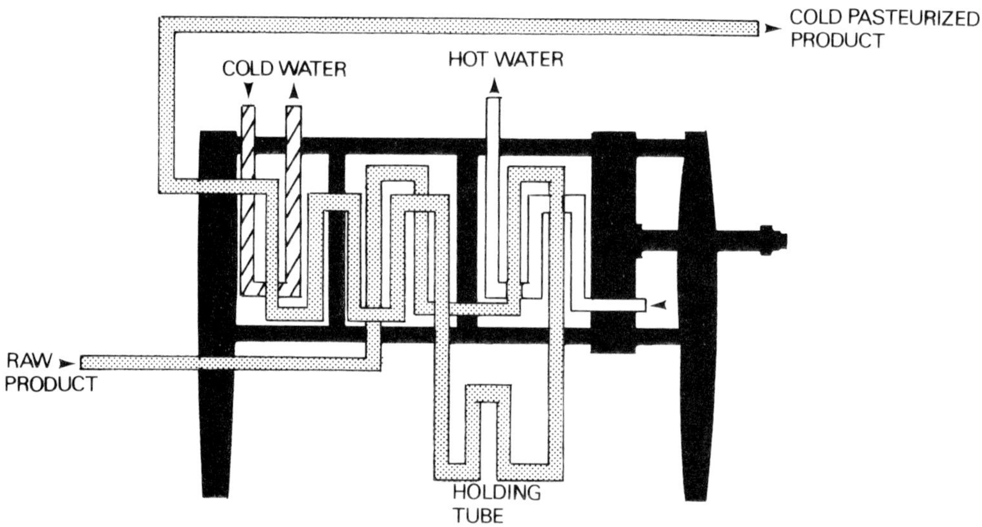

Fig. 3.6 – Plate heat exchanger pasteuriser.

1. Soft drinks – Pasteurization

Soft drinks are based on sugar and fruit juice, and depend on pasteurization and chemical preservatives for a satisfactory shelf life. As is well-known, heat treatment in food processing consists of a temperature–time exposure. In an in-line continuous process where pasteurization is often achieved by a plate-type heat exchanger with heating, temperature-holding, and cooling sections, fouling of the plate surfaces can lead to a falling-off in heat transfer and consequential difficulties in reaching the required temperatures. See Fig. 3.6.

It was found that when processing particularly concentrated products at high volume flow rates, the plate heat exchanger rapidly became blocked, with a rise in back pressure and fall-off in heat transfer. This led to the possibility of not achieving pasteurization conditions, which would then call for either stripping of the machine or back-flushing, with the inevitable interruption of production.

The solution to this hygiene hazard was to fit reasonably coarse duplex changeover strainers to the upstream side of the pasteurizer which in effect transferred the problem from the heat exchanger to the strainer but with the result that the cleaning could be easily carried out on the strainers. In addition, back-flushing has been introduced which will remove any secondary deposits passing the strainers and enables the machine to be run for long periods without dismantling and manual cleaning, and yet ensures effective hygiene conditions.

2. Sparkling wine filtration

Sterilization is usually achieved in a process flow either by UHT treatment or, as in the case with our sparkling wine product, by using sterilization filter sheets which physically remove micro-organisms from the liquid without damaging the flavour. It is then vital, of course, that recontamination does not occur after filtration, and that all succeeding pipelines, valves, and vessels must be pre-sterilized This means, of course, that all pipework and valves must be of a high crevice-free hygienic standard.

3. Fine wines – Contamination

During the filling cycle, as a precaution against the risk of wild yeasts entering the filler bowl, sterile inert gas (carbon dioxide or oxygen-free nitrogen) under low pressure is pumped into the filler headspace. This has proved to be very effective in practice. At one time the bottle neck used to be 'flamed' immediately before corking, but this proved unnecessary. (See Fig. 3.7).

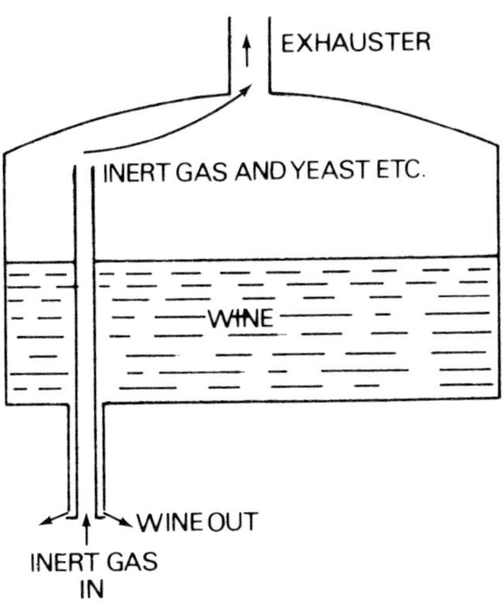

Fig. 3.7 – Wine filler vessel.

Where pressure gauges are fitted in product pipelines we have found it beneficial to operate them through the medium of a suitable flexible diaphragm and glycerin bank, thus avoiding the risk of any contamination from the gauge parts. (See Fig. 3.8.)

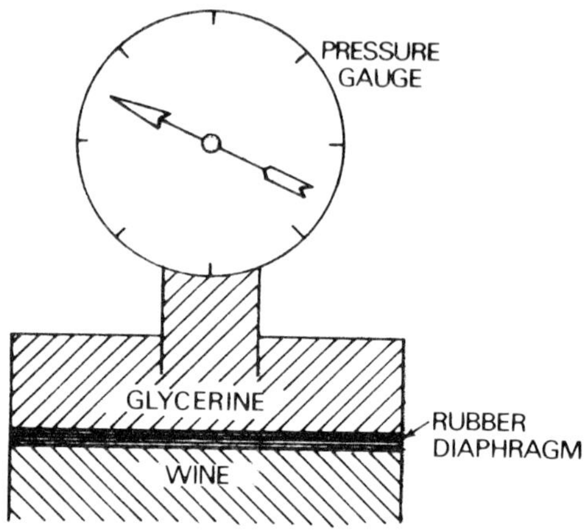

Fig. 3.8 – Use of diaphragm in food product pressure gauges.

4. Baby foods – Wet contamination

a) In a roller dryer system (Fig. 3.9) used for manufacturing baby food products hygiene hazards did occur owing to partly-dried materials from the ends of the dryer drum leaving the drum and entering the main dry-product collecting stream. This is more noticeable when 'outboard' dam plates bear on the *ends* of the drum and feed rolls, rather than inboard as shown in Fig. 3.10. To overcome this a reciprocating doctor knife was used to ensure the discharge of a continuous dried product sheet in combination with short end and face scrape which remove the partly-dried material before it reaches the doctor knife and the dried product stream. The applicator rolls are manufactured from 316 SI6 stainless steel, and the main drum is hardchrome plated to ensure that hygienic operating conditions are maintained.

b) Where slurries are fed to the dryer it may be desirable to take steps to prevent survival of micro-organisms by increasing the overall heat treatment so that, apart from the heat exposure on the drum itself, the slurries are preheated before transfer to the applicator rolls. For thick slurries which contain starch this can also be achieved by using a scraped surface heat exchanger or a steam injector.

c) Other slurries for roller drying which are at temperatures which would be near optimum for microbial growth are made up with ice at the milling stage to keep the slurries at low temperatures in the holding tanks before processing.

5. Prepared mustards

One of the products in this range is English ready-mixed mustard in which the starch is gelatinized and cooled in a scraped surface heat exchanger. The manufacturing plant is difficult to clean because of the nature of the cooked material.

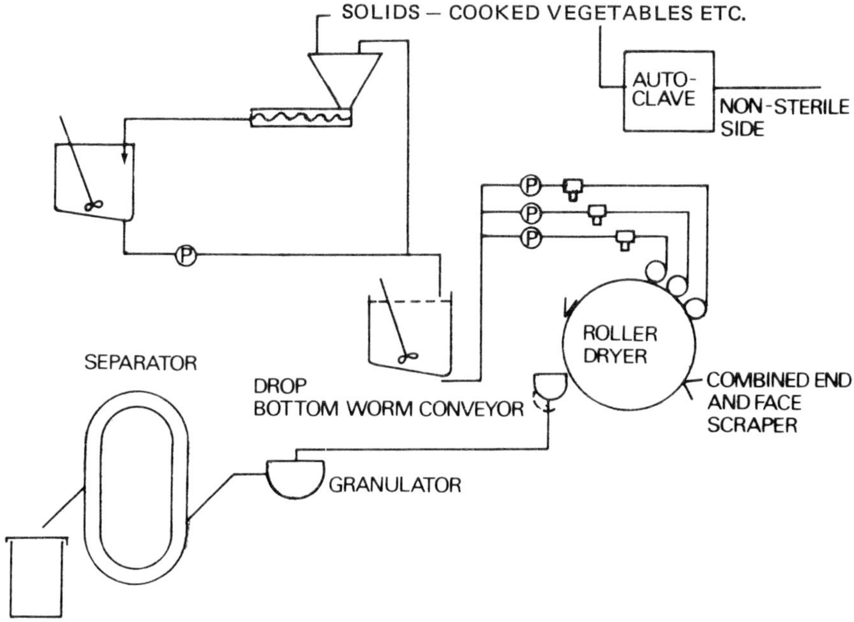

Fig. 3.9 – Arrangement of baby food production.

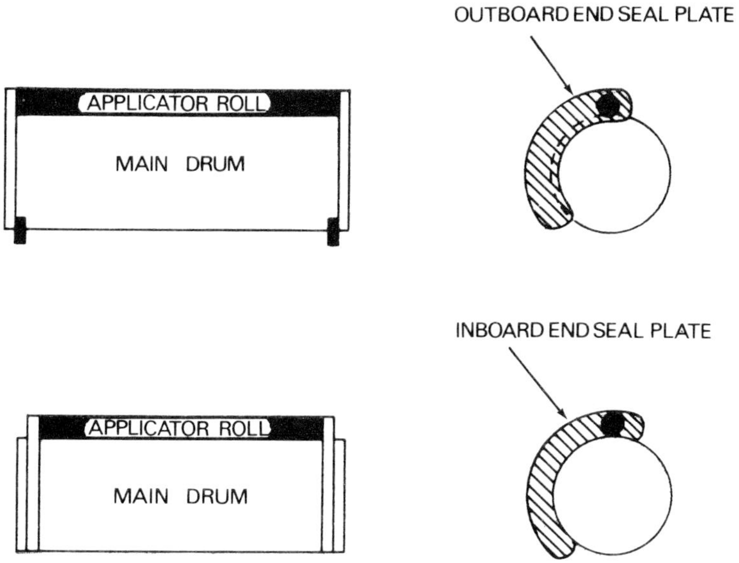

Fig. 3.10 – Roller dryers.

Because this material is not bacteriostatic, salt is introduced into the plant at the end of a production run, which allows production to be suspended until the next day with the system full of self-preserving product. A full regular plant clean can then be deferred until the weekend.

6. Wet sauces

Where products containing large particles in suspension which would be damaged in a scraped-surface heat exchanger have to be cooked/pasteurized, a form of falling-film heater is used in which the product is transferred to the inner wall of a vertical tube supplied with steam at a suitable pressure (Fig. 3.11). High rates of heat transfer are then possible from the direct condensation of steam.

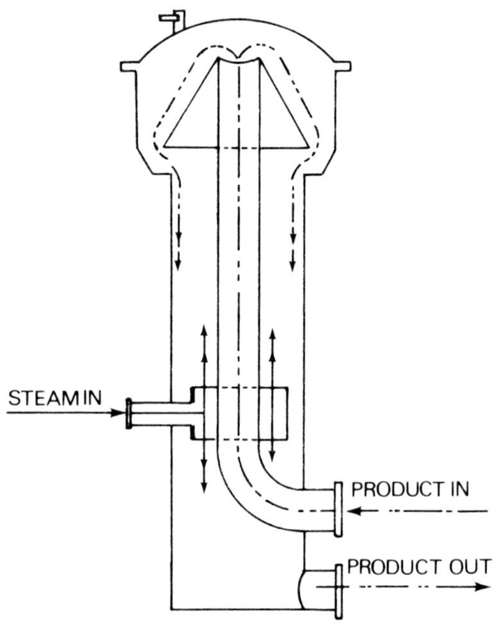

Fig. 3.11 – Live steam heater.

A cold filling process is used for filling wet sauces, and for low-acid varieties provision is made for sterilization of pipework between the above-mentioned cooking unit and the bottle filler. The filling machine can be steam sterilized, and the filling heads have been redesigned to give a smooth easily-cleaned shape.

7. Beer kits

In the filling of hopped wort extract into cans for beer kits a hygiene hazard in the form of 'dead legs' (Fig. 3.12) in the process pipeline layout was encountered. Such 'dead legs' can allow dilution of product to occur, and they provide conditions under which fermentation can take place. The problem had been compounded by the fact that the holding time in the pasteurizer had been reduced by an accidental change in holding tube size.

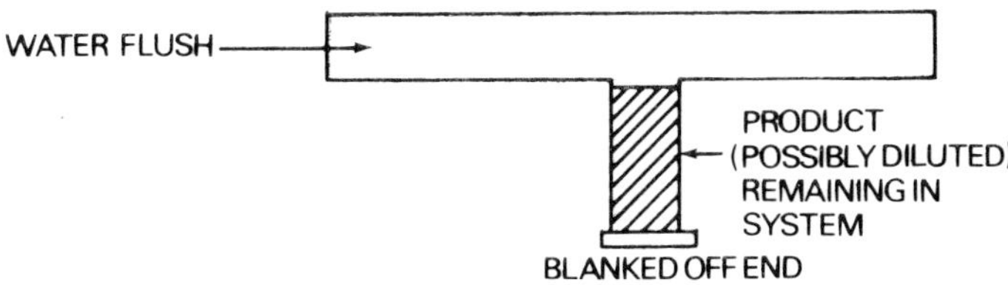

Fig. 3.12 – Example of bad hygiene standard caused by 'dead-leg'.

The solution, of course, was firstly to remove the examples of poor pipeline design and then to install a holding tube of the correct dimensions.

To provide the required residence time at the required pasteurizing temperature it is usual to introduce into the heat exchanger, between the heating and cooling sections, a holding tube of the correct volumetric capacity in relation to flow rate. This company uses an efficiency factor based on holding times achieved by empirical measurements, and these consist of figures arrived at by injecting colour or acid into the entry point of the holding tube and measuring the time to reach the exit. Efficiency factors have been determined for fluids of different density and vicosity.

CLEANING IN PLACE

CIP is regarded as a particular solution to a specific hygiene problem by process design. Although it has been used in dairies and breweries for many years, increasing use of this technique is anticipated, as hygiene standards are increased in the future, either in simple form or in fully automatic schemes.

CIP techniques are capable of achieving the highest standards of hygiene in process plant, equivalent to that obtained by dismantling and cleaning all the pipework and plant by hand. A simplified typical CIP circuit is shown in Fig. 3.13. This shows a common arrangement of batch tanks, pipelines, heat exchangers and storage tanks; the addition of CIP features permit cleaning of the tanks by use of spray balls and of the pipelines and general plant items by high velocity detergent and water which is recirculated. This scheme is used, for example, in the soft drinks plant. A common cycle for cleaning a plant of this type would include a water rinse stage (hot or cold as required) to remove product and gross contamination, followed by a detergent wash to remove the remaining contamination and then a final rinse to remove the detergent from the system. The complete cycle is as follows:

CLEANING IN PLACE (CIP) SEQUENCE

Operation	Function
1. Preliminary rinse	Remove gross soil
2. Detergent wash	Remove residual food etc.
3. Rinse	Remove detergent
4. Sterilise	Destroy residual micro-organisms
5. Final rinse	Remove any CIP solutions

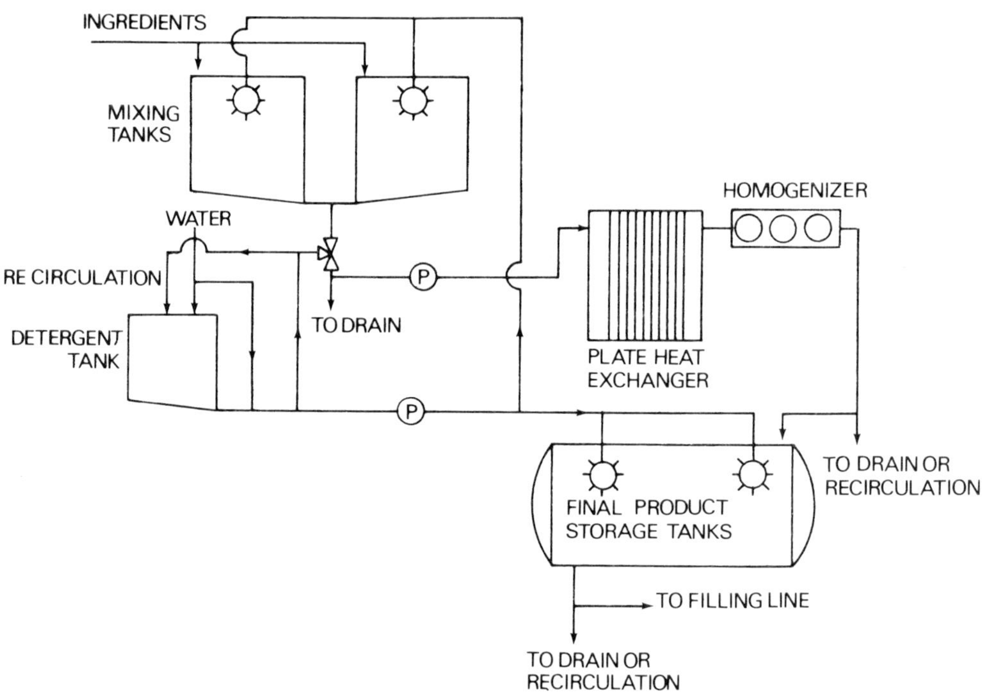

Fig. 3.13 – Simplified CIP system.

The plant layout for CIP is very important since a feature of the system is that dismantling of the process and plant is not necessary. Pipework must therefore have crevice-free joints, and all tanks must be designed so as to be enclosed (incorporating the features referred to hitherto) and with smooth walls capable of being cleaned by liquid spray. The spray balls can either be fixed or rotating and either design can produce a high velocity jet of liquid in a 360 degree pattern which covers the interior walls of the tank and thoroughly cleans away any remaining product or other contamination. Another paper deals in detail with this subject (see p. 183) but the following table lists the advantages and disadvantages of CIP compared to manual cleaning.

ADVANTAGES OF CIP

1. Cost savings – better use of water, detergents, heat.
2. Better plant use – less downtime.
3. Less manual work required – no need to dismantle plant.
4. Greater comfort and safety for operators – no need to crawl into tanks or come into contact with detergents/sterilants.
5. Better hygiene – cleaning schedules followed exactly and consistently. Less risk of recontamination.

DISADVANTAGES

1. Not suitable for all applications.
2. High capital cost.

PACKAGING

It is utterly useless to spend a great deal of effort, time and money in manufacturing a product satisfying all the criteria laid down for perfect hygiene quality if the packaging does not reflect the same standards and at the same time ensure the consumer appeal and shelf life demanded. This is true of wet or dry products, whether preserved, pasteurized, or sterilized, and in whatever form. This demands critical monitoring right through the whole operation from the basic ingredient stage through to the finished package on the shop or supermarket shelf: half-measures are doomed to failure.

BUILDINGS

In conclusion, a few pointers on processing and packaging building standards which reflect the hygiene standards perceived as essential for this company's product range might be helpful, particularly when remembering that one is catering for home and export markets subject to EEC as well as United Kingdom regulations.

The floors, walls, and roof should be of solid construction, preferably in concrete or brickwork, thereby avoiding cavities which attract vermin or provide breeding grounds for bacteria. For this reason it is not possible to provide thermal insulation or acoustic materials on internal surfaces, and where these are found necessary it is best to apply them on the outside of the structure directly beneath the external weather protection material. The floors and lower wall surfaces need to be finished in a material that is impermeable, durable, non-staining, and non-dusting, and which will withstand heavy mechanical wear, attack from acids, alkalis, oils, etc., and yet provide a non-slip floor surface.

The ingredients used in food manufacture such as sugar, fruit juices, vinegar, and sulphur dioxide can attack and cause rapid deterioration of cement-based materials. Hot liquid sugar, for instance, if allowed to penetrate into a void or hair crack in concrete, will, on cooling, crystallize and cause the break-up of the concrete by mechanical action. To avoid this, vitrified ceramic floor tiles jointed in epoxy resin are used. They are one of the few materials possessing the required properties which at the same time give a clean and hygienic appearance and working environment.

Structural members that will create dust ledges are avoided, and service line runs and duct work are grouped so far as possible into a central services bay. Natural lighting is minimal to avoid solar heat gain, and the windows have no opening lights in order to exclude birds, insects, dust, etc. Ventilation and heating is by a filtered air supply discharging at high level, with the main duct runs as far as possible outside the building. The floor generally is well-drained to gullies having removable silt baskets, but the really wet processing areas are isolated by continuous kerbed surrounds. Any dividing walls are of solid construction, since timber and moveable partitions are highly unsuitable for production areas.

Although such a building may be more expensive initially, it will subsequently require little maintenance, and in the case of wall tiles it is only necessary to apply them up to working height. Above this and over the ceiling the surfaces may be subject to sulphur dioxide- and moisture-laden vapours discharged during processing and which can percolate into the substrata of the building and (if paint is applied) create the risk of paint flakes falling into the product. For this reason a polymer such as 'Plastapak' is highly suitable for all such areas. When sprayed on walls and ceilings it provides a flexible, continuous, impervious barrier having the capacity to bridge minor cracks, etc., thereby reducing the risk of mould and bacterial growth.

DISCUSSION

Mr George Heighton (Geo. Bassett & Co Ltd.): You have shown, Mr Charlish, auger screw feeders of various types. We have encountered some problem in ensuring that these are clean. Is there an easy way of getting over this?

Mr Charlish: There is not. I think that is the answer. We are achieving success by using CIP systems. Of course it depends absolutely on the material you are augering and what sort of consistency it has, but CIP systems, if properly applied, will, in our experience, remove extraneous matter. If not, it's a case of stripping and cleaning down.

Mr W. E. Whitman Leatherhead Food RA): I would like to ask for a little more information about the system of filling the heat exchangers (as I understood it) with salt solution overnight to preserve the thing for use again the following morning. What quantity of salt is required?

Mr Charlish: We have found it expedient with ready-mixed mustards to charge the last batch which is sufficient to fill the processing vessels and the pipelines with a heavily-salted mustard which can then be mixed-in the following morning to give a standard product and guarantee adequate preserving overnight.

Mr Warman: Certainly it is not satisfactory if we have to put about three day's production through subsequently to eliminate the overfeed! It doesn't need a very heavy overdose of salt to ensure sterile conditions for a period which is adequate for our purposes. It is a high-solid product, and the amount of salt added is relatively little and can easily be mixed out during the first batches of the next day.

Mr T. C. Tamplin (APV): I think I should just draw attention to the hazards of acid chloride conditions in stainless steel equipment. I hope that everybody is aware of this when putting the saline solutions through their equipment for bactericidal purposes.

Mr R. Jowitt (National College): Just to complete that picture, Mr Chairman, what is the pH of this sterilizing product?

Mr Charlish: The pH is above 5.5.

CHAPTER 4

Hygienic Design of Plant Exterior

G. R. Ridgway and **R. Coulthard**, Baker Perkins Ltd.

INTRODUCTION

At the concept stage of any machine, the designer is faced with a total set of problems. Each has to be solved, but not at the risk of incurring other problems or upsetting the balance of features which are to be provided. For example, consideration has to be given to the actual process and function of the machine – its compatibility on cost – the economics for ease of operation; reliability and maintenance requirements; and last, but not least, the overall hygienic and safety features.

The exterior of the machine is not something that can be tackled in isolation. It is an integral part of the complete design. It is no solution to put easy-to-clean boxes around dirty machines.

However, this paper concentrates on the various hygiene aspects of a machine's exterior.

First a definition of what we mean by exterior. The exterior of a machine, or plant, is those parts of the equipment for which the operator, or cleaning staff, would normally be responsible. This includes not only the outer surfaces of the machine, but also the product areas, for which the operator has responsibility.

The general philosophy in tackling hygiene is three-fold:

1. If a basic process is, in itself, one which creates dirt, dust, and unhygienic conditions, attempt to replace that process with a cleaner one.
2. If a basic process change cannot be made, then separate the product zones from the non-product areas.
3. Position operator controls so that the operator does not have to touch the product.

THE PROBLEM

The food industry covers a vast spectrum of activities – the author's company serves principally the biscuit, bread, cake, and chocolate and confectionery sectors, both in the UK and in other countries. There are certain unit machines such as mixers and creamers, but in the main we deal with lines of plant which present additional problems.

A typical biscuit plant would consist of :

1. Ingredient storage and handling for flour, sugar, fats, water, etc. This is a potentially unhygienic area owing to dust leakage, fat spillage, etc.
2. Mixing – this is potentially unhygienic owing to dry ingredient leakage and product spillage.
3. Dough forming machinery, consisting of either moulders or cutting machines which shape and size the biscuit dough piece. These are potentially unhygienic owing to surfaces becoming either greasy or sticky.
4. Baking ovens, cooling conveyors, and wrapping machines. Here there is potential dust and crumb accumulation.

Coupled with all the above items, the problems of heat and noise must be dealt with.

HYGIENIC SOLUTIONS

The following illustrations are typical examples of how one may deal with the fundamental problems associated with the hygienic design of plant exterior.

Fig. 4.1 shows a machine in which moulding starch contained in trays and imprinted, may be used for the manufacture of sweets. This is an extremely dusty operation which contaminates the complete department, as well as the exterior of the machine. It results in dust, as well as scrap product, being deposited fairly liberally over the surfaces of the machine.

Fig. 4.2 shows the alternative – a starchless moulding plant. Changing the process has eliminated dust. The result is a more hygienic plant exterior. The equipment is designed so that all the material in the product area is unaffected by the product, or by cleansing agents. It is abrasion-proof, corrosion-proof, and has a hard, smooth, non-porous surface. The depositor has easily removable pistons and hopper, and likewise each mould can easily be detached.

Fig. 4.3 shows the mould circuit on the same plant, and indicates the avoidance of any absorbent or organic-based materials.

Where it is not possible to change the process for a cleaner one, it is advisable to separate the product-zone from the non-product zone.

Fig. 4.4 shows a Baker Perkins rotary moulder drive. It is housed on the outside of the machine under guards which facilitate maintenance without risk of dirt contaminating the product area.

Fig. 4.5 shows another view of the rotary moulder. It can be clearly seen that the product area has been separated from the driving mechanism of the machine. It also shows the hopper tilted back for easy access to, and for removal of, the moulding rolls. If hoppers are too large either to be hinged or to remove, they should be supported in a way which does not restrict access to the product area.

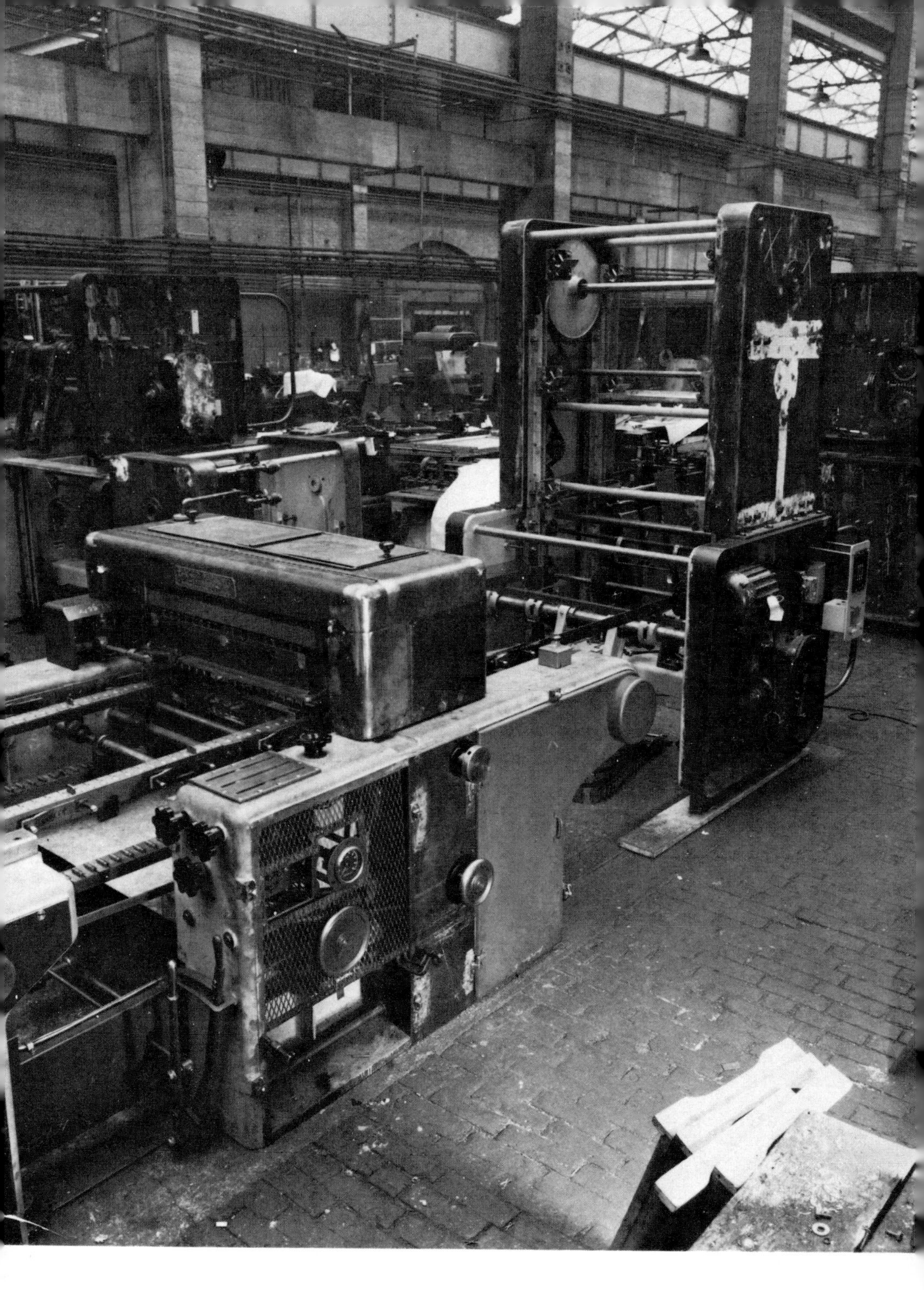

Fig. 4.1

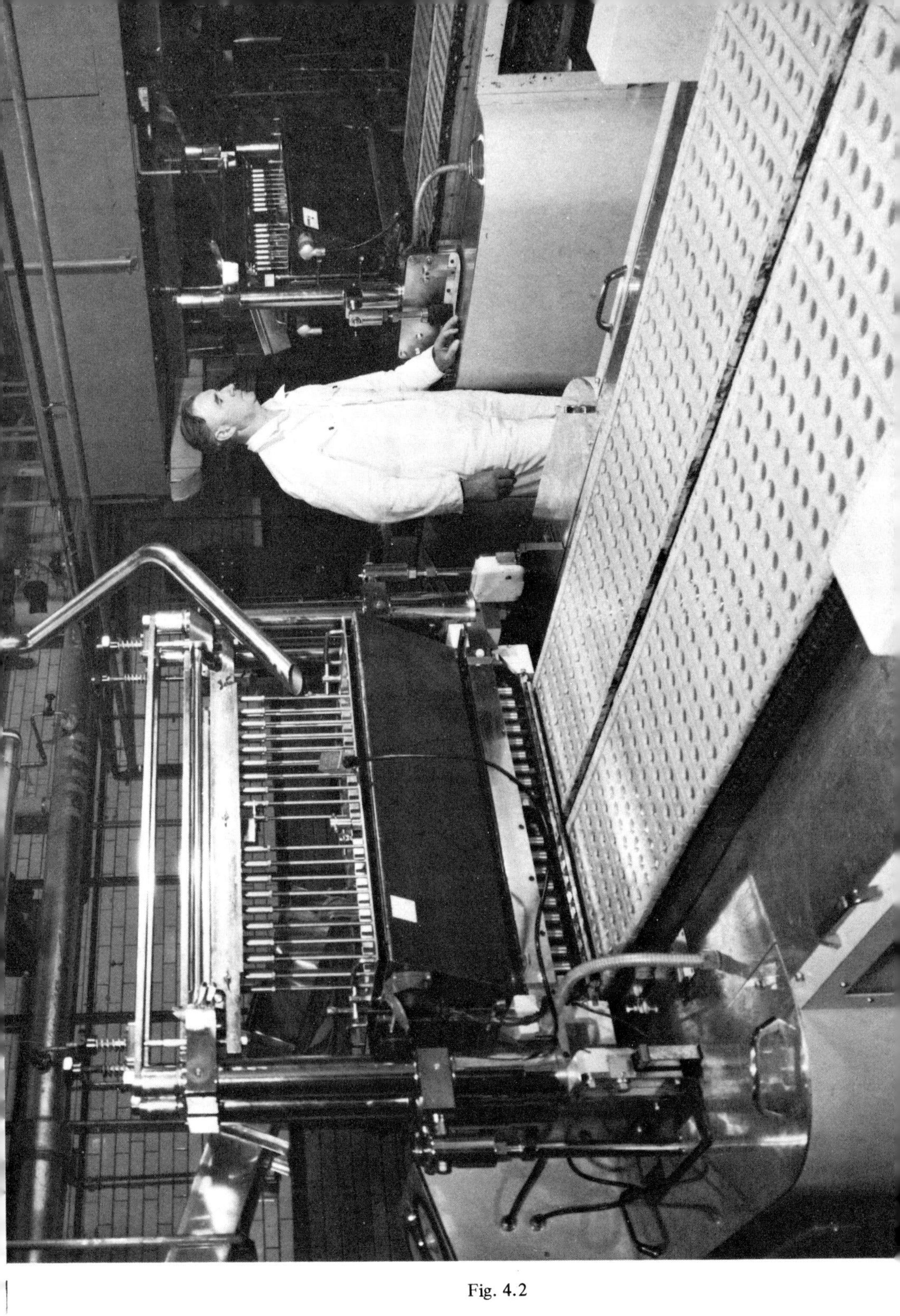

Fig. 4.2

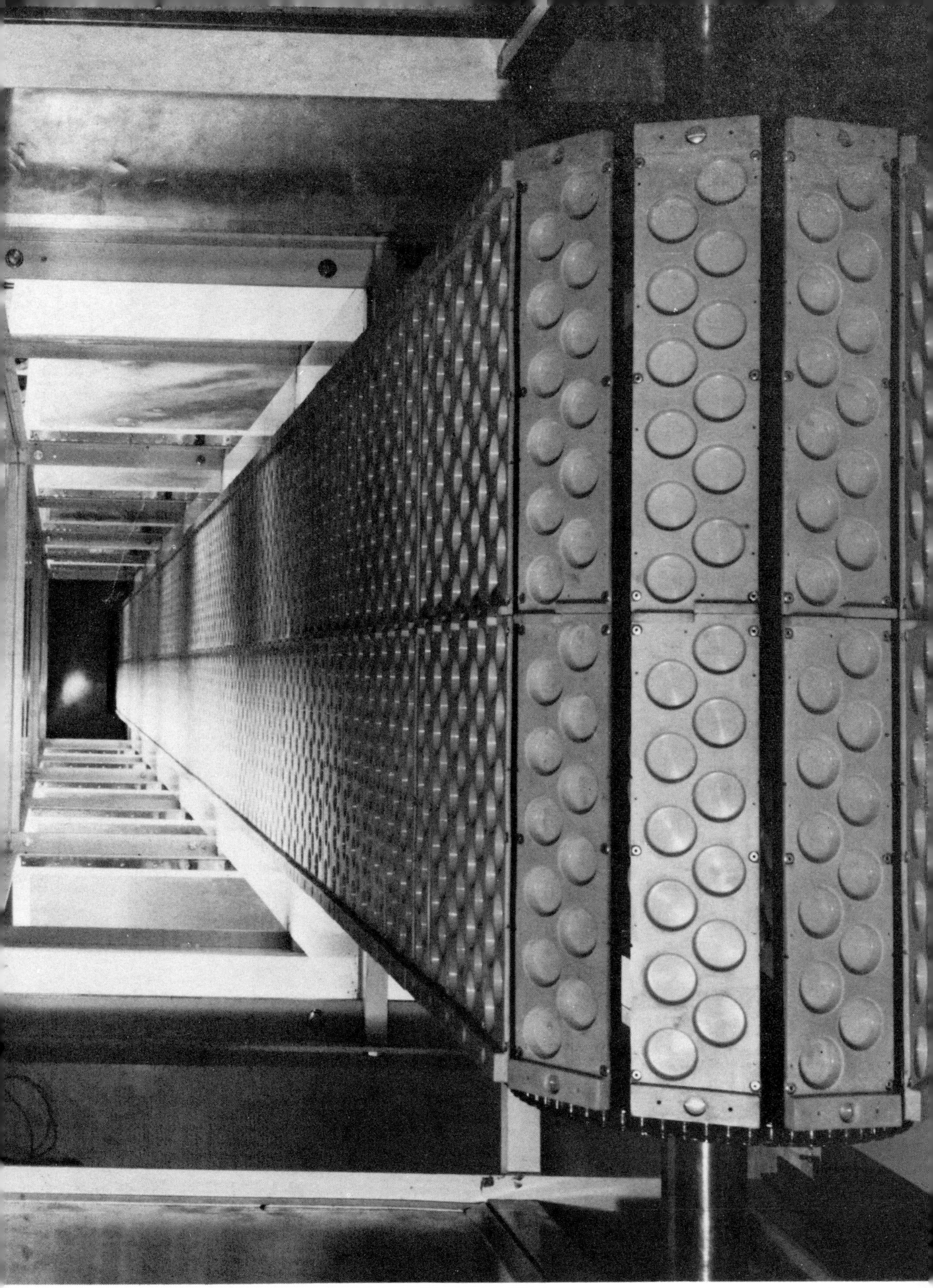

Fig. 4.3

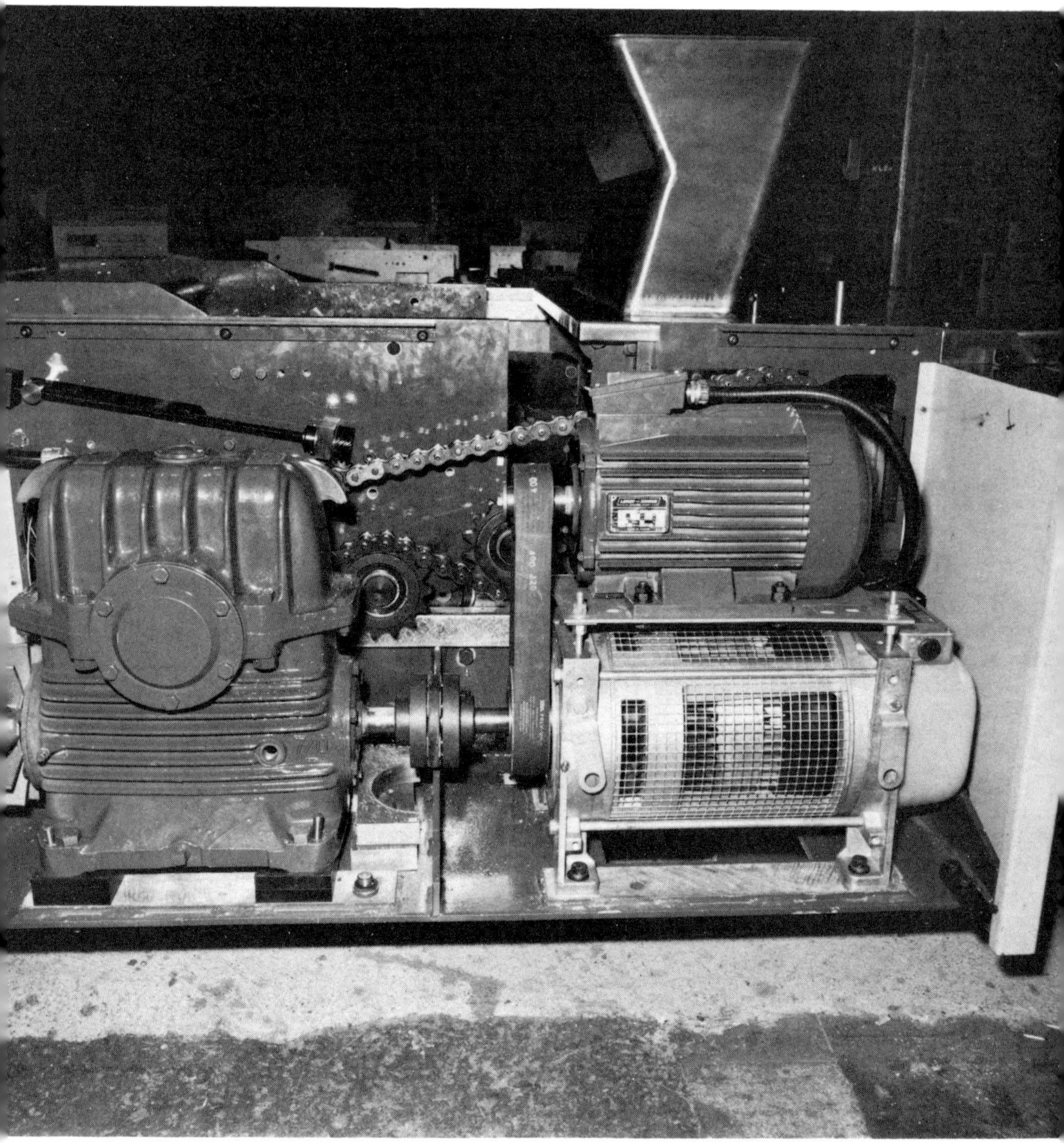

Fig. 4.4

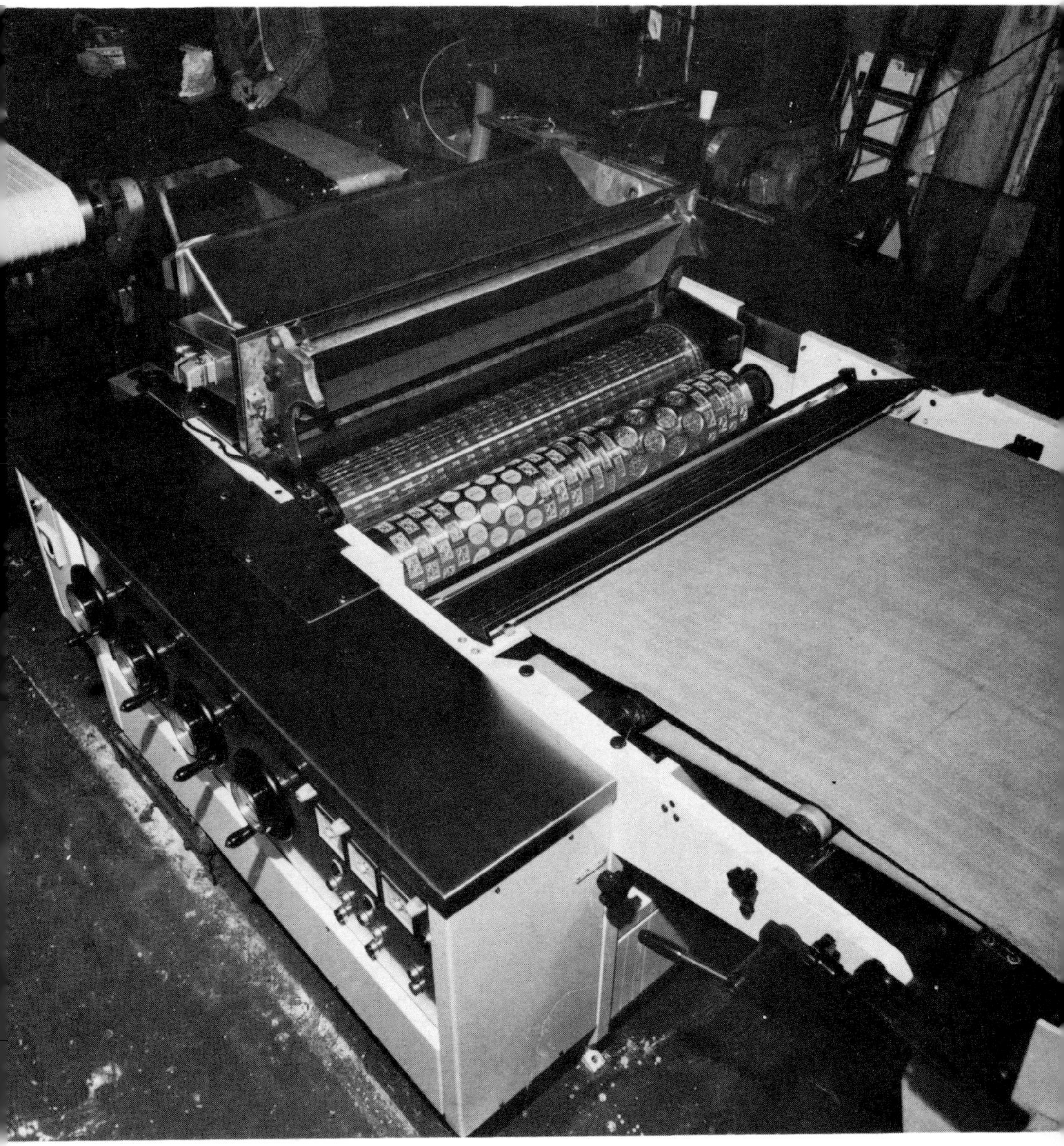

Fig. 4.5

The controls on this machine are located so that the operator does not have to lean over the product area when operating the machine. Also illustrated here is the use of non-painted or plated materials in potential 'wear' areas. These areas are ones that are likely to be leaned on, stood on, kicked, knocked, or handled. In this particular case stainless steel is used on the tops of the side covers and aluminium on the fascia of the control panel.

Fig. 4.6 shows the old design of biscuit forming line where, from an external hygiene point of view, the difficulties facing an operator in keeping the plant clean can be readily seen.

Fig. 4.7 shows the current approach where all surfaces are easily and quickly wiped down. The clustering of controls at one centre, of course, is one of the major factors that makes this possible. Large horizontal surfaces, which harbour debris, should be avoided wherever possible.

Fig. 4.8 shows a Baker Perkins 850 kg high-speed mixer. Here it was not possible to eliminate completely the large, near-horizontal surfaces, as a box construction is necessary for strength and stability. In this case a sloping top to the box section – with a smooth, hard surface – provides both robustness and accessibility. In this illustration, note also the crevice-free surfaces near the mixing bowl, made possible by the use of thick flat plate, in place of the old ribbed castings. This use of bold, simple-form, clean, white frame and stainless-clad mixing bowl should encourage an operator to keep a 'clean machine'.

Fig. 4.9 shows a vertical spindle mixer where the mixing bowl is a removable tub. This leaves a completely accessible area for wiping down. It shows also how the operator is well away from the product area when operating the controls. It also clearly indicates the separation of the product-zone from the drive-zone, which is located at the top of the machine.

There are occasions when spillage within the product-zone is unavoidable. To prevent contamination of the product, catch trays should be provided. Fig. 4.10 shows catch trays on a vertical laminator. This, and Fig. 4.11, the underside of a cutting machine, illustrate some guidelines for 'inside of frames' construction. By our definition this is also a part of plant 'exterior'.

One should avoid:

1. Ledges and dirt traps (use round rather than rectangular stretchers).
2. Recessed corners.
3. Sharp edges.
4. Unfilled seams.
5. Uneven surfaces and hollows.
6. Projecting bolt threads, screws, and rivets.

In general, avoid creating inaccessible spaces where product may accumulate. This illustration also demonstrates the necessity to provide adequate space for cleaning between linked machines in a line of plant. This is an area where the designer does have a specific problem in getting the right compromise between hygiene and safety.

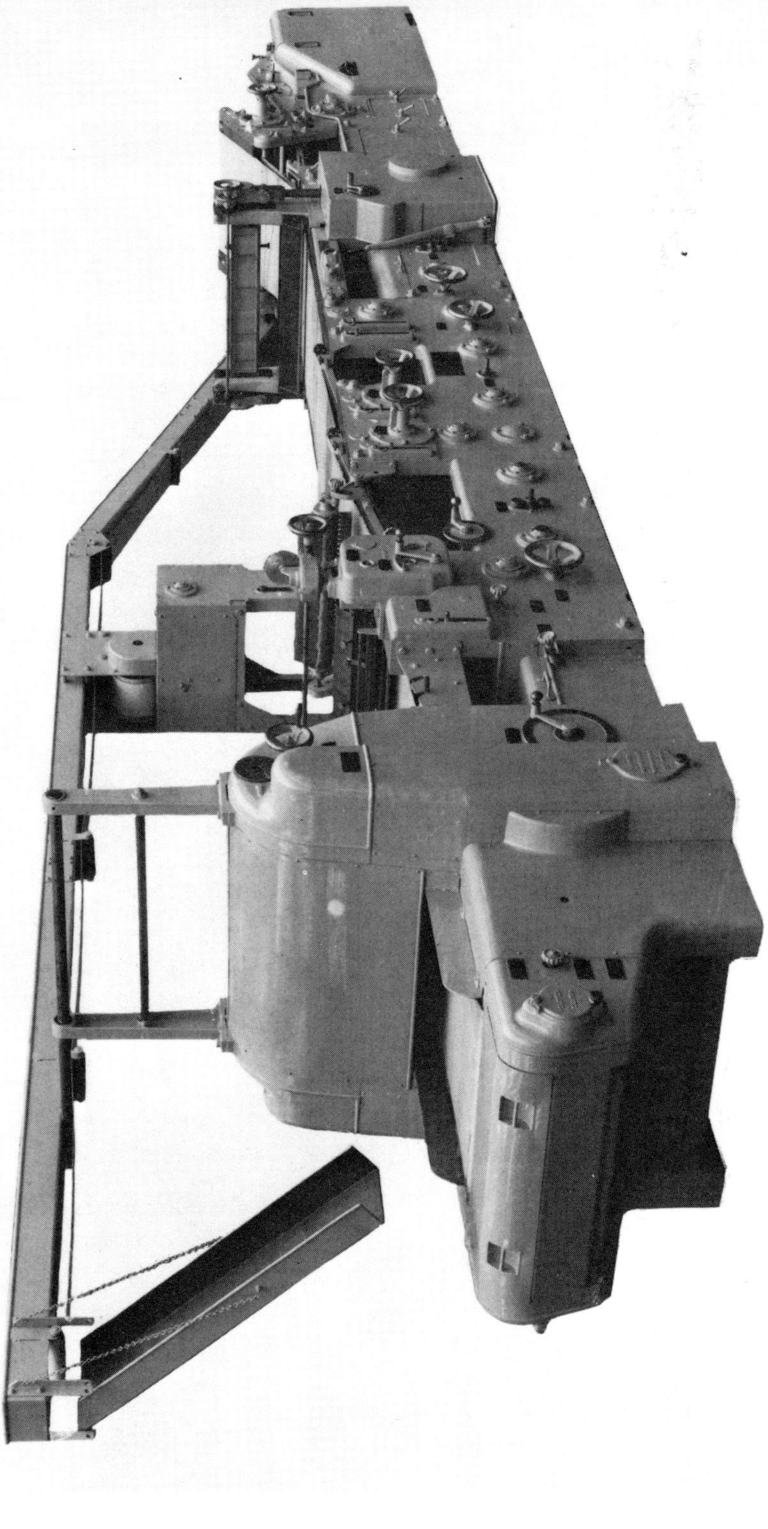

Fig. 4.6

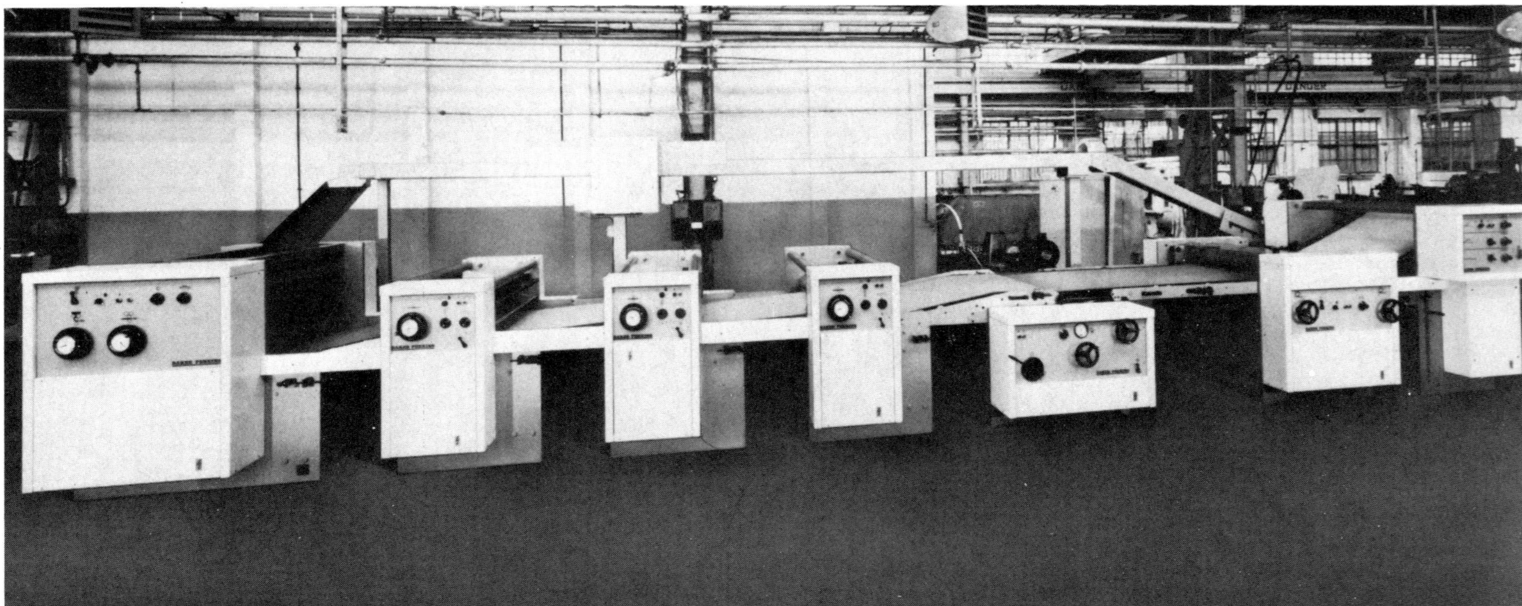

Fig. 4.7

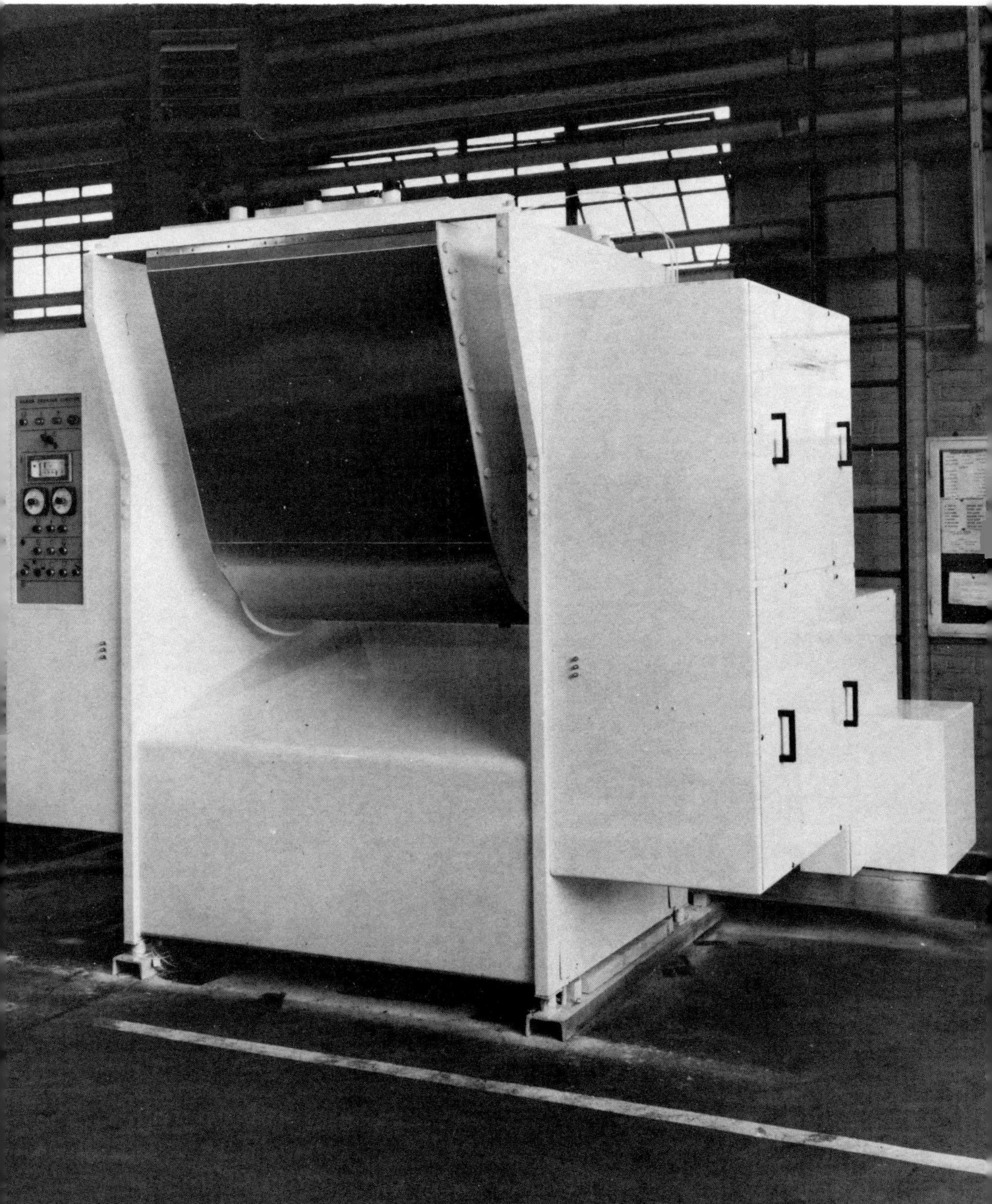

Fig. 4.8

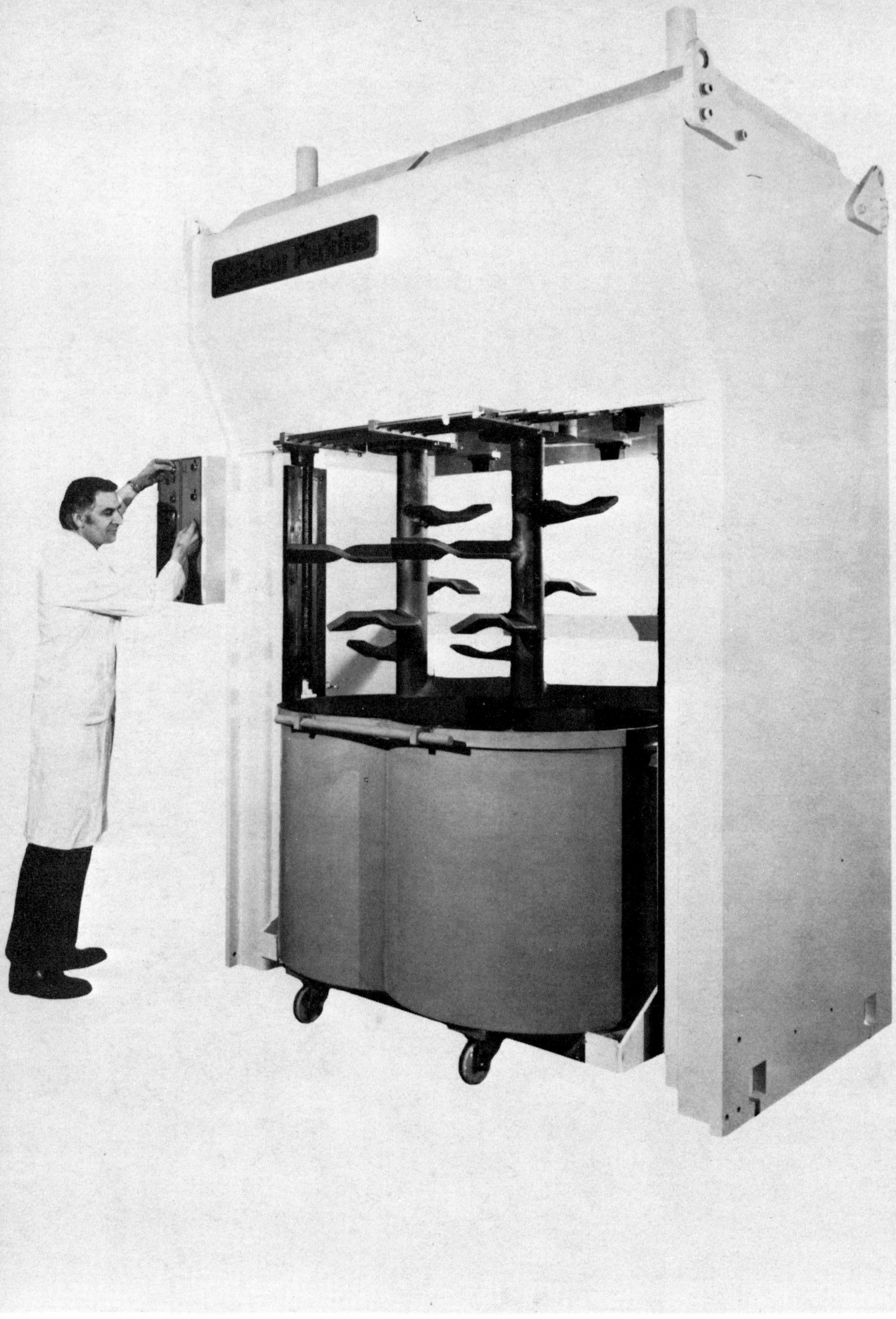

Fig. 4.9

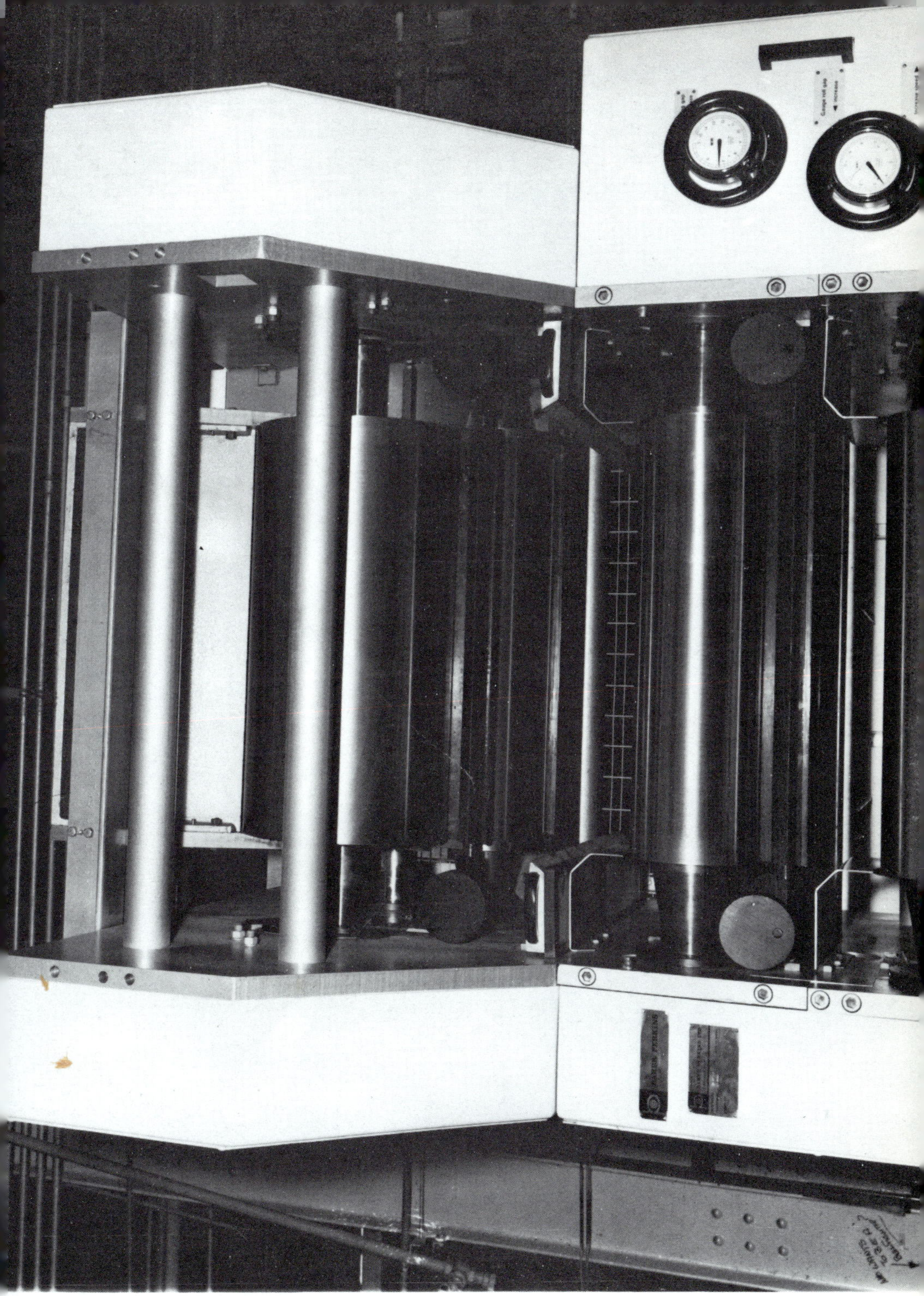

Fig. 4.10

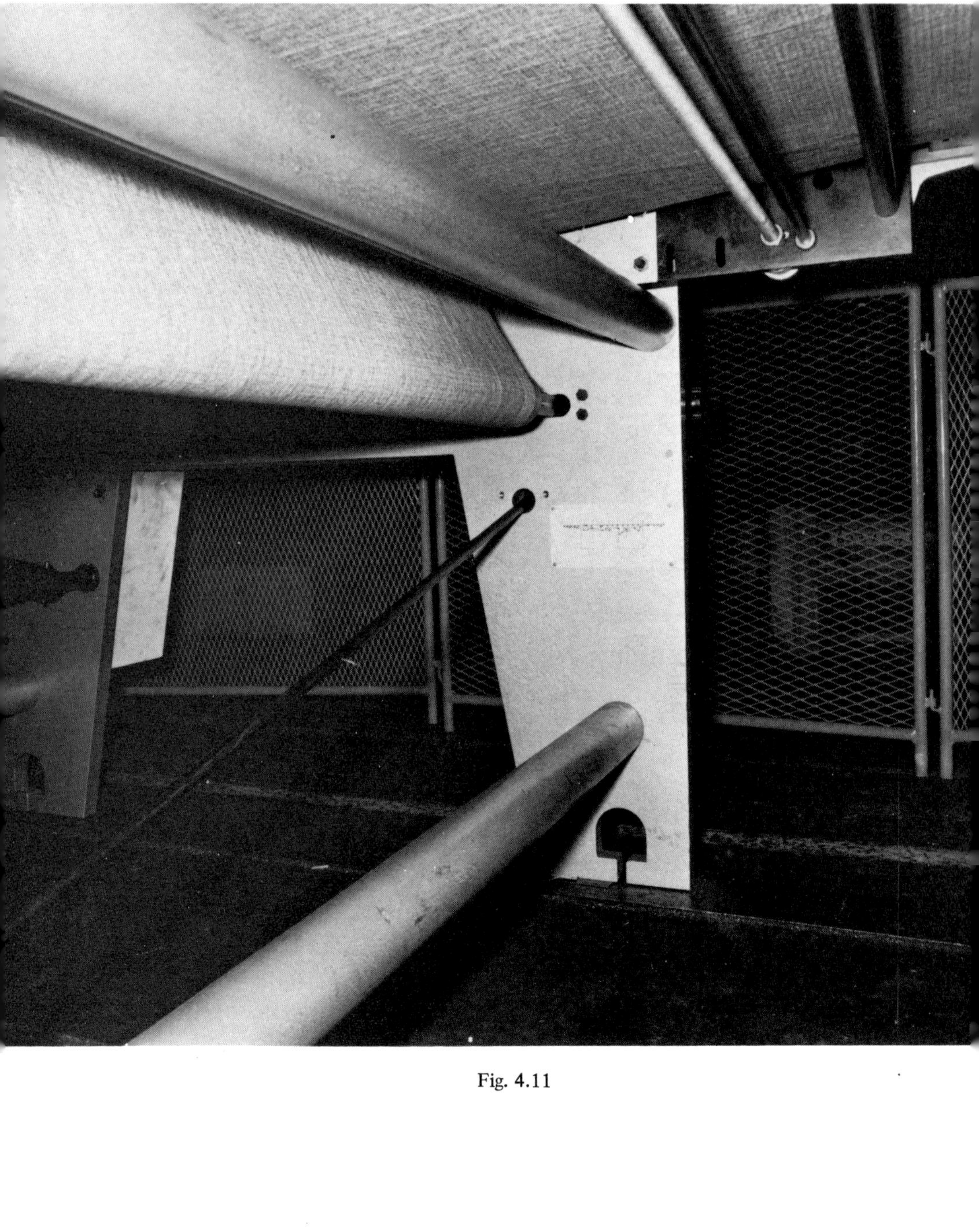

Fig. 4.11

The 'big box' machines present particular hygiene problems. Fig. 4.12 shows a continuous oven standing clear of the ground and having a generous number of access doors for cleaning out the product area. These frequently-used doors are made of a self-finished material; in this case, stainless steel.

Fig. 4.13 is a section of a cooler under construction. It is a good example of how machines should, where practicable, be well clear of the floor. Sufficient height to enable a brush, held at 30° to the horizontal, to reach the machine's centreline allows the complete floor to be cleaned, without stooping, from both sides of the plant. Of course, the fewer supports to the floor there are, the better.

Fig. 4.14 shows the same cooler and the access to the product-zone. Hinged doors are better than lift-off panels, and the hinges are of a take-apart type without cracks or crevices. The doors are Melamine-faced polyurethane foam construction, and completely sealed. They are light enough to fold down or lift off easily, but they also function as insulation panels; they are rigid and extremely hygienic owing to the simple and completely flat surfaces. A further point is that on this machine all upward facing flanges have been avoided, since they may retain debris.

The cooling drum, Fig. 4.15, is part of a line of plant used to make fondant creme for confectionery products. It demonstrates some of the attributes already mentioned, plus:

> It has a simple, bold form, with smooth, easily-wiped surfaces. Round-section, chromed stretchers are used between the plate frames; self-finish material surrounds the control area, and the machine is well clear of the floor. Additionally, the product area is self-cleaning, being equipped with a steam spray, scraper blade, catch tank, and drain point.

Automatic cleaning is most desirable, and all wash-down areas should be self-draining.

No difficult-to-clean components should be situated where there is the probability of product spillage. If practicable, such components should be resited. If not, they should be shielded – as is the motor on the machine shown in Fig. 4.16. Note the catch-tank drain point and self-finish materials in the product zone, as well as the smooth-finished motor shield. Hollow components, like the legs of this machine, should be sealed to prevent infestation.

Chocolate coating is a primary confectionery process, or a secondary process in biscuit production. Fig. 4.17 shows a recent design of chocolate enrober. The external form reflects the close attention to hygiene. The overall form is simple, with no awkward projections, and the product zone is easily accessible. The pump and tank assembly are completely removable from the coating head and band. No tools are needed to reach the product-zone. This, of course, is a prime aim.

Fig. 4.18 illustrates the pump on this enrober, and how it can be entered without tools. For complete dismantling of the pump rotor, tools are required, but this is outside our definition of operator function.

Access should always be quick and easy – or the job won't be done. Reassembly must also be easy, with no danger of fouling the product-zone.

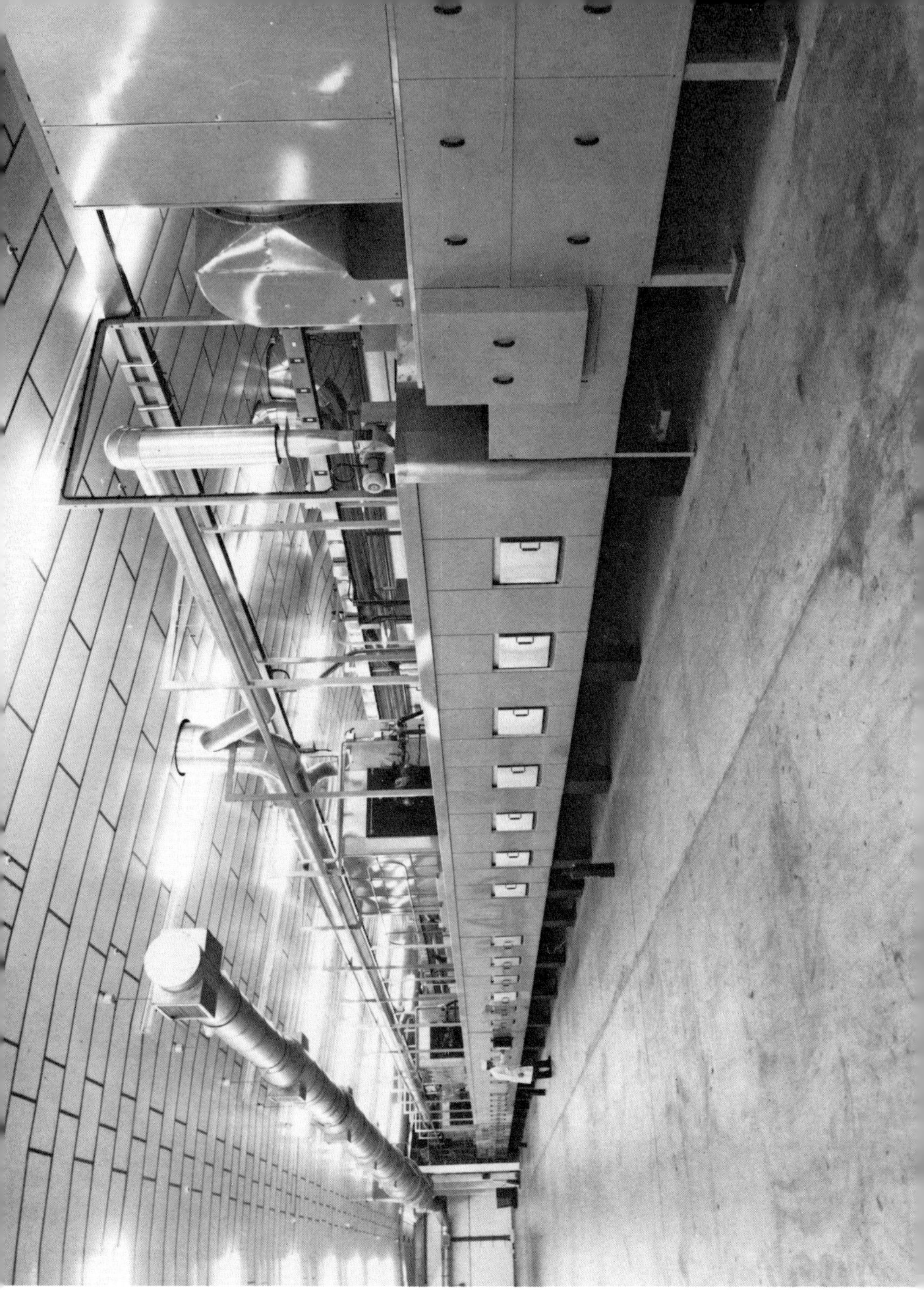

Fig. 4.12

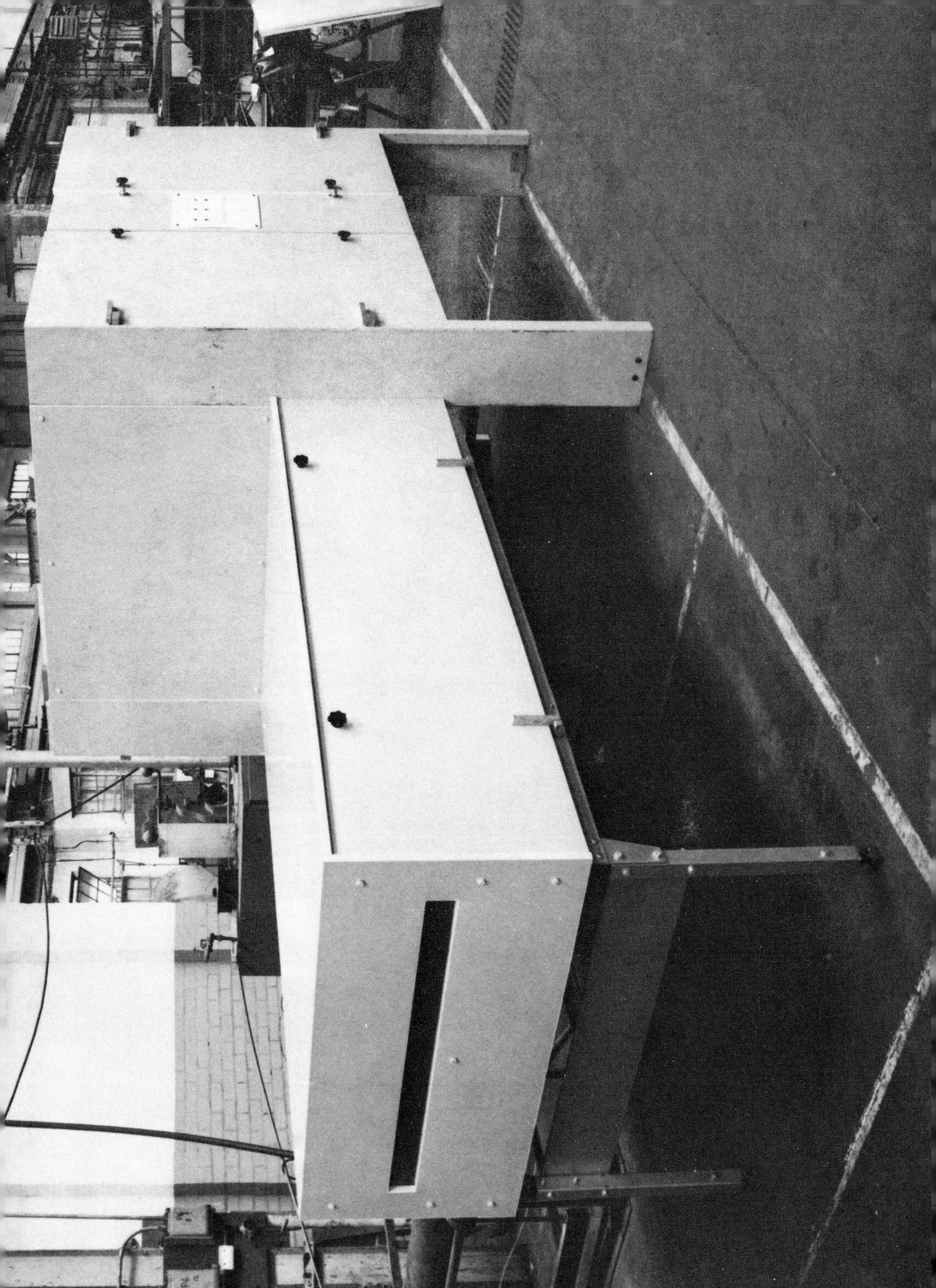

Fig. 4.13

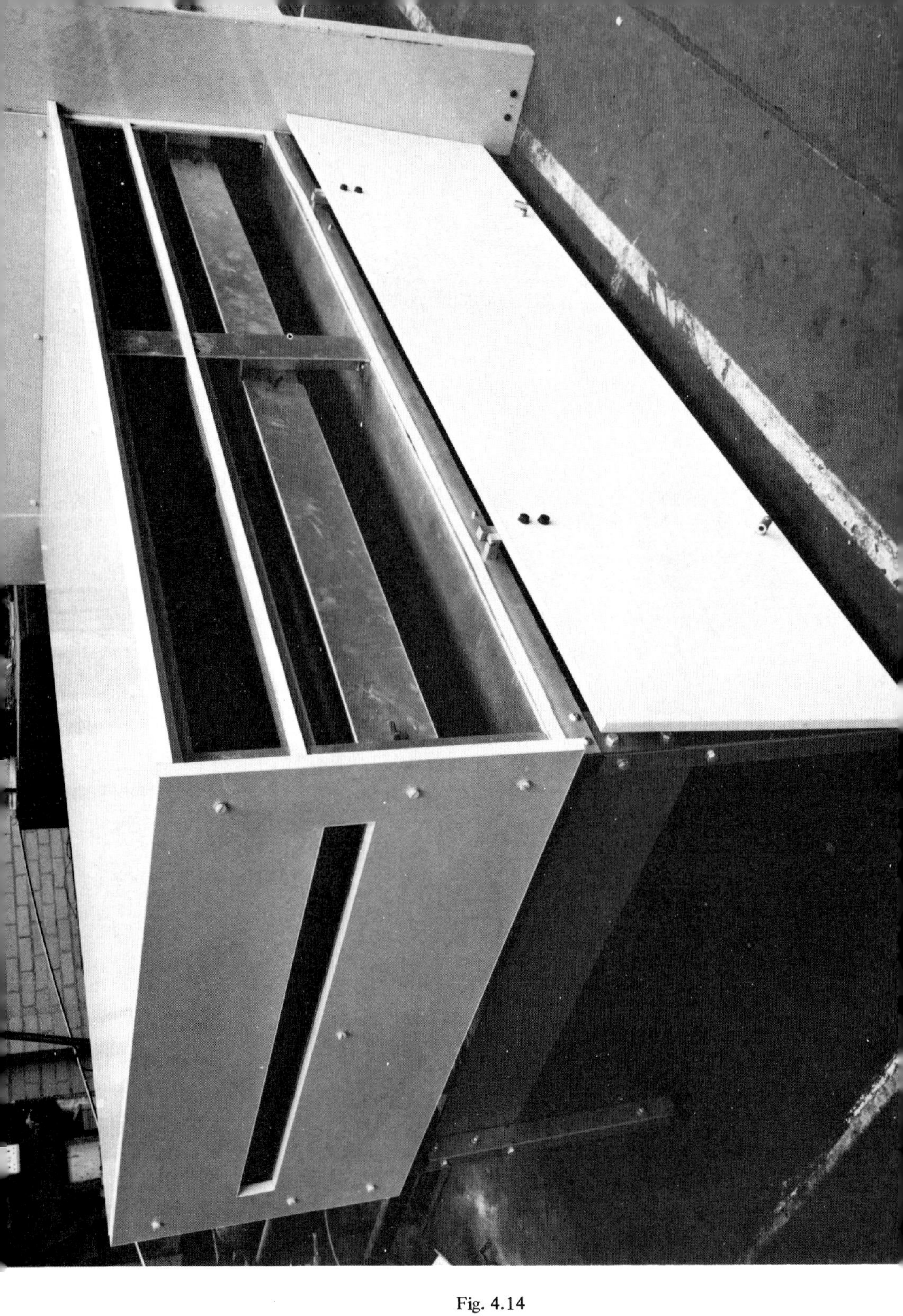

Fig. 4.14

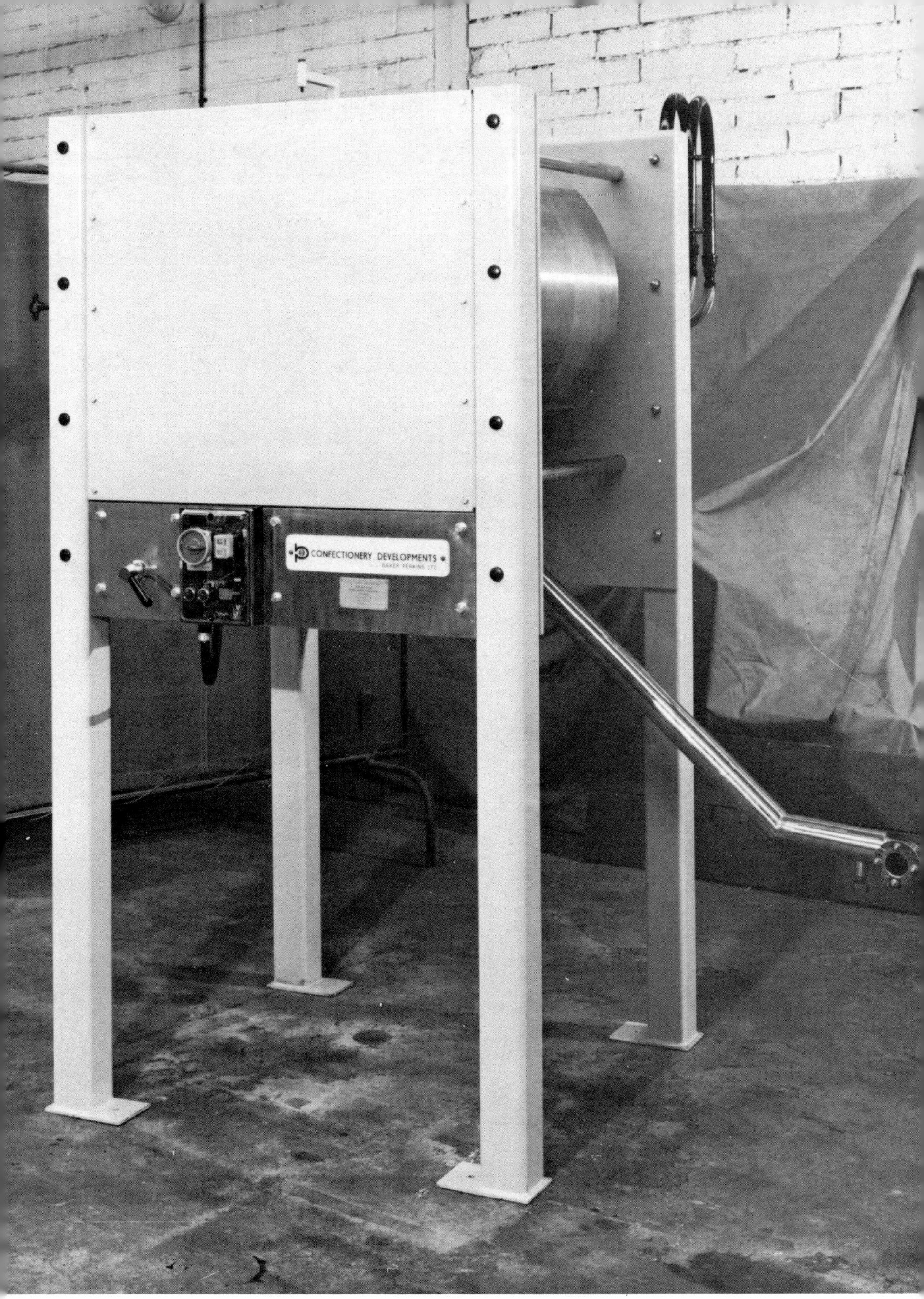

Fig. 4.15

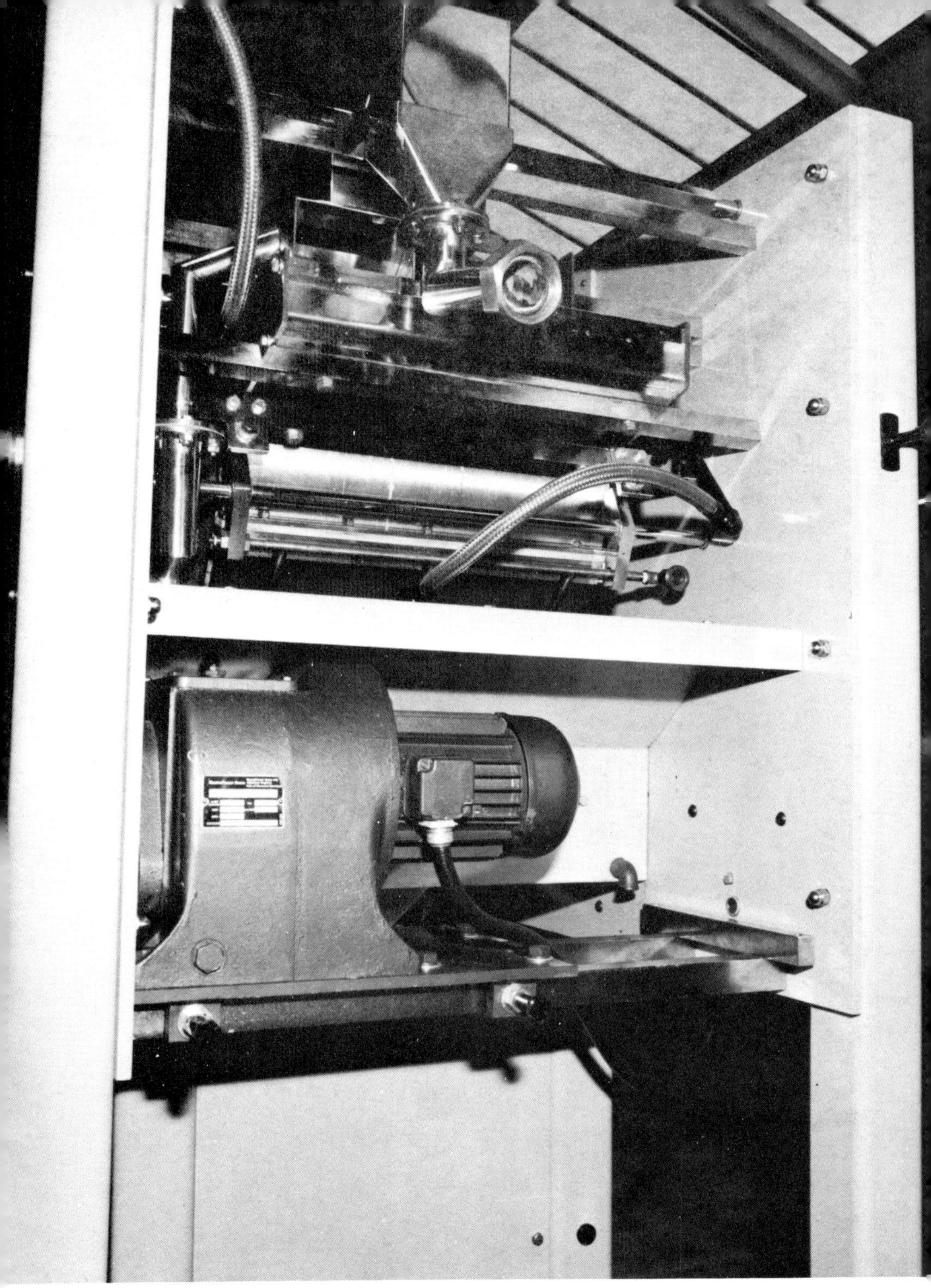

Fig. 4.16

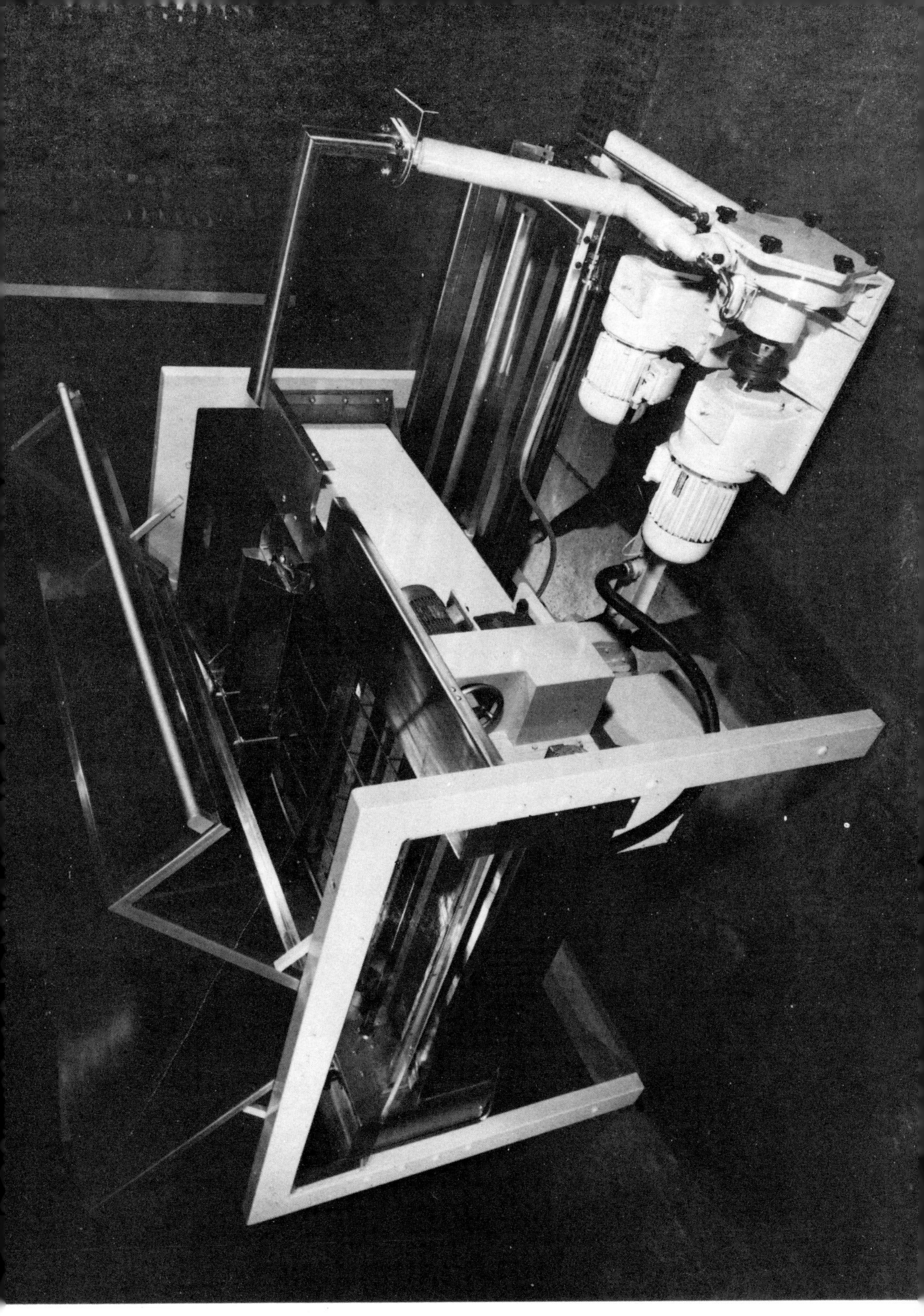

Fig. 4.17

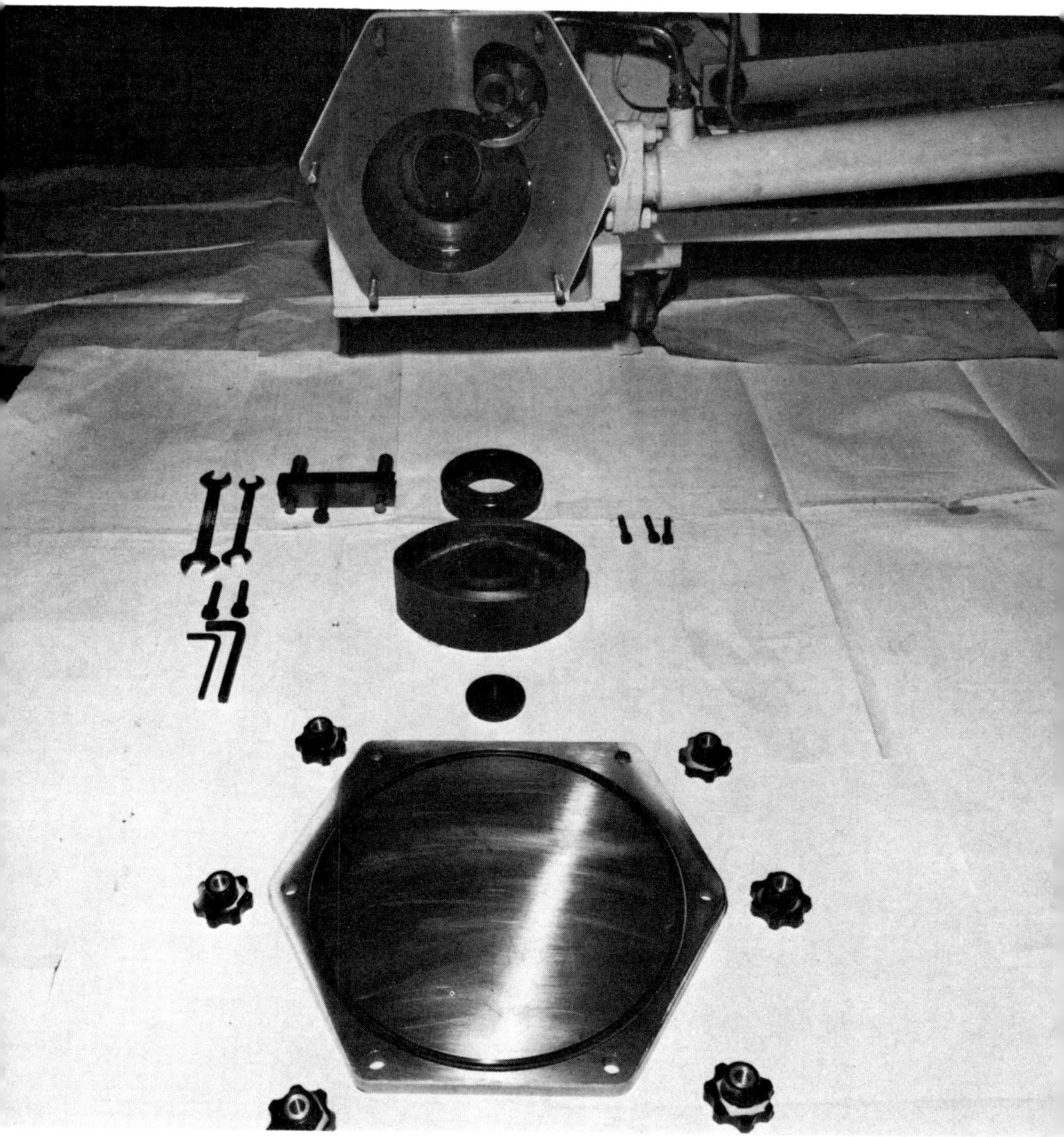

Fig. 4.18

SUMMARY

Summarizing, therefore, one must conclude that hygienic plant exteriors can be achieved only if sufficient thought is given to the problems at the functional specification/design stage of any machine or plant. Hygiene is not an 'add-on' feature.

Consideration must be given to configurational and process changes; to styling which will generate pride and operator care; and to the use of the latest materials and constructional techniques to help avoid nooks, crannies, and inaccessible ledges.

DISCUSSION

Mr W. E. Whitman (Leatherhead Food RA): Although I found Mr Ridgway's equipment very impressive, I wonder if he would say a few more words about the problem of contact between the machinery and the floor. Perhaps he might like to refer particularly to the high-speed mixer that he showed on one slide.

Mr Ridgway: The machine that I showed (Fig. 4.8) was one being manufactured in the Peterborough works. It was mounted on channels because that is our lining-up device for doing so. Of course, those surfaces will go directly down to the floor and one would grout in that particular base.

Mr D. J. Halliday (Unilever Engineering Division): On the same pieces of equipment you have gone to great lengths from the machine's point of view in sloping the surface of the box section and yet (presumably) the gearbox is in the box on the side with the flat top! It's not meant as a criticism, but it is very often a point which our electrical engineering friends tend to forget. We design a piece of equipment and they come along and stick a square box on the side of it which is just above eye level at the top surface which collects dust!

Mr Ridgway: All we can say about that is that that is part of the compromise. We do accept that is a problem with that particular machine. In mitigation it is a very smooth flat surface and it's beautifully finished!

Mr J. Brentnall (Mars Ltd.): On the electrical component side I wonder what you feel, Mr Ridgway, about pushbuttons? It always strikes me that this is unfortunate, especially on a flat panel when they often use shroudings presumably to prevent inadvertent actions. Have you thought about proximity buttons which we can now fit to improve this aspect.

Mr Ridgway: We are still using the type of equipment which you saw – the straightforward pushbutton, and thought is being given to the proximity type. I think one has to be very careful. When using proximity type buttons it is more easily accidentally operated and it is rather a novel thing. A lot of equipment suffers from what we call 'knob-twiddlers'. You know you can set a client up and somebody comes along and twiddles, and I think there could be a danger with proximity type switches. Having said that I don't think that is the end of the line, because developments are always coming along. There is the dirty area between the button and the shroud – I agree entirely. We do occasionally provide special type panels which are hose-proof which do cater in a more hygienic way than the ordinary standard press button which does have the crevice around the actual button. A good question: it will make me go back and think!

Mr John Milledge (National College): I noticed that all the motors had exposed fins and that you didn't use very many cap nuts. Could you comment on this?

Mr Ridgway: I think here we are dealing with component suppliers. It's a chain of events, and I think there is no doubt that the suppliers to the machinery manufacturers are improving. They are once removed, and I think things like motors and gearboxes in the food industry compared with the late 1950s are great improvements: there are smooth surface motors available. Motors themselves are getting smaller, and the old theory behind all these things is to get rid of the heat. So the British tradition of solid engineering and old principles is gradually changing, and we are certainly putting pressure on bought-out gearbox manufacturers, on motor suppliers, to take note; and I think if the code we were hearing about this morning does come into effect it will be up to the machinery suppliers to make sure copies of that do go to the basic components industry, whatever they might be. They have got to realize that these types of industry are demanding a certain standard, and certainly we will do what we can.

Mr E. A. Guthrie (United Biscuits): Mr Ridgway showed some examples of stainless steel in the immediate proximity of the product. Can he comment on what alternatives there are to paint on larger surfaces where stainless steel would be prohibitively expensive?

Mr Ridgway: I think we have a problem in large areas where it is desirable but impractical to use stainless steel throughout. You have to sit down and analyse just which parts are going to be knocked, kicked, leant on, and generally handled, and you have just got to draw the line somewhere. You know you have to go through every bit of the plant and say which bits are going to suffer damage and which are less likely to and design accordingly.

Mr Guthrie: I was wondering whether metal spraying would take the place of paint.

Mr Ridgway: Where we have used it we felt it has not always been entirely satisfactory. The question of cost comes into it, and appearance. It is possible in a lot of areas to what we call 'Armourmax' or 'Armourcoat' metals, and this is a molybdenum-type of spray with PTFE. They are sintered together, and it is a very durable surface and we do put this on certain machines. The net appearance is a very dark brownish, blackish surface which I think would not be acceptable in general practice. It is used on certain strategic parts. The second approach is that you can use more and more and more stainless of a domestic type. You know it doesn't have to be the terribly expensive 316 type, not for this class of machinery. It's a question really what, when you walk into your factory, you want to see. If we were doing a fat spray, for example, we would probably say 'all stainless'. If you were doing a complete biscuit line with big ovens I think the whole environment for your work force (those that are still on the floor, not in the control rooms!) would not be conducive to keeping that particular department so bright and perhaps clean. I appreciate that in talking this way I am talking again bakery type products. One couldn't apply these remarks, I am sure, to the fish and meat industry.

CHAPTER 5

Test Rigs for Evaluation of Hygiene in Plant Design

D. A. Timperley and **G. B. Lawson**, Unilever Research Ltd.

INTRODUCTION

Until recent times, little thought was given to the subject of hygienic design applied to food processing plant. It was only when a piece of equipment was running in a factory that people realized that an important consideration, in addition to the normal performance criteria, was how the equipment was to be cleaned. And again, usually, cleaning meant hosing until the visible surfaces looked clean, and little thought, from unskilled operators at least, was given to the hidden parts of machinery. The result was that many pieces of standard equipment, in widespread use in our industry, have never been designed with hygiene in mind, and little objective scientific information on hygienic performance exists in the literature.

With increasing use in general food processing of techniques of in-place cleaning, which were developed in the first instance for the dairy and brewing industries, it was considered that a study should be made of the *principles* of cleaning food equipment.

It was appreciated that, ideally, such a study should take place on actual production plant, using typical operating conditions so as to take into account important effects of the build-up of product in dead spaces during a run, or residual product on start-up. It was realized, however, that to obtain objective and widely-applicable data, it was necessary to work under laboratory conditions, and so, some time ago, a test rig was designed and built for the investigation of the effects of design on in-place cleaning efficiency. This work was extended to include flow visualization studies on selected pipe fittings. More recently, a test rig has been developed for the evaluation of the cleaning of hard surfaces.

In this paper, the test rigs will be described and examples of applications will be presented.

CLEAN-IN-PLACE RIG

A test rig was designed and commissioned which is capable of pumping a liquid or semi-solid food through tubes, test pieces, and valves. The rig is so designed that cleaning solutions can be circulated over a wide range of flow rates and temperatures. The whole rig is now capable of being cleaned to a very high standard.

Description

The rig was designed so that various liquids (water, detergents, sanitizers, etc.) could be pumped through a test section at various flow rates and temperatures to determine the optimum conditions for cleaning and sanitizing a particular item.

A schematic diagram of the rig as originally built is shown in Fig. 5.1; this was later modified at the commissioning stage. Cleaning fluids are drawn from any one of three 180 litre stainless steel vessels; the outlet from each vessel is

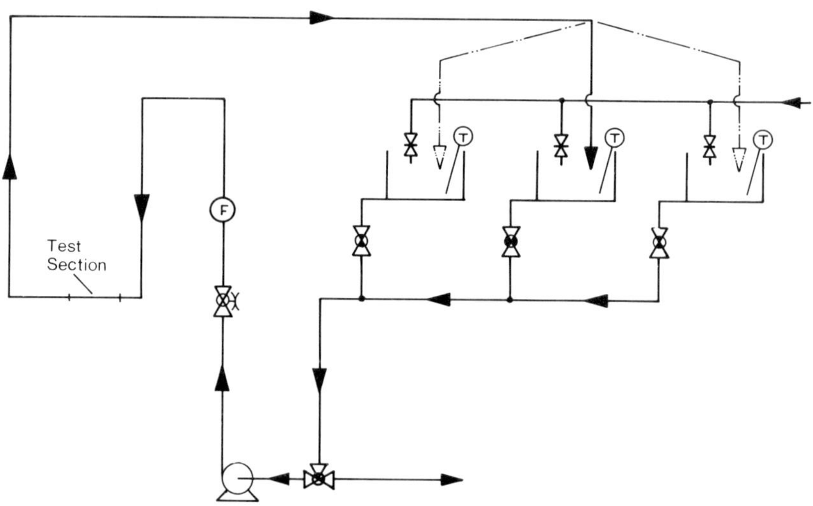

Fig. 5.1 – Original CIP circuit.

fitted with a 2-way plug cock. A 3-way plug cock is fitted in the suction line to the pump so that the system can be drained. The pump, capable of delivering up to 19 000 l/hr, is a centrifugal type of crevice-free design and stainless steel construction; all product surfaces are either of polished stainless steel or of synthetic rubber. A water-cooled seal is fitted to protect the seal faces should caustic soda solutions be circulated, as these would crystallize on cooling. The fluid is discharged from the pump, via a pinch valve for flow regulation and 45–225 l/min hygienic orifice rotameter, to the test section which may be up to 1.5 m in length. Following the test section the pipework is raised to ensure that the test section always runs full. The fluid may be returned to any of the three vessels, as the end of the pipe has a flexible section. Standard, mechanically-polished inside and outside tubing of 38 mm outside diameter is used throughout.

This size was chosen as it was considered to be an average size and would permit velocities of up to 5 m/s to be attained. All pipe fittings are of the crevice-free I.D.F. type. The grade of stainless steel used for the vessels and pipe-work is Type 316 S16 as it has superior corrosion resistance to other chromium-nickel steels and in particular to pitting corrosion.

The vessels may be filled with either hot or cold water; as temperatures of up to 85°C are required a thermostatic steam/water heater is fitted in the supply. Clips are attached to the rim of each vessel to support a thermometer.

Commissioning

During commissioning several features were found to be lacking, and some difficulties arose with certain parts of the system. The rig was therefore modified to correct these, and the system is now as shown in Fig. 5.2.

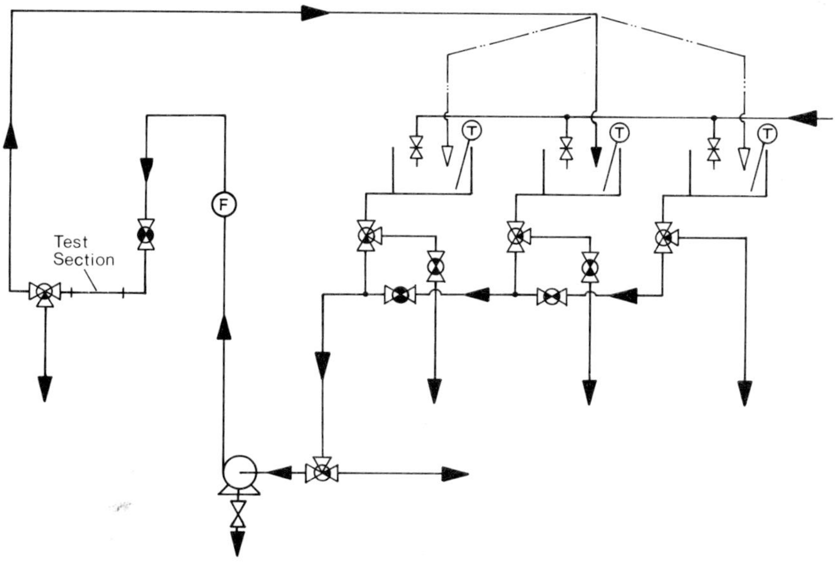

Fig. 5.2 – Modified CIP circuit.

When running at low flow rates, that is, at a high discharge head, the pump surged, and this was attributed to flexing of the rubber sleeve in the pinch valve as it was subjected to a high pressure drop. The valve was replaced by a diaphragm type, and although this was an improvement surging did sometimes occur. As the head on the discharge side of the pump is quite low it was decided to replace the original 5¼ inch diameter impeller by one of 4 inch diameter which gave a flow of more than 14 000 l/hr at lower heads and eliminated the surging. This gives a maximum mean velocity of flow of 3.5 m/s through the 38 mm o.d. tube.

Additional plug cocks have also been fitted so that (i) each vessel may be independently drained while the other vessels are in use, (ii) the suction pipe from the vessels may soil only the pipe leading from the particular vessel in use, and (iii) the test section may be flushed through to drain to avoid excessive soiling of the return system.

The pump could only be completely drained if the housing was removed, and to avoid this a drain plug was fitted.

When these modifications had been completed the rig was cleaned, using the basic cleaning schedules and, in addition, a biocide was circulated to sanitize the rig. A soiled test piece was inserted and subjected to the basic cleaning schedule. The rig was then stripped and critically examined for dead areas.

With one exception, the various parts of the rig appeared to be clean, and it was considered suitable for the type of investigations proposed. The rather important exceptions were the plug cocks. These can only be cleaned completely by either dismantling or loosening the top cover during sanitation so that fluid leaks from the cock. In practice very little soil should be circulating during cleaning, but on a production line the plug cocks would certainly cause problems. Air-operated diversion valves which can be cleaned in place would be preferred but on a cost basis they could not be justified.

Our final check of the rig showed that the temperature of solutions fell on circulation. As this has a marked effect on the Reynolds number, thermostatically-controlled immersion heaters were fitted to each vessel.

Applications

Having built a rig with which the cleaning-in-place of soiled equipment could be studied, it was decided that the optimum flow rate of the cleaning solution should be determined firstly, as this was of fundamental importance to the cleaning of a closed system.

In addition to using the correct cleaning velocity, it is most important to select the correct surface finish to ensure the minimum deposition of soil and to obtain maximum cleanability. As the pipework forms a considerable part of a closed system, the effect of surface finish on soil retention was investigated.

The range of items of food equipment is in most cases very wide, and the selection of a particular piece of equipment which may be available from a number of manufacturers may depend upon price and delivery. However, as more types of food products are made which are not microbiologically stable and are not sterilized in the pack, the bacteriological requirements for the equipment are becoming increasingly more important. Not only must much of the equipment be suitable for cleaning-in-place, in which case surface finish and the absence of crevices are important, but it must be suitable for steam sterilization as well as being bacteria-tight.

A wide range of equipment is being examined for these requirements, and of this range mention will be made of pipe couplings, welded pipework, valves, and T-pieces.

Closed systems often, of necessity, include dead-ends. Pipework T-pieces are used to mount instrument probes and valves, and it is the blanked-off T-piece which can cause a microbial hazard during production or prove difficult if not impossible to clean in-place. A dead-end can contaminate product in two ways. Soil in which organisms can grow may be left in a dead-end after cleaning, or on start-up product will fill the dead-end and if conditions are suitable there will be microbial growth during the run.

Flow velocity

The mean velocity of flow for cleaning is widely quoted as being of the order of 1.5 m/s, but this has not been substantiated by published data. It has also been stated that the greater, and hence the more turbulent, the flow of detergent solution over the soiling film, then the greater will be the chances of penetration, solution, and emulsification. It was, therefore, of interest to study the effect of Reynolds number on cleaning because when the Reynolds number for two geometrically-similar systems is the same, then dynamic similarity exists and the flow pattern is the same.

Two sizes of stainless steel pipe were used for these experiments, 38 and 76 mm o.d. The internal surfaces were coated with a tenacious soil containing micro-organisms. After cleaning at each velocity, swabs were taken from the internal surface and the count of residual organisms obtained.

The results are shown on Fig. 5.3. It is seen that the residual level of organisms for both sizes of pipe decreases rapidly with increase in velocity before levelling off at about 1.5 m/s. It is also interesting to note that all velocities the results for the two sizes of pipe are very similar. Whilst higher velocities would result in increased turbulence they would have little effect on the residual soil level.

The results are now shown on Fig. 5.4 plotted versus Reynolds number and show that increasing Reynolds number does improve cleaning, but, at constant Reynolds number, cleaning is most efficient in the smaller pipe where the mean velocity of flow is higher. This effect was rather surprising because, as stated earlier, better cleaning would be expected at higher Reynolds Numbers.

These tests showed that pipes of different size are cleaned to the same degree if the same mean velocity of flow of the cleaning solution is used. The same degree of cleaning of pipes of different size is not achieved at equivalent Reynolds numbers. Based on our findings it is inferred that the level of residual bacteria on a surface for the soils used, is reduced to a minimum if the mean velocity of flow is about 1.5 m/s.

Surface finish

Whilst there are British and ISO standards for the surface finish of stainless steel tube for the food industry, there is little published information on the relationship between surface finish and residual soil levels. The existence of adhesion can be ascribed to intermolecular forces, but mechanical adhesion makes a significant contribution to the strength of a bond through the physical interlocking of the soil into the irregularities of the surface.

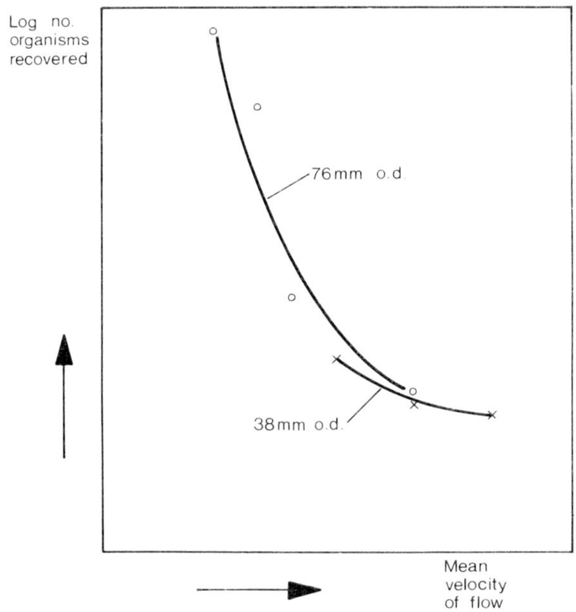

Fig. 5.3 – Effect of mean velocity of flow on removal of organisms from pipes.

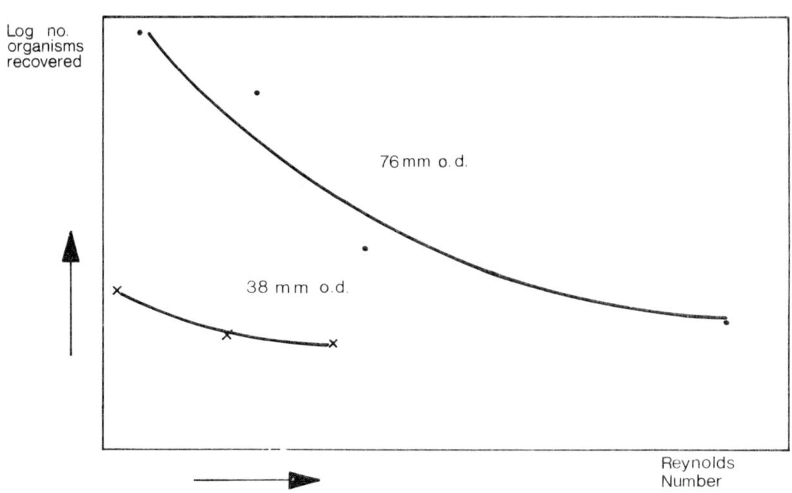

Fig. 5.4 – Effect of Reynolds number on removal of organisms from pipes.

The samples of tubing used for the experiment had different surface finishes which had been produced by different processes. All manufactured surfaces depart to some extent from absolute perfection, and in order to specify surface requirements, instruments have been developed to measure surface texture on a numerical basis. The main measuring parameter which is recognized internationally has the designation Ra and is identical to that known previously as CLA (centre-line-average). The Ra value is a quantifying concept and bears no physical resemblance to the profile. It can give an indication of the amplitude of surface irregularities, but it takes no account of their spacing.

After subjecting the samples to the same soiling and cleaning techniques, swabs of the internal surfaces were taken at different times, and the results are shown in Fig. 5.5. The tube having the smoothest surface was mechanically polished, the next was electropolished, and the remaining three were descaled.

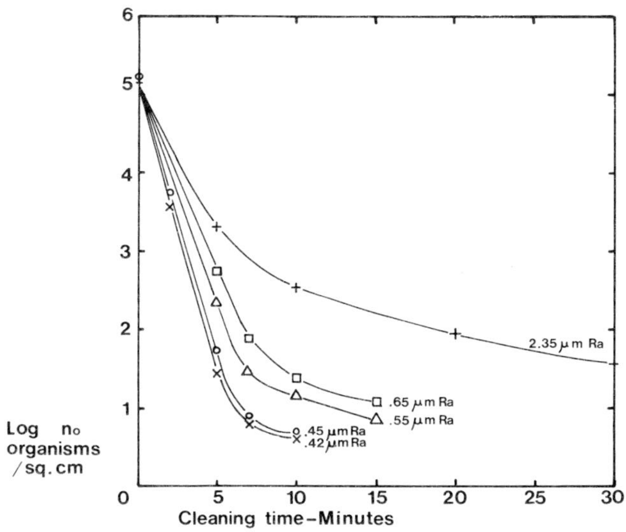

Fig. 5.5 – Residual counts from different pipe surfaces.

If a residual count of 10 organisms/square centimetre is taken as a reasonable value for a clean surface, then for this experiment which was designed to be comparative, only surfaces having a surface finish of up to 0.5 μm Ra can be cleaned in 15 minutes. The residual count after a cleaning time of 10 minutes is shown as a percentage of the initial level and plotted versus surface finish in Fig. 5.6. This is a linear relationship. The time taken for a 99.99% removal of soil is shown plotted versus surface finish, Fig. 5.7, and it is seen that it takes twice as long to clean a surface of 1.0 μm Ra as it does one of 0.5 μm. The figure of 99.99% removal results from the difference between the initial inoculum level of 10^5 and the final count of 10^1. It is reiterated that this was a comparative test, and it does not necessarily follow that surfaces having high Ra values cannot be cleaned with stronger detergent solutions or over longer periods; but the results clearly indicate that the rougher the surface finish, the more difficult it is to clean.

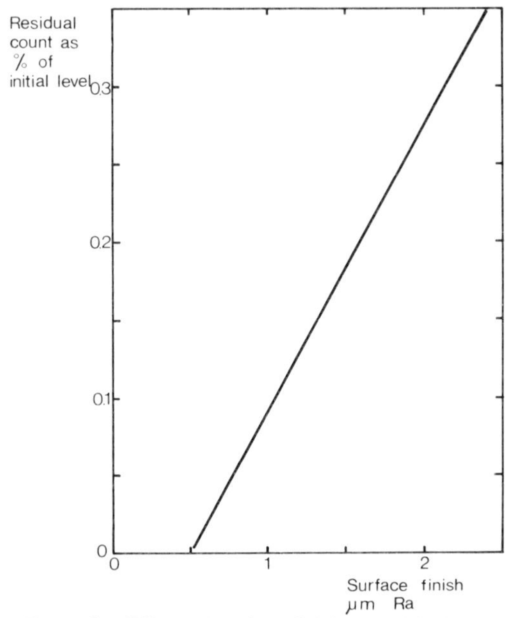

Fig. 5.6 – Effect of surface finish on residual count.

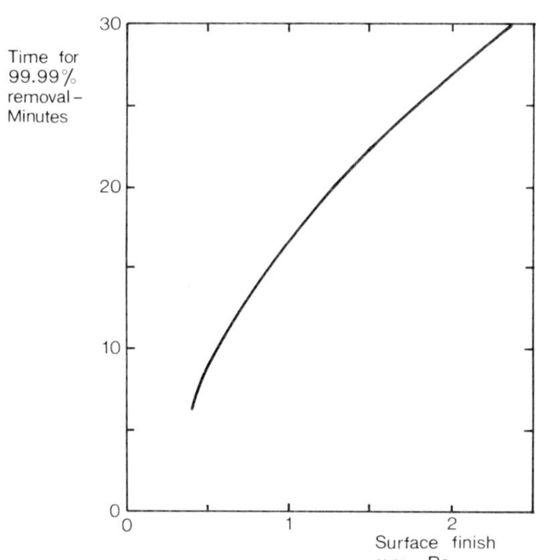

Fig. 5.7 – Effect of surface finish on cleaning time.

The effect of electropolishing the internal surface of a descaled tube is shown in 5.8. This is a more economical way of reducing the Ra value than by mechanical polishing. It is interesting to note that not only has the Ra value been almost halved, but the frequency of the irregularities has been reduced, the peaks rounded off, and the valleys widened. The Ra value has, however, been shown to give good correlation with the bacteriological assessment of the cleanability of the internal pipe surfaces. The scale has been included because cocci, which are common food poisoning bacteria, are merely 0.5 to 1.0 microns in diameter, and these actual traces of pipe surfaces show how great the peak to valley heights are in comparison.

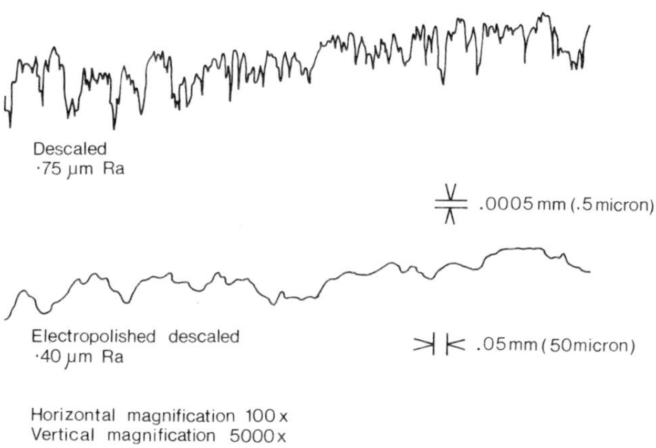

Fig. 5.8 – Effect of electropolishing on a descaled surface.

Pipe couplings

The range of couplings available is so wide that selection is most difficult. Although there is an ISO standard, many countries have their own standards, and many manufacturers their own particular version. Basically, there are two types – those which are attached to the pipes by expanding and those by welding. In most cases a seal ring is clamped between the two ferrules which are drawn together by a nut or by a split clamp. Couplings are designed for breakdown cleaning or in-place cleaning, and some for both. For most expanded couplings the grade of the ferrule material is relatively unimportant, but for the welded coupling it is essential that the coupling and pipe materials are compatible.

A coupling designed and widely used for breakdown cleaning in this country is the RJT, the Ring Joint Type, Fig. 5.9. It is a simple robust fitting which can withstand a degree of misalignment and is based on British Standard 1864. It suffers from two faults; one, it has a crevice, and two, the 'O' ring is difficult to remove for cleaning.

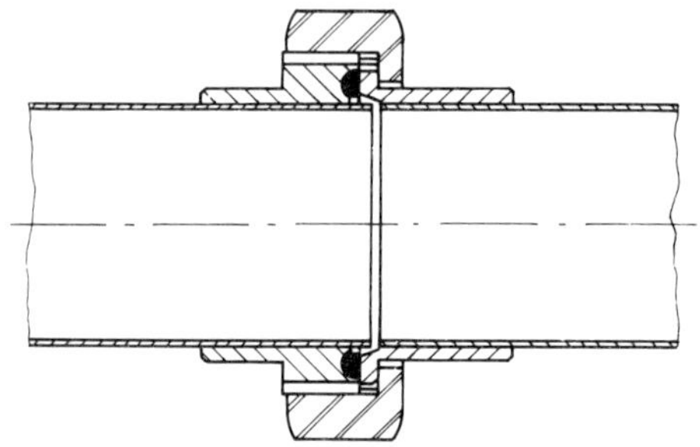

Fig. 5.9 – RJT coupling.

The IDF coupling, which is based on the International Dairy Federation paper No. 14/1960, is becoming widely used in Europe. It is designed for in-place cleaning and is available in both expanded or welded form, (see Fig. 5.10). In its welded form it can be seen that a smooth, continuous surface results, but in its expanded form, because the same seal ring is used, there is a step, and soil particles may remain on the downstream side of the seal after cleaning. This is a fault common in many of the couplings tested. If the bore is flush, then the coupling will be satisfactorily cleaned in-place, and if the seal material is suitable,

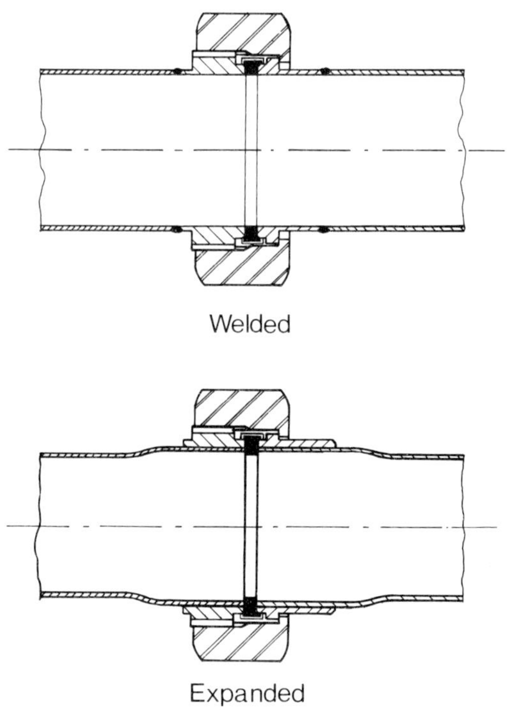

Fig. 5.10 – IDF coupling.

then it can be sterilized; but unless the nut is tightened correctly, the coupling will not be bacteria tight. Whilst the nut may be tightened sufficiently to make the coupling leak-tight, it was found that bacteria can penetrate unless a minimum torque is applied. Excessive tightening will result in the extrusion of the seal ring with resultant cleaning problems.

Welded pipework

Orbital welding of pipework has been used for a number of years in the dairy and brewing industries to join sections of pipe as an alternative method to couplings. It is particularly attractive for large installations where there are long runs of piping which will not require rearranging for long periods. There are a number of machines on the market, and the welding heads are such that they are used easily in situ. The machines are basically TIG torches which rotate around the pipe. The wall thickness of tube used in the food industry is thin enough not to require filler metal. An orbital weld is shown on Fig. 5.11, and a cross-section, Fig. 5.12, shows little change in the wall thickness.

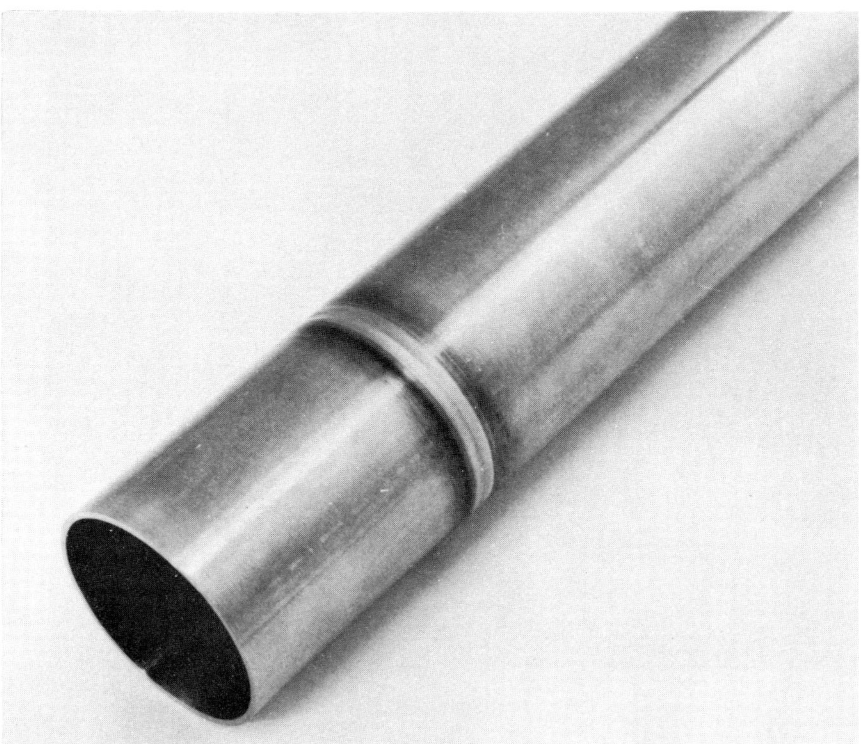

Fig. 5.11 – Orbitally welded pipe.

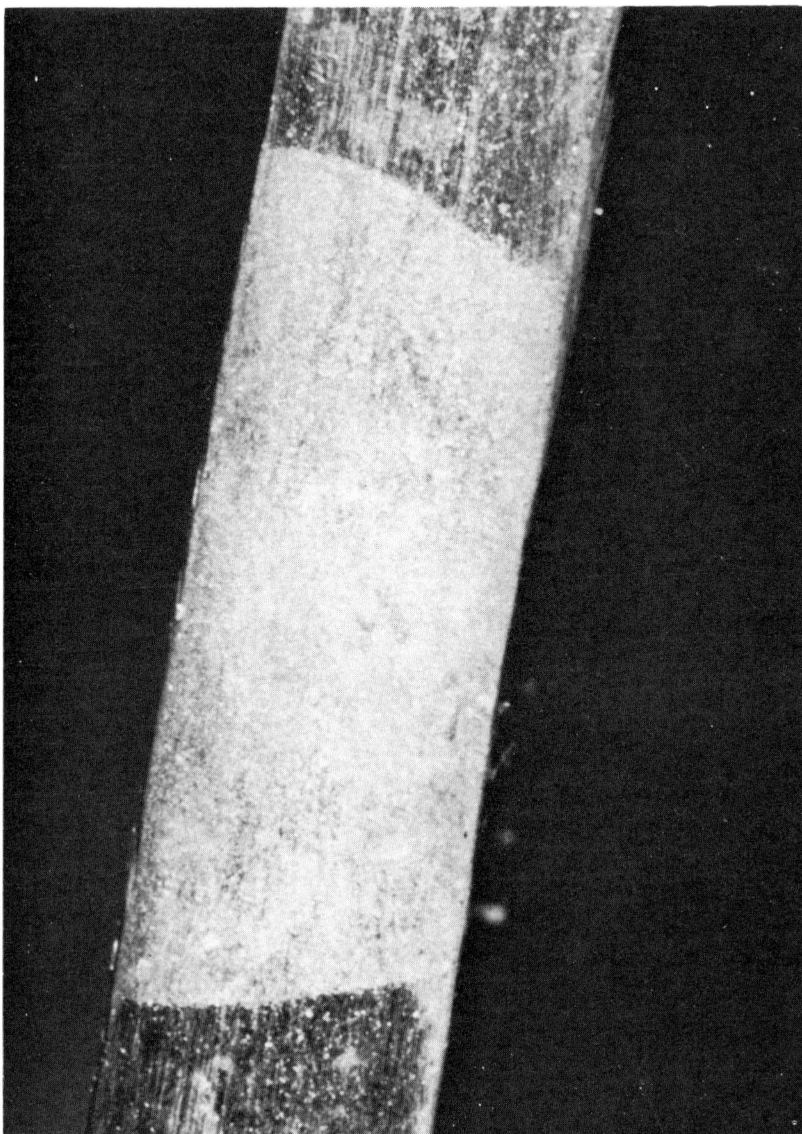

Fig. 5.12 – Cross-section of an orbital weld.

Samples of orbitally-welded pipes were obtained from various manufacturers worldwide, and the in-place cleanability of them compared with the best coupling. They all equalled it and have the added advantage that they are bacteria-tight.

Orbital welding is an automatic process, and if properly programmed it gives consistently good welds which do not require polishing.

Valves

The range of valves also is very wide, and they cannot all be examined for their hygienic aspects. There are, however, three main types – the membrane or diaphragm valve, the plug and stem valve, and the plug cock. There is a great variation in the number and size of dead-ends in each type of valve so that in addition to the bacteria-tightness aspect, the cleanability and sterilizability also may vary to a great extent.

The membrane type shown, Fig. 5.13, is a good example of a valve which is cleanable in-place, can be steam sterilized at 140°C, and is bacteria-tight. The design is such that the annular space is completely swept by product so that build-up during production is avoided. The membrane requires regular inspection depending on conditions of use. The example shown is hand-operated, but it is also available with air-operation for remote control, and a diversion valve, Fig. 5.14, is also available. This particular type of membrane valve is especially suitable for aseptic process lines.

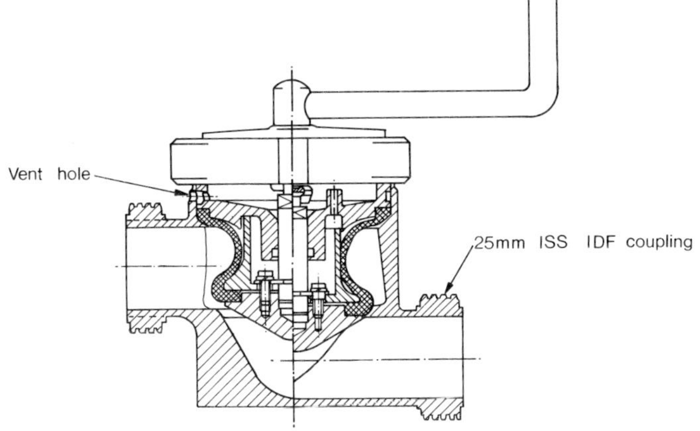

Fig. 5.13 – Membrane valve.

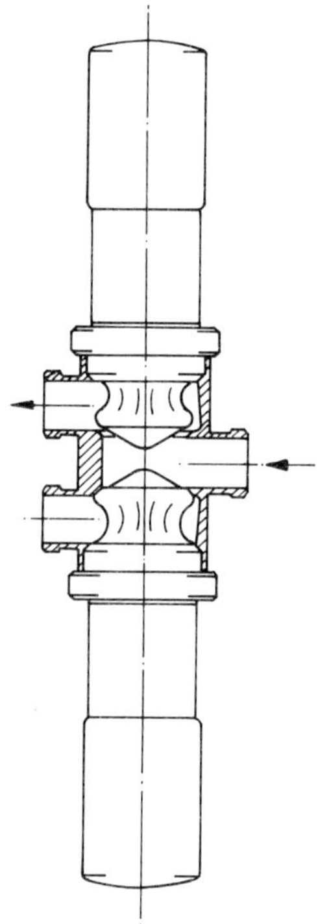

Fig. 5.14 – Flow diversion valve.

The next type of valve is that which has a stem passing through the body, Fig. 5.15. It is available from several manufacturers with a variety of ports; that shown is a simple on/off with a single valve head which is actuated through the stem by a pneumatic cylinder. The stem of the version on the left is sealed by a diaphragm and that on the right by a lip seal. Both are suitable for c.i.p. and for steam sterilization at 140°C, but only the left-hand version is bacteria-tight, making it suitable for aseptic process lines.

Plug cocks, Fig. 5.16, which are widely used are not suitable for in-place cleaning because of the retention of product in the tapered seat and in the plug when it is in the 'off' position. This valve can only be cleaned by dismantling, and then the valve seat is prone to damage.

Tee-pieces

Experiments have been conducted using the contaminated dead-end of a T-piece. In all three arrangements of the T-piece the product became contaminated to some degree. If samples taken immediately production starts are contaminated, then this could indicate a contaminated dead-end, and it is likely that subsequent production will also be contaminated but to a lesser degree. On the other hand, if contamination occurs during production owing to microbial growth in the dead-end, then this may well determine the duration of production before cleaning operations have to be carried out.

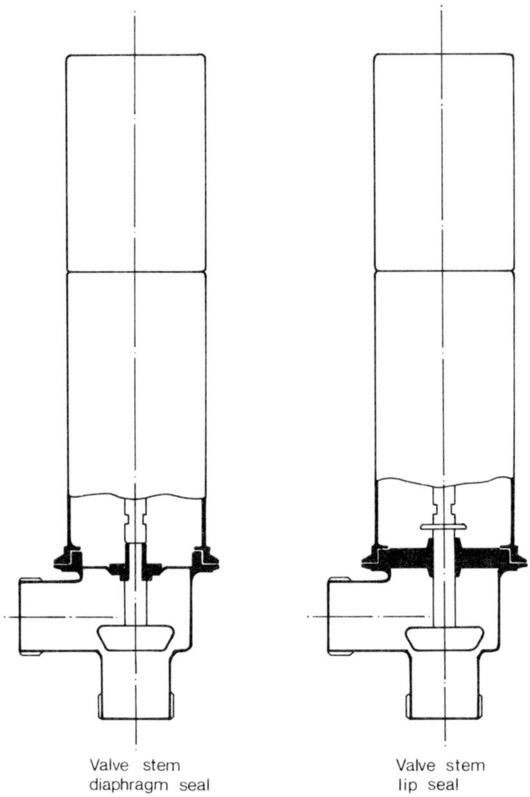

Fig. 5.15 – Plug and stem valve.

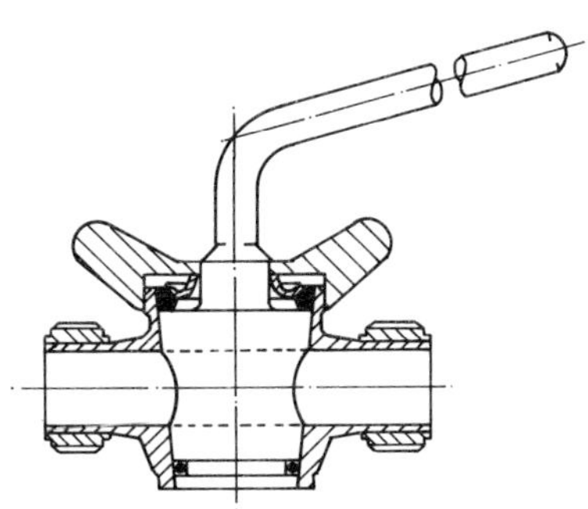

Fig. 5.16 – Plug cock.

Although it has been shown that dead-ends can be a source of contamination we did, however, investigate the cleaning of dead-ends, using a standard pipework T-piece. Various soils containing organisms were used to fill the dead-end, the depth of which could be varied. The T-piece was tested in the rig in all three positions; flow into, flow past, and flow from the dead-end. The results showed that, as would be expected, the shorter the dead-end the easier it is to clean. Equally important is the position of the dead-end relative to the direction of flow, and this should be such that the cleaning solution flows into it, as in Fig. 5.17. The ideal solution is to eliminate dead-ends completely as we have found that spoilage of large batches of product can result from comparatively small quantities of trapped contaminated material. As this is often not possible, when T-pieces are employed, then the dead-end leg should be reduced to a minimum (a stub of about 7 mm is sufficient for welding a coupling on) and the fluid should be directed into the dead-end when cleaning.

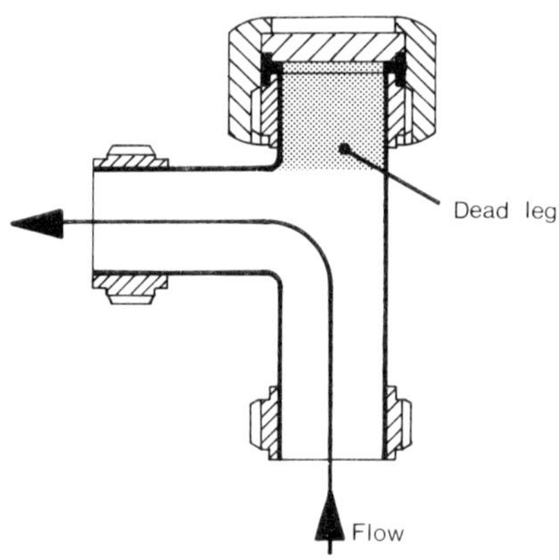

Fig. 5.17 – Modified pipe tee-piece.

FLOW VISUALIZATION RIG

Flow visualization techniques have been developed to enable the simulation and study of a wide range of flow problems. In particular, this technique was used to study the flow patterns in a pipework T-piece when one leg is blanked off. The results explained the findings of the bacteriological investigation.

Technique

An optical tracer technique using aluminium particles suspended in a transparent flow medium was selected for the study. The particles follow the slow patterns of the fluid and with suitable illumination their motion may be recorded by still or high-speed cinephotography or by video tape recording. The video tape method provides a complete record with the advantage of slow motion or stop replay where single frame photographs may be taken from the monitor screen, each frame representing 0.02 seconds. In this case particle velocities were suitable for the video tape method to be applicable.

Description

The test section was a standard QVF T-piece (13.6 mm internal diameter) encased in a rectangular perspex box. A close-fitting, stainless steel plug designed

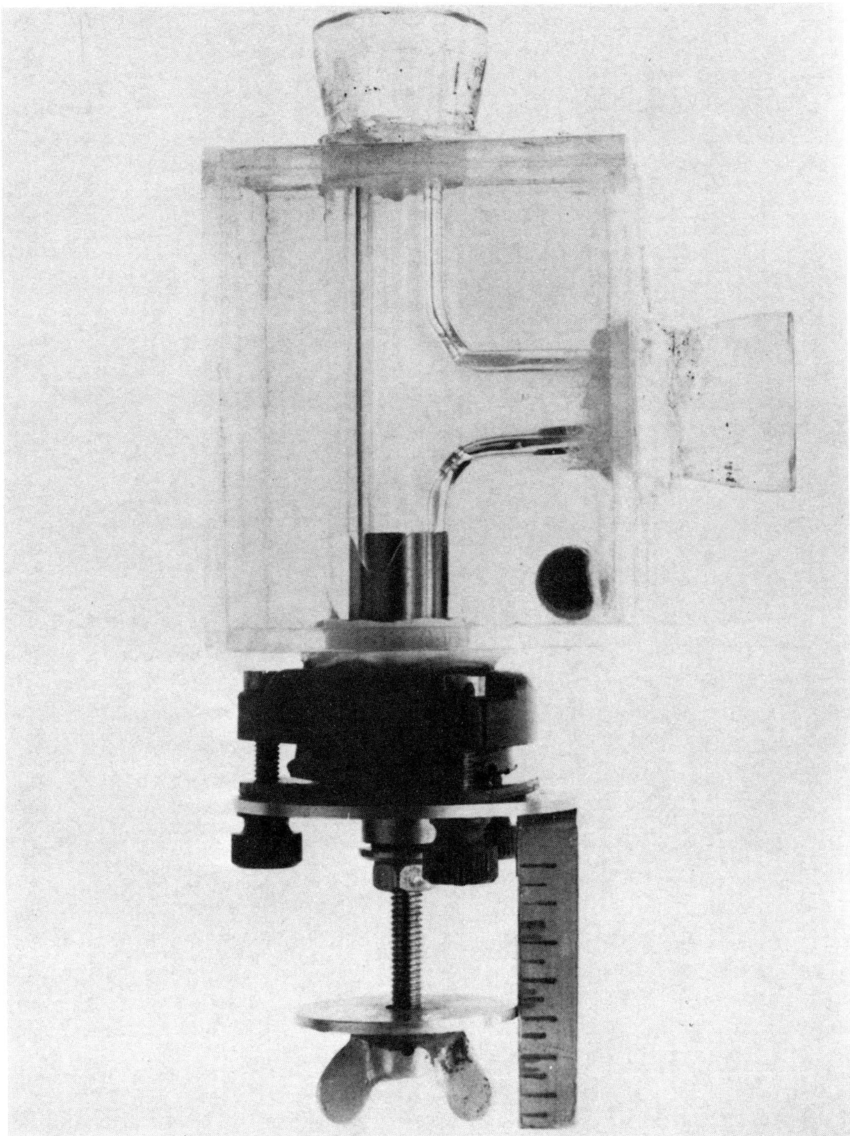

Fig. 5.18 – Tee-piece test section.

to fit any arm of the T-piece was attached and adjusted to give the required depth of 'dead-leg' or distance between plug and mainstream flow. Fig. 5.18 shows the test section and Fig. 5.19 the flow diagram of the system. Connecting pipework was also QVF throughout to facilitate alterations in direction of flow through the T-piece. In all tests flow was turbulent, so no extended entrance lengths were needed to stabilize flow.

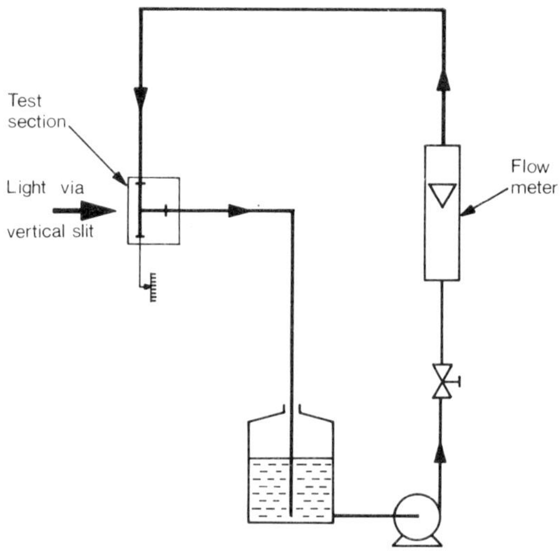

Fig. 5.19 – Flow visualization circuit.

The flowing medium had the same refractive index as the glass T-piece. The Perspex box surrounding the T-piece was filled with a fluid which also had the same refractive index as the glass, so that an undistorted view of flow within the T-piece was obtained when viewing normal to the plane of the perspex.

Two concentrations of aluminium powder were used: a) a relatively large amount to show up gross flow effects, and b) a very small amount to show individual particle traces. The powder was less than 0.074 mm diameter (200 mesh) so that settling effects were negligible. Actual concentration levels were determined visually by trial and error.

The aluminium was illuminated by a floodlight via a 3 mm wide vertical slit which was set 40 mm away from the centre of the T-piece so that a curtain of light approximately 5 mm wide was projected through the major plane of the T-piece. The test section was viewed at right angles to the curtain of light, and flow was recorded on video tape.

Results

Traces of the motion of individual particles in the dead-leg were made at different main flow velocities with the blanked-off leg in the three positions. They were compiled from consecutive frames of video tape where each frame represented motion in 0.02 sec.

Typical traces for the three positions are shown in Fig. 5.20, for a mainstream velocity of 1.5 m/s. When the flow is directed into the dead-end the highest velocities in it are obtained. They increase with increase in mainstream velocity. Flow past the dead-end gives a much reduced velocity in it, and an increase in main flow velocity has little effect. Mass transfer from the dead-end is even lower. The motion becomes increasingly more random with increasing main flow velocity.

These traces illustrate the direction and velocity in two dimensions only but do confirm that the condition where fluid flows into the dead-end gives the best soil removal.

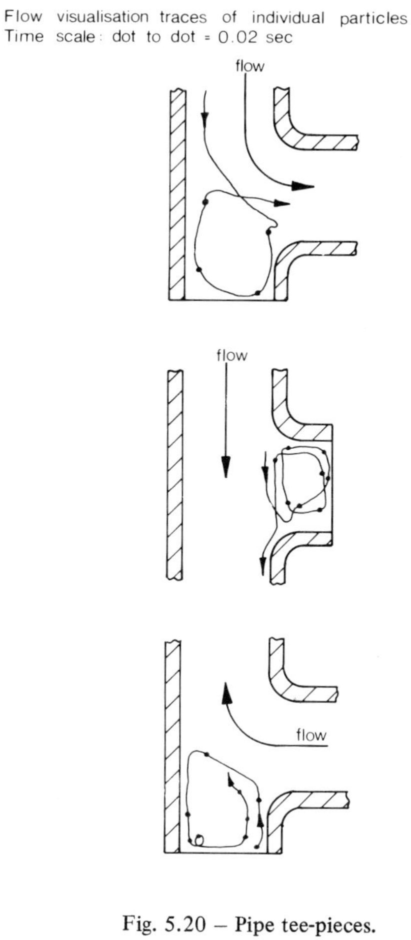

Fig. 5.20 – Pipe tee-pieces.

HARD SURFACE CLEANING RIG

Much equipment used in the food industry cannot be cleaned in-place, and cleaning has to be carried out by applying detergent to the soiled surfaces followed by washing using hand-held hoses or lances. Dismantling of the equipment is often necessary before cleaning. There are many spray cleaning units on the market, and there are many arguments as to the effectiveness of high-pressure /low volume or low-pressure/high-volume systems, although there may well be other considerations, such as a water shortage or effluent problems. Food contact surfaces should be smooth and non-porous, but how smooth, and how many conveyor belts are non-porous? The principles of cleaning with jets are so different from those for cleaning in-place that, in order to gain a better understanding of the subject and to establish criteria for surface finish, a rig for this purpose has been designed and built.

Description

The rig, shown diagrammatically in Fig. 5.21, consists basically of a variable speed conveyor to which samples under test can be attached and sprayed by a variety of cleaning fluids at different temperatures, pressures, and flow rates via a nozzle, the distance and angle of which can be varied.

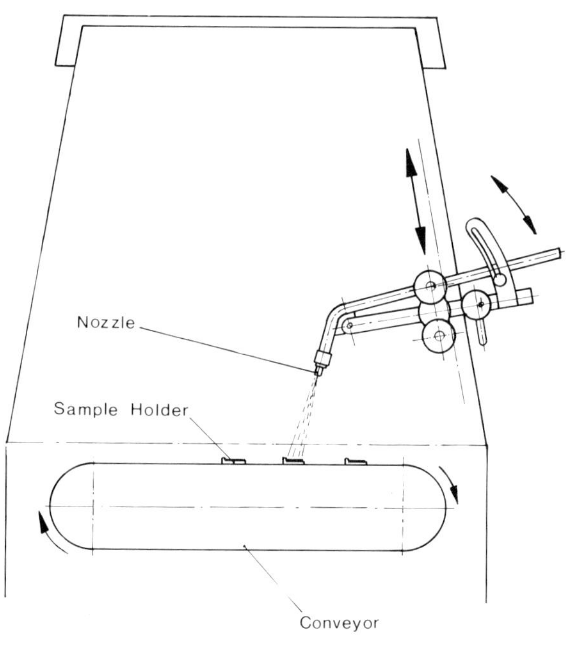

Fig. 5.21 – Diagramatic arrangement of spray cabinet.

It comprises a free-standing frame containing the conveyor, tanks, pump and controls, above which a hood is mounted to house the spray head. A general view is shown in Fig. 5.22. The base section with the front cover removed is shown in Fig. 5.23.

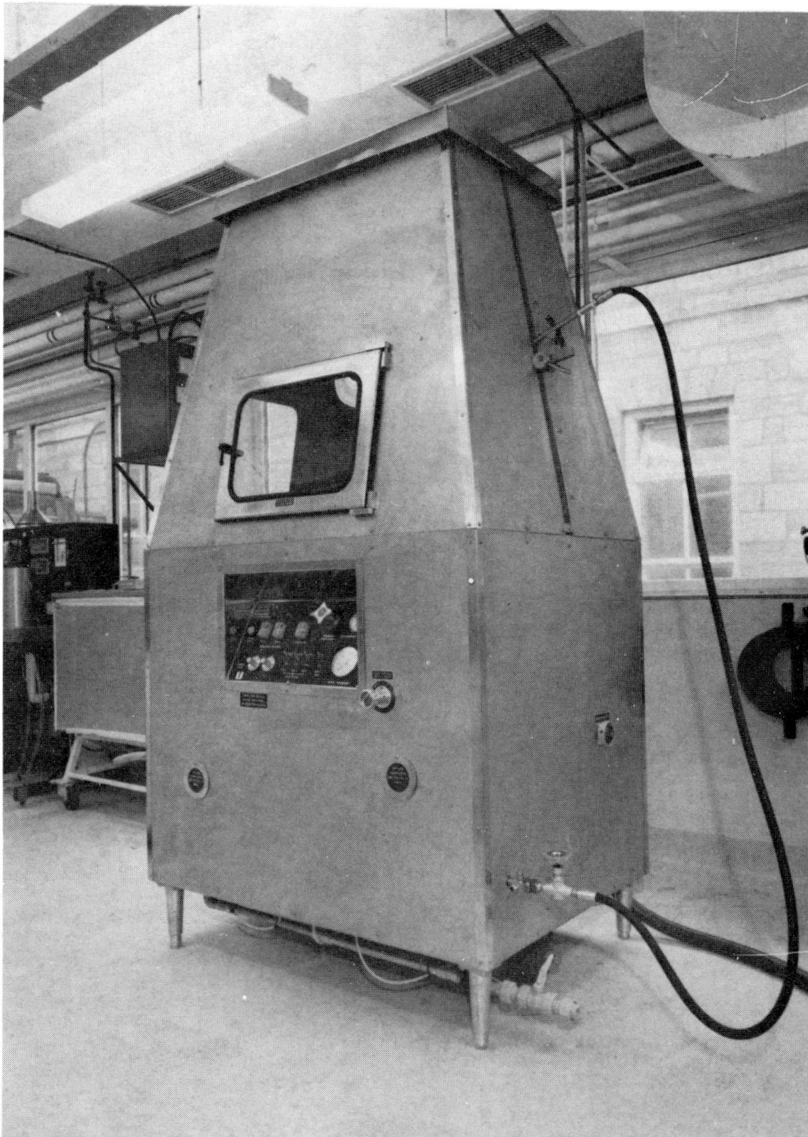

Fig. 5.22 – Spray cabinet.

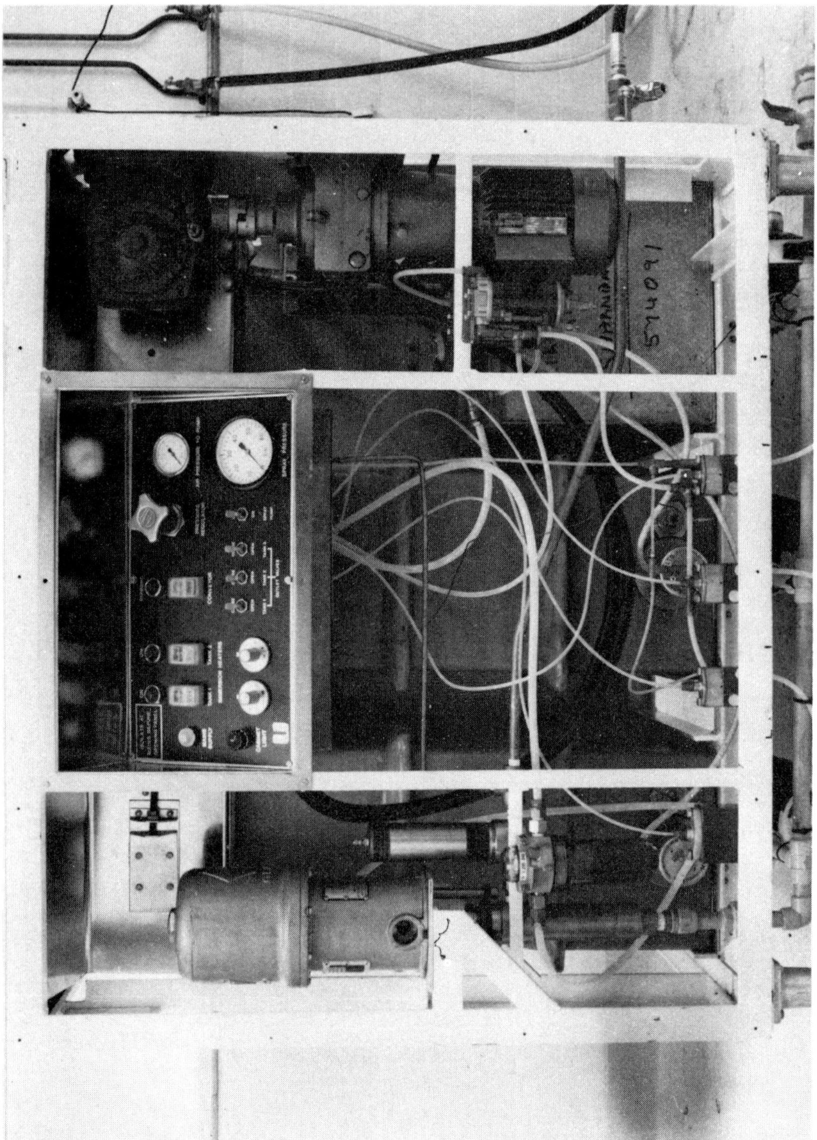

Fig. 5.23 – Spray cabinet with front cover removed.

An air-operated piston pump which can deliver fluids at pressures of up to 70 bar and flows up to 12 l/min draws fluid from one of three tanks, the selection being made via air-operated diaphragm valves. Two tanks, each having a capacity of 120 l, are of g.r.p. and are fitted with thermostatically controlled heaters. The third tank of 80 l capacity is of galvanized steel and is for the supply of cold water only. An air vessel is fitted to the discharge side of the pump to damp pulsations. Flow rate is controlled by a needle valve, and the high-pressure fluid is fed up to the nozzle by a flexible hose. A stainless steel trough runs the full width of the frame and is mounted above the tanks. This contains the conveyor which is driven by a variable speed motor via a right-angle gear box at speeds from 0.05 to 0.6 m/s. Fluid collected by the trough is led directly to drain; it was decided not to recirculate cleaning fluids so as to avoid the possibility of recontamination. The control panel is also mounted in the base frame. The circuit is shown in Fig. 5.24.

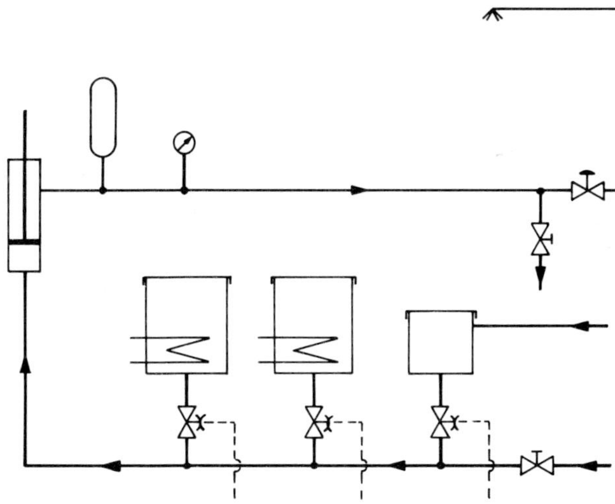

Fig. 5.24 – Spray circuit.

The hood which is secured to the top of the base section houses the spray head. An access door is fitted to the front and a light inside the top of the hood. Observation panels are positioned in the door and one end to check the nozzle setting. The spray head, Fig. 5.25, is attached to a carriage so that the height of the nozzle above the sample may be varied from 85 to 960 mm.

The jet angle may also be readily varied by up to 20 degrees from the vertical. Two of the twelve sample holders attached to a polyacetal slat conveyor can be seen.

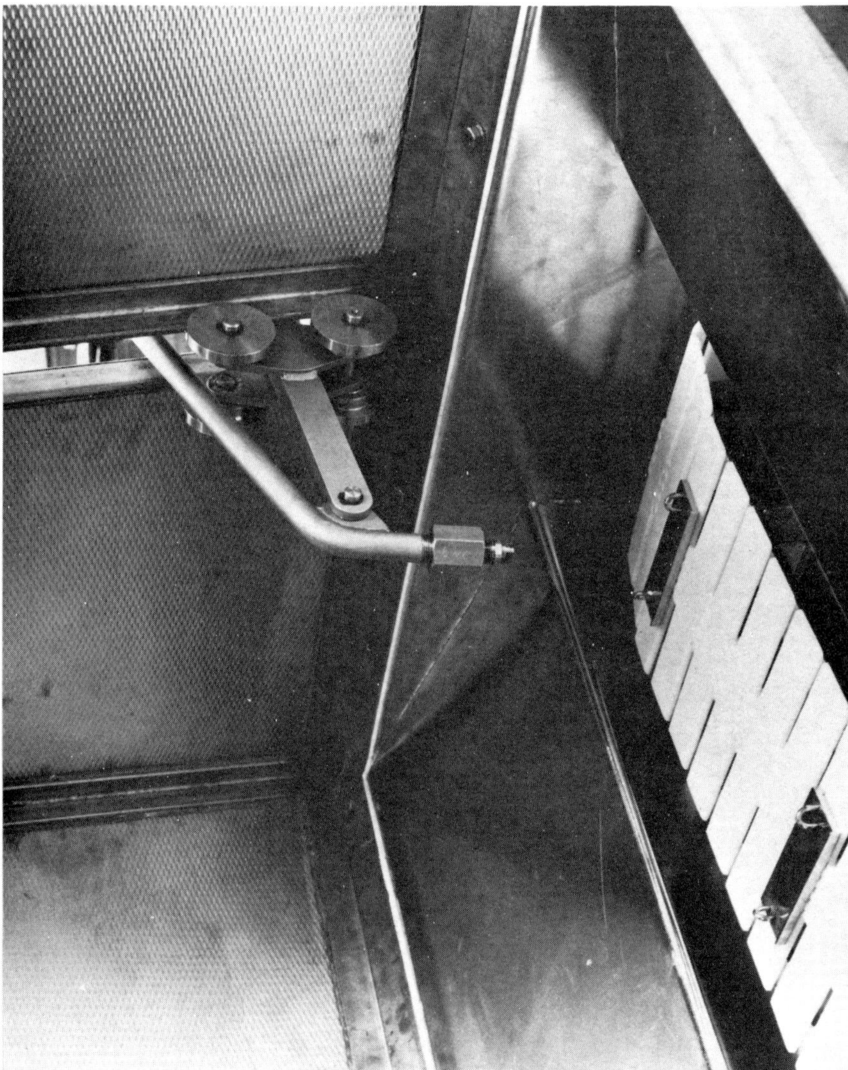

Fig. 5.25 – Spray head.

Commissioning

The major problem encountered was the rapid build-up of foam in the bottom of the conveyor trough. The return run of the conveyor with the samples attached passed through the foam and introduced another variable. Three spray jets were fitted in the opposite end of the trough to the drain to flush the foam away. The existing discharge pipe was, however, unable to cope with the increased flow so the entire end of the trough was cut out and a chute fitted, as shown in Fig. 5.26. It was also observed that there was some splashing from the jet which could cause cross-contamination. A deflector plate was fitted between the top and bottom runs of the conveyor to prevent contamination of the return run of the conveyor from the spray and to reduce splashing; the slats between those carrying the sample holders were cut back, as shown in Fig. 5.27. The pulsations in the pressure of the pump output were considered to be too great, and as this too would be another variable an additional air vessel was fitted.

These modifications have all proved to be satisfactory.

Programme

As this rig has only recently been commissioned a test programme has not yet been embarked upon. Stainless steel is probably the most widely used contact material in the food industry, so that initial investigations will be made on this material to determine the relative cleanability of different finishes.

Conveyor belts can present cleaning problems. Selection is difficult, as a recent survey showed. Some 140 different samples of 'food quality' belting have been collected, and it is proposed to evaluate them for cleanability.

There is also a wide range of stainless steel conveyor belting and non-metallic surfaces to be examined as well as the nozzles themselves, the angles, distances, fluid pressures and temperatures, detergent strengths, and other factors which all contribute to the total effect.

CONCLUSIONS

This paper has described the work done in Unilever Research using test rigs in an attempt to understand objectively and quantitatively, if possible, the factors which are important in the hygienic design of certain pieces of food plant.

It is easy to fall into the trap of 'if it looks clean, it is clean'. It is only when one gets down to actual measurements of surface soil before and after a cleaning procedure that it becomes possible to make reliable judgements about a procedure's effectiveness and to make meaningful comparisons between different procedures.

From this study of hygiene by multidisciplinary teams of mechanical and chemical engineers and bacteriologists, the principles involved in some hygienic design situations have begun to emerge. Good hygiene is expensive, but the lack of it may cause not only financial loss to the company through spoilage but the spread of food-borne disease.

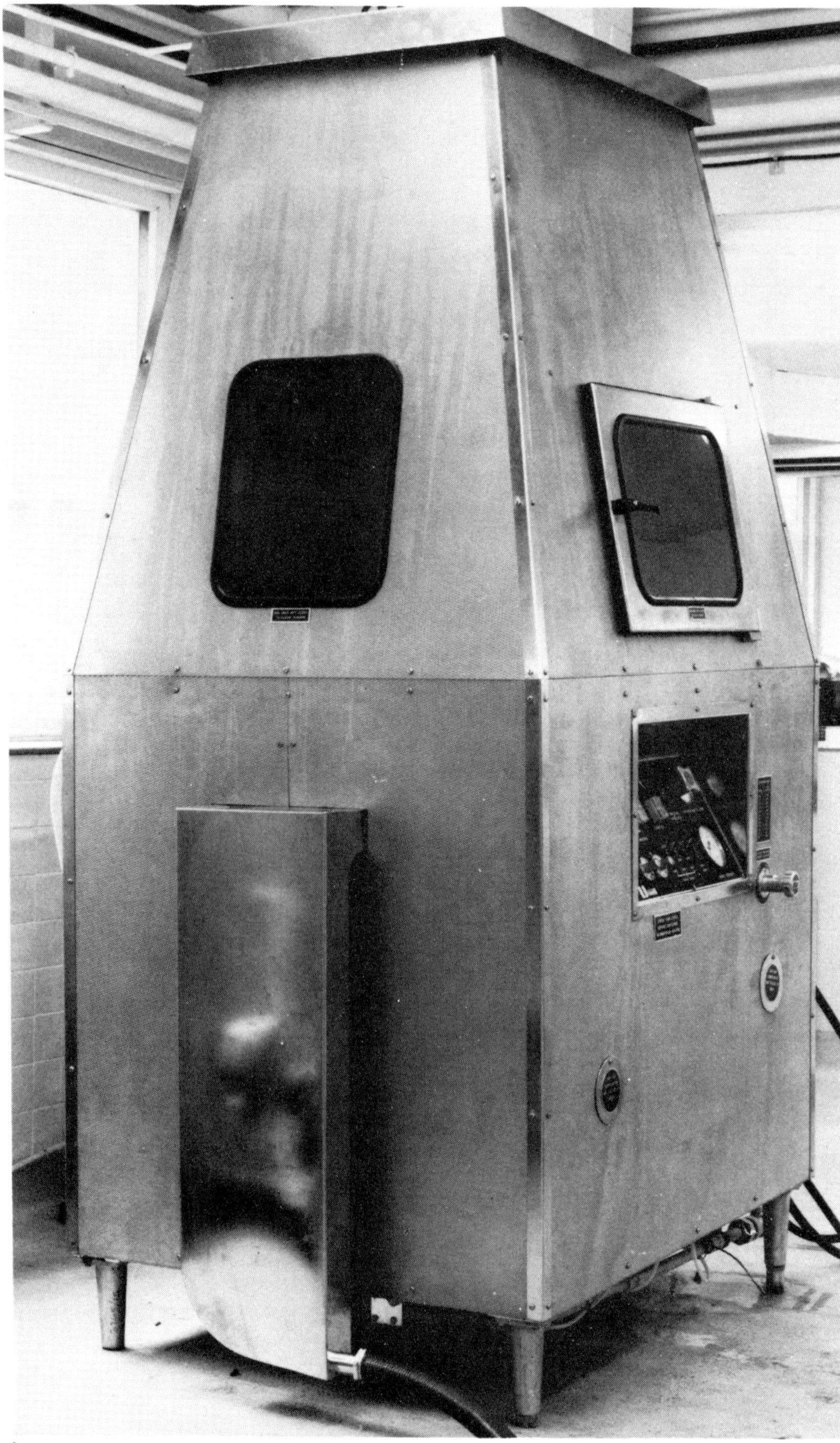

Fig. 5.26 – Modified trough discharge.

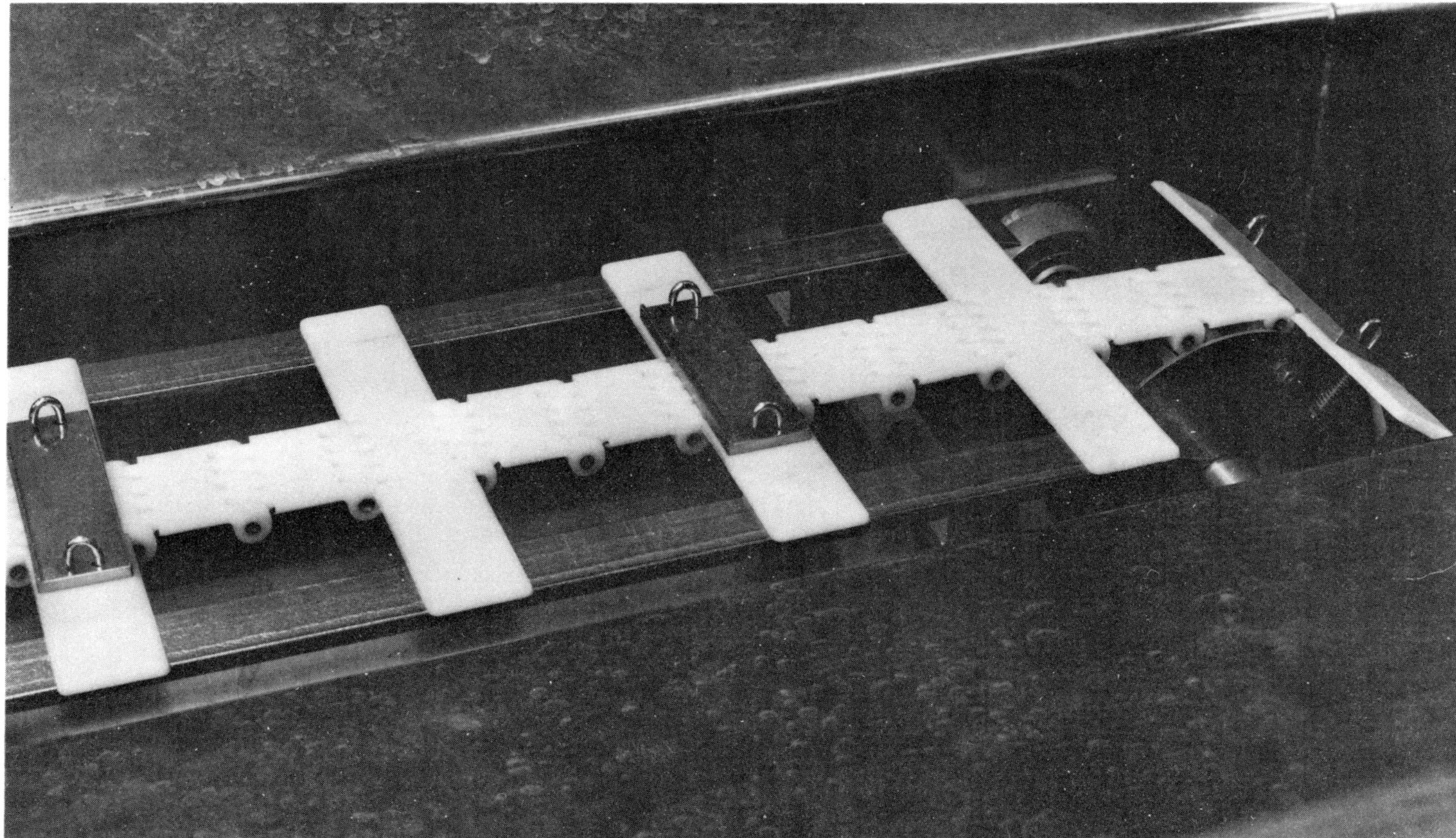

Fig. 5.27 – Modified conveyor.

The evaluation of the hygienic design of equipment is a lengthy and costly exercise and one which is likely to continue for some considerable time, but it is considered that in the long term it will yield a good return in product quality and a reduction in plant cleaning costs.

DISCUSSION

Mr V. R. Charlish (Colman Foods): I was intrigued, Dr Lawson, with the slide illustrating the deposition in a descaled pipeline and an electroplated one. Assuming the ordinates of the graphs were the same, how do you account for the fact that the peaks and the valleys were different? Was it something to do with some particular feature of the pumping process itself, or was it, in fact, inexpert electroplating? There was quite a significant difference in the pitching of the peaks and valleys.

Mr Timperley: First of all it was electro-*polished* tubing. It was of the same length of pipe, two pieces cut off consecutively. One was taken and measured on the talysurf, the other was sent away for electropolishing, and then that was measured as well, so that it wasn't exactly the same length of pipe.

Mr A. G. Cleather (APV Company): I was fascinated by your reference to the expanded IDF pipe coupling concerning the extrusion of the rubber joint ring into the tube, and I presume that your tests were performed under controlled conditions and all the fittings you used were at the recommended torques. Are you able to give some quantifiable measure of how much this really came into the tube? The implication of what you said was that it was certainly a bacterial hazard.

Dr Lawson: I can't give you the actual data in torques and so on used for tightening the various nuts. All we were trying to illustrate with that example is that certainly there is more than one way to make up any fitting. If you do it correctly then you don't normally have a problem in that particular case. If you tighten too much – and a great tendency, of course, is for operators to tighten rather more forcefully than they need to – in such an instance you can then get the ring extruding into the pipe and the possibility to have material trapped behind the surface, the edge that is opposite to the direction of flow.

Mr Cleather: You are talking about actually tightening the nut up by the operator rather than when the fitting is expanded on to the tube?

Dr Lawson: Yes, I mean when the joint is made up in use.

Mr T. C. Tamplin (APV): I just want to make a note – it may be explanatory for people who aren't familiar with these surface finish measurements that the actual measurement is taken by a needlelike probe which traces across the surface of the metal and drops into crevices on the surface, and this is amplified and produced as a trace on a chart so that you can actually receive an indication of the surface irregularities. Another thing that concerns me which is of great interest because we have also been working on similar problems is how did you achieve a 'British Standard' soil, because this is the one that has plagued us for some considerable time – how regularly and consistently for experimental purposes to produce a 'British Standard' soil which is satisfactory for all times?

Dr Lawson: I am sorry I have to dodge the question. We were limited in the amount of experimental technique that we were given permission to publish in this particular work, and unfortunately the answer to that question was one of the paragraphs we had to take out from the paper.

Mr J. J. Milledge (NCFT): What was the basis for selecting the swab method for assessing hygiene, and how were these results arranged and analysed, remembering the incompleteness of removal of bacteria by swab methods, variations between operators, and that bacterial distribution on a surface is not Gaussian but log-normal?

Mr Timperley: We have done a lot of work over some ten years on this, using the swab method (over 90% removal of organisms), and our bacteriologists consider the swab method to be very reliable, and better than the contact methods to remove organisms from the surface, which can leave some behind. We take a large number of swabs, and we find that we can go back after a period of years, do the same tests, and get repeatability; so we are in fact very happy with our method, which has taken us a long time to develop. Unfortunately, we can't publish it.

Dr Michael Hoare (University College, London): I was wondering whether you had attempted to correlate your results for the pipe-cleaning experiment using high velocity flows with the flow properties at the surface of the pipe (for example, wall shear stress) rather than with the bulk flow properties such as Reynolds number or mean flow velocity.

Dr Lawson: We have done some work where we have looked at some boundary layer experiments, as well as the bulk flow which you mention. We have a whole set of information on boundary layer activity and the relationship between the structures of the boundary layer and the conditions within it. Those results are not included in this paper but might be the subject of an additional publication some time in the future.

Mr R. Jowitt (NCFT): Centre-line-average roughness doesn't take into account the longitudinal or lateral distribution, does it? It just takes account of the vertical displacement of the stylus which is used. So that a piece of surface could have the same CLA or Ra value but with the peaks and valleys stretched out very much more, and this almost certainly would be the case with an electropolished surface whether you start off with the same roughness measurement or with some other starting material. Have you been able to compare surfaces with the same CLA or Ra average roughness, the one produced by electropolishing, the other produced ostensibly of the same Ra value but with ordinary mechanical polishing?

Mr Timperley: The answer is 'Yes we have'. We have looked at mechanically-polished finishes and electropolished, both having the same Ra value, and in fact they do have the same cleanability. This led us to state in the paper that in our opinion the cleanability is related directly to the CLA value or the Ra value.

Mr D. Carver (H. J. Heinz Co Ltd.): Although you cannot disclose your standard soiling technique, was it a relatively good simulation of the real thing?

Dr Lawson: Yes, and the one thing that we were able to do, as I hope came out, is that we were able to carry out an experiment and then at some later date repeat it and get the same answer. We have therefore a great deal of confidence that, whether you like the procedure or not, the actual results we get do allow us to conduct sensible scientific experiments.

CHAPTER 6

Health and Safety at Work and Hygiene Requirements

G. G. Daniels, The Health and Safety Executive

The law's objectives

In Britain the object of the various statutes applying in the food and pharmaceutical industries is, as regards public health, medicines, food, and drugs, to protect the *consumer,* whilst, as regards the Factories Act 1961, the Offices Shops and Railway Premises Act 1963, and the Health and Safety at Work Act 1974, the object so far as the items discussed in this paper are concerned is to protect the *employee.* To protect the consumer it is necessary to ensure that all parts of the machinery coming into contact with the product are capable of being cleaned and sterilized, and that it is not possible for contamination to occur owing to foreign bodies dropping into the product, or through cross-contamination between one product and another. To protect the factory operative, and others working in or visiting the premises, dangerous parts of the machinery must be guarded so that contact with them is not possible while such parts are in motion or use. At first sight it appears that these two requirements are incompatible, one requiring open and free access for cleaning, the other aimed at preventing access. However, with a little thought and goodwill, the two can be made to dovetail together quite satisfactorily.

The need to clean and sterilize is, of course, self-evident. The raw material is often, by the very nature of its origin, heavily contaminated, as it comes mainly from animals or the earth. It is also frequently an ideal medium in which, under appropriate conditions, the micro-organisms responsible for food poisoning can multiply. Cross-contamination of one product with another can also, in some instances, create serious problems and hence must be avoided by rigorous machine stripping and cleaning schedules. The extent to which cleaning needs to be carried out is normally well-established within a particular section of manufacturing industry. It is, however, desirable that product manufacturers and their outlets are given adequate guidance to enable them to comply with their legal and moral obligations.

Who is responsible?

The question of how to achieve machinery safety while still allowing adequate cleaning to take place therefore becomes the predominant issue. For new machinery, consideration of the guarding requirements commences with the machine designer and maker. The Health and Safety at Work Act 1974, Sections 6(1)(a) (see Appendix) makes it plainly a responsibility of the manufacturers, designers, and others defined in the section to produce a machine which can be used safely and without risks to health. For the industries under discussion this should include a facility for the machine to be safely cleaned.

The Factories Act 1961, at Section 17, sub-sections 1 and 2 (see Appendix) also places obligations concerning the guarding of machinery on machine makers and others involved in the supply of new machinery.

Many machine makers have worked hard to comply with their legal requirements, but regrettably a number of machines still reach the user in an unsatisfactory condition. It is, therefore, suggested to British machinery makers, designers, and suppliers, and the agents and suppliers of imported machines, that they check their machine designs for operator safety when in use and for safety of the machine sanitation personnel while it is being cleaned.

In those sections of the food industry where a survey of machinery accidents has been possible it appears that some sixty per cent of the accidents occurred during cleaning and the clearing of blockages.

The relevant Acts

The ultimate destination of the machine is a manufacturer of a product who in the main will lack the engineering facilities to be found in the premises of the machinery manufacturer. He will, therefore, have a piece of machinery with which he must manufacture his product in a manner which satisfies the law. As stated earlier, provided that he complies with the various hygiene requirements relevant to his product, he will then be left to comply with the legal safety requirements. These are to be found in Section 12 (prime movers), 13 (transmission machinery), 14 (guarding of other machinery), 15 (unguarded machinery), and 16 (maintenance of guarding) of the Factories Act 1961, and Sections 1, 2, and 3 of the Health and Safety at Work Act 1974. There are premises other than factories (such as offices, shops, and warehouses) in which food machinery is used and to which the Factories Act may not apply. In these instances it may well be that the Offices, Shops and Railway Premises Act 1963 applies, in which case Section 17 of that Act (see Appendix) will be relevant together with Sections 1, 2, and 3 of the Health and Safety at Work Act 1974.

The requirements of Sections 12, 13, 14, 15, and 16 of the Factories Act 1961 and Section 17 of the Offices, Shops and Railway Premises Act 1974 are absolute, and no relaxation is allowed unless the Secretary of State makes specific regulations for particular machinery. As regards food machinery, no regulations relaxing guarding standards have been made.

Section 2 of the Health and Safety at Work Act 1974 introduces requirements for a reasonably practicable standard of safety when the machine is properly used, and a safe working system: but as Section 14 of the Factories Act has not been repealed the user is still required to fence securely his machine, and it is this standard together with a safe working system which the Factory Inspector is required to enforce.

Clearing blockages

There is an impression in industry that a fitter or some other duly certificated individual may, without question, remove a guard to carry out setting, cleaning, or other preparatory operations and then set the machinery in motion to ensure its correct working. The instances, extent, and conditions under which this type of operation can be carried out are defined in Sections 15 and 16 of the Factories Act, the Regulations referred to in these sections being the Operations at Unfenced Machinery Regulations 1938 (SR and I 1938 No 641).

In Section 15 of the Factories Act no reference is made to cleaning or to clearing of blockages. It therefore follows that machinery must not be in motion under power while the guards are removed for the carrying out of these operations. As the law does not allow the cleaning of machinery in motion under power or the clearing of blockages while the machine is in motion under power with the guards removed, the Regulations referred to above are irrelevant to the matters under consideration.

Interlocks

It is very rare for the management of a company to be able to guarantee the complete isolation of a machine from the power supply at all times during a cleaning operation. This is the very time when some or all of the guards will of necessity be removed from the machine processing areas to allow the sanitation crew to gain access. It is the time when access is needed for removal of residues and the cleaning of parts in contact with the product. It has therefore, over the years, become the practice to provide interlocks to ensure that a machine cannot be set in motion if a guard which has to be removed for cleaning or clearing blockages is removed. Factory Inspectors are often consulted as to the acceptability of this type of arrangement, and while the principle of ensuring that dangerous parts of machines are not moving and cannot be set in motion while a guard is removed has proved in practice to be generally satisfactory great care must be taken in the design of the arrangements if they are to prove themselves in time of need. The failure of an interlock can result in much suffering for an employee and can be very expensive for the firm.

British Standard 5304: 1975, *Safeguarding of Machinery,* contains many examples of interlock using direct mechanical, electrical, and other methods which isolate a machine from its power supply. It also contains information on various interlocking systems and a paragraph on the risk assessment of machinery. On the outcome of risk assessment will depend whether the interlocking needs to be designed to high or normal risk standards. If the machine is driven directly by an electric motor, then the interlocking would normally be by means of electrical limit switches which directly control the drive motor contactor. These limit switches should be capable of withstanding the rigours of the industrial environment. Similarly, if the motion is generated by pneumatic of hydraulic power then the interlock should, as far as possible, be by means of a pneumatic or hydraulic valve as appropriate, and operated as described in the Standard.

Stored energy dangers

Care must be taken with pneumatic interlocking to ensure that trapped air under pressure in the machine cannot cause unintended movement due to leakage past seals or enable the machine to move dangerously after the freeing of any jams or blockages. The possibility of a dangerous gravity fall must also be taken into account.

Accidents are on record in which an employee working at one end of a long machine has received injury while cleaning a part of a machine with the interlocked guard open, when an operator has touched a sensing probe further along the machine, causing the part of the machine the person is working on to operate Guard interlocks must therefore protect employees in all circumstances, so that the dangerous parts can never move under power when the guard is open.

In a further case an article became jammed in a very large machine. After the unit had been switched off the side panel was removed and the jam freed, whereupon the residual air in the machine operating system caused it to operate, trapping an employee who was reaching through the gap opened up by removal of the side panel. In this case the injuries proved fatal. When an accident or incident reveals a weakness, as in this case, the units are normally so modified as to prevent a recurrence. At this machine, after an accident, the controls were modified, and the panel was interlocked, so that the act of switching off the machine or removing the panel exhausted residual air pressure. It would, however, be far better if the designers of new machines, or the chief engineers of companies using old machines, asked themselves in each case whether cleaning and the clearing of blockages can be done safely. If they have any doubts as to the machine's safety, they should remedy the defects to prevent employees being injured.

Interlocking is, therefore, not just a simple matter of providing a suitable switch or valve properly operated, but an operation that must be followed through to the very heart of the machine. Failure to provide correct interlocking can result in injury or loss of life to the operator or some other person and could result in legal action against the machine maker or designer for failing to carry out the requirements of Section 6 of the Health and Safety at Work Act and against the occupier and his management for failing to securely fence a dangerous part of machinery.

A factor which must be taken into account is the possible overrun of a machine after it has been switched off and the guard removed. It should not be possible for a person to gain access to a machine for cleaning or other purposes until the dangerous parts have come to rest. Here again, BS 5304: 1975 contains a useful section on overrun protection.

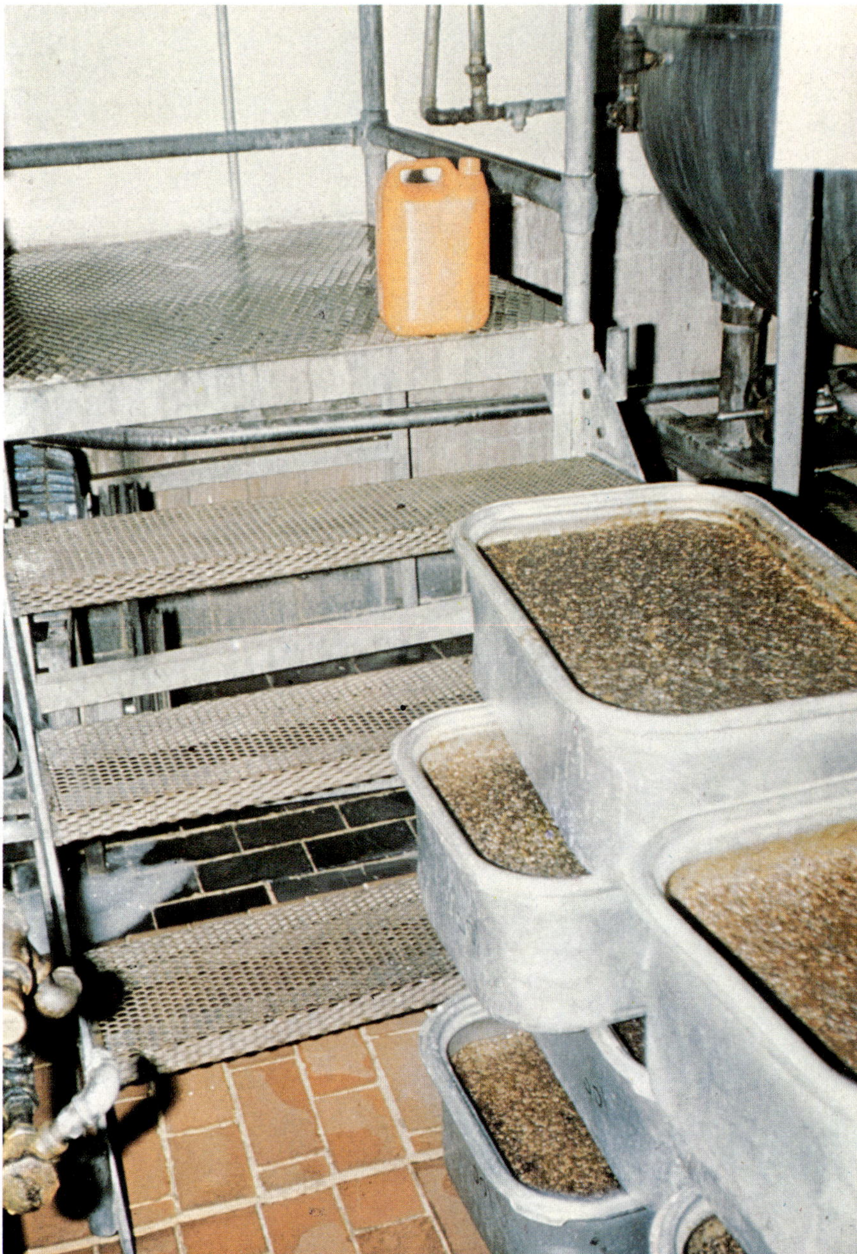

Fig. 7.1 – Plastic detergent container without label or cap stored over open trays of prepared meat.

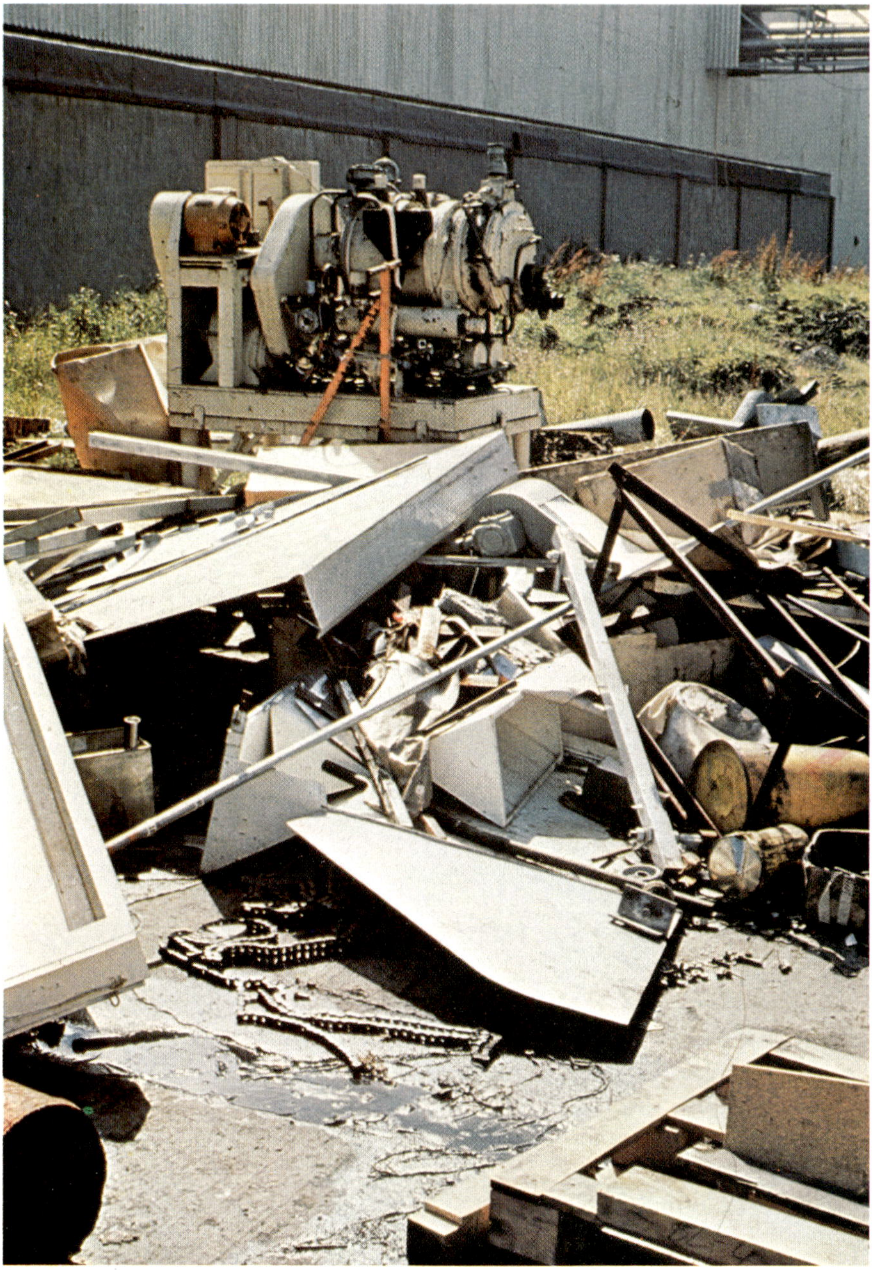

Fig. 7.2 – Surplus or useless equipment stored untidily on factory perimeter area. Often such equipment is not properly cleaned, and frequently harbours infestation.

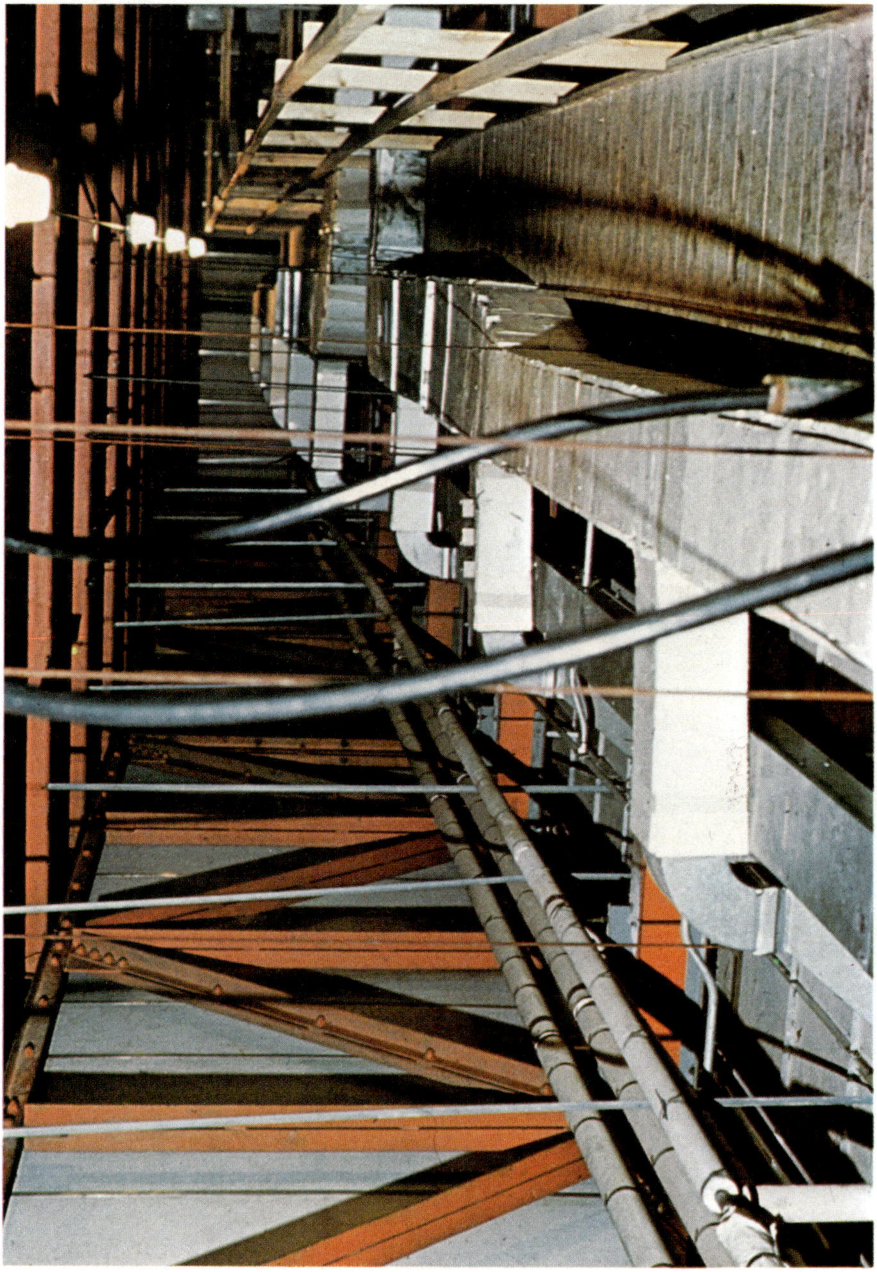

Figs. 7.3 and 7.4 – Principal services can be located with advantage in a separate overhead floor, which should be fully accessible for servicing and hygiene purposes.
(Continued next page)

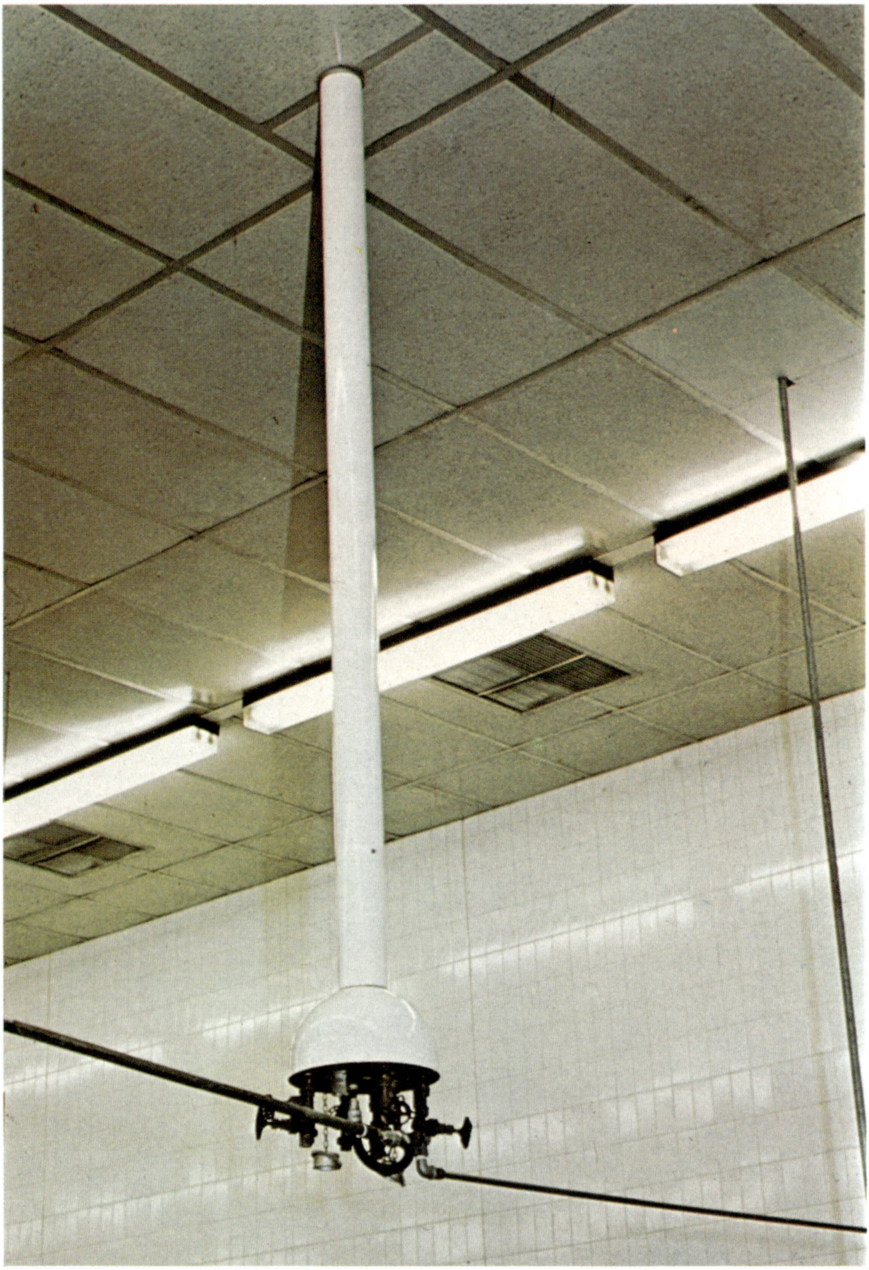

(Continued from previous page)
A single channel then passes through the ceiling of the production area, and provides overhead service feed to the equipment. This arrangement also permits ceiling, lighting, and air conditioning vents to be clear and free from pipework, girders, and conduit, all of which may collect dust and pests.

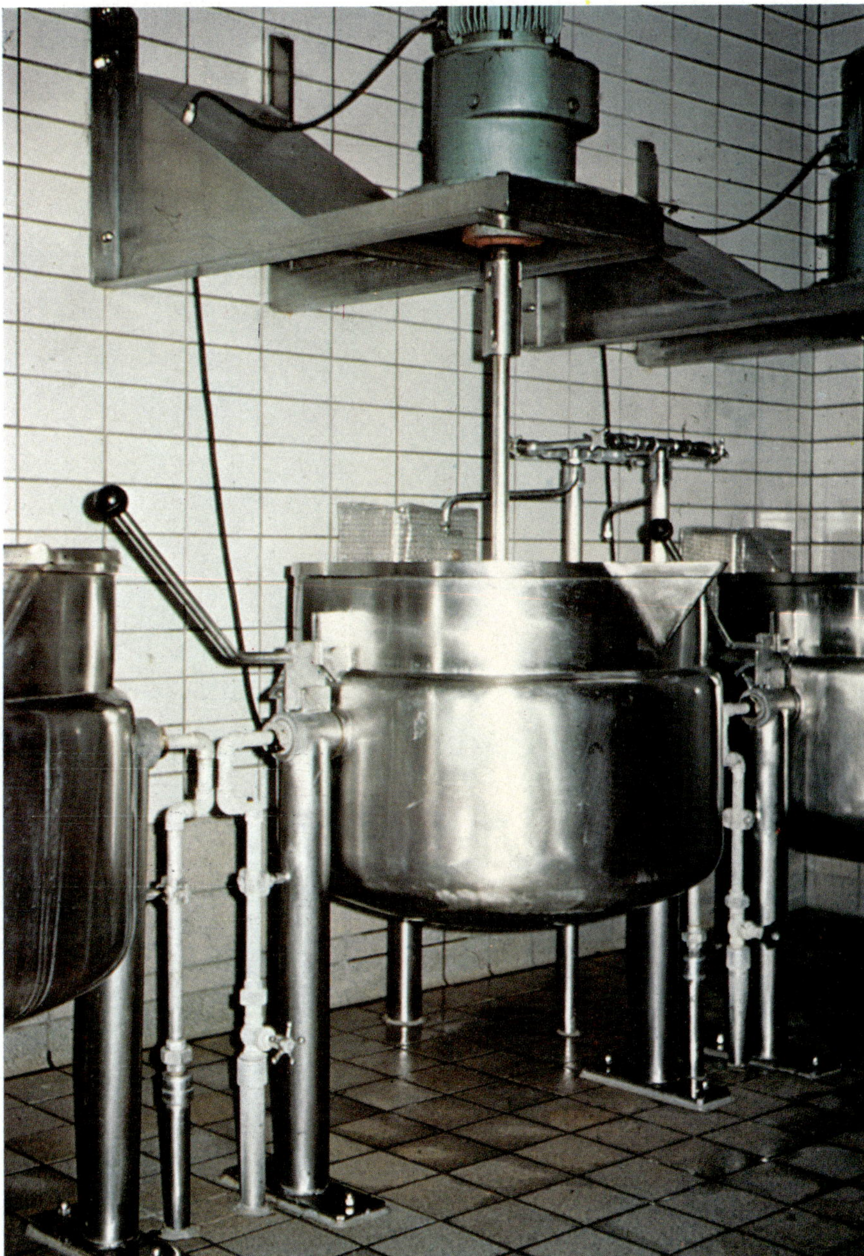

Fig. 7.5 – Clean stainless steel equipment, sited well off the floor, away from walls, with steam removed via extract fans and cowls. Note the stirrer motor located above the cowl, protecting the contents of the bowl from the motor, and the motor from the steam.

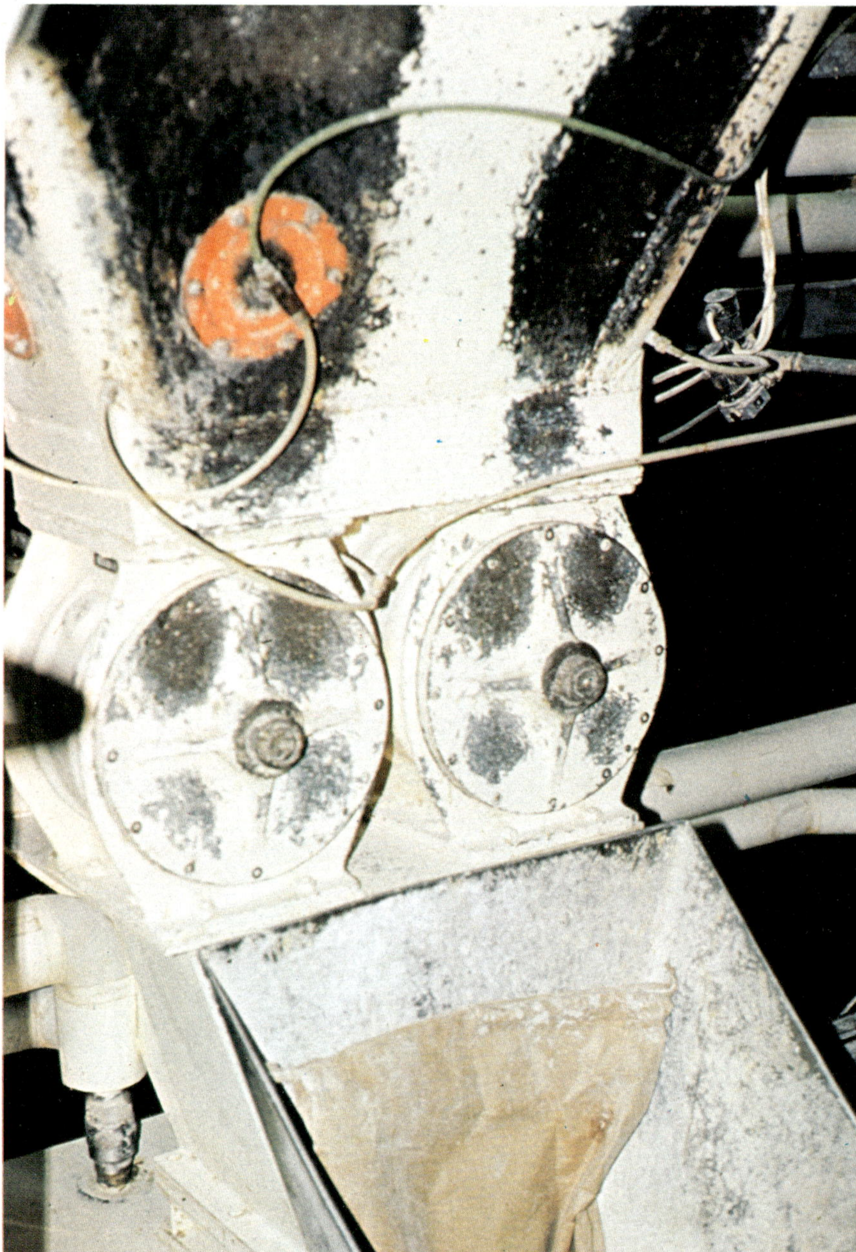

Fig. 7.6 – Badly designed flour hoppers, with the exterior surfaces painted. Flour clogs at the bottom of the hoppers; it can be released only by hammering on the outside metal surface, and this causes the paint to flake off and fall into the flour container below.

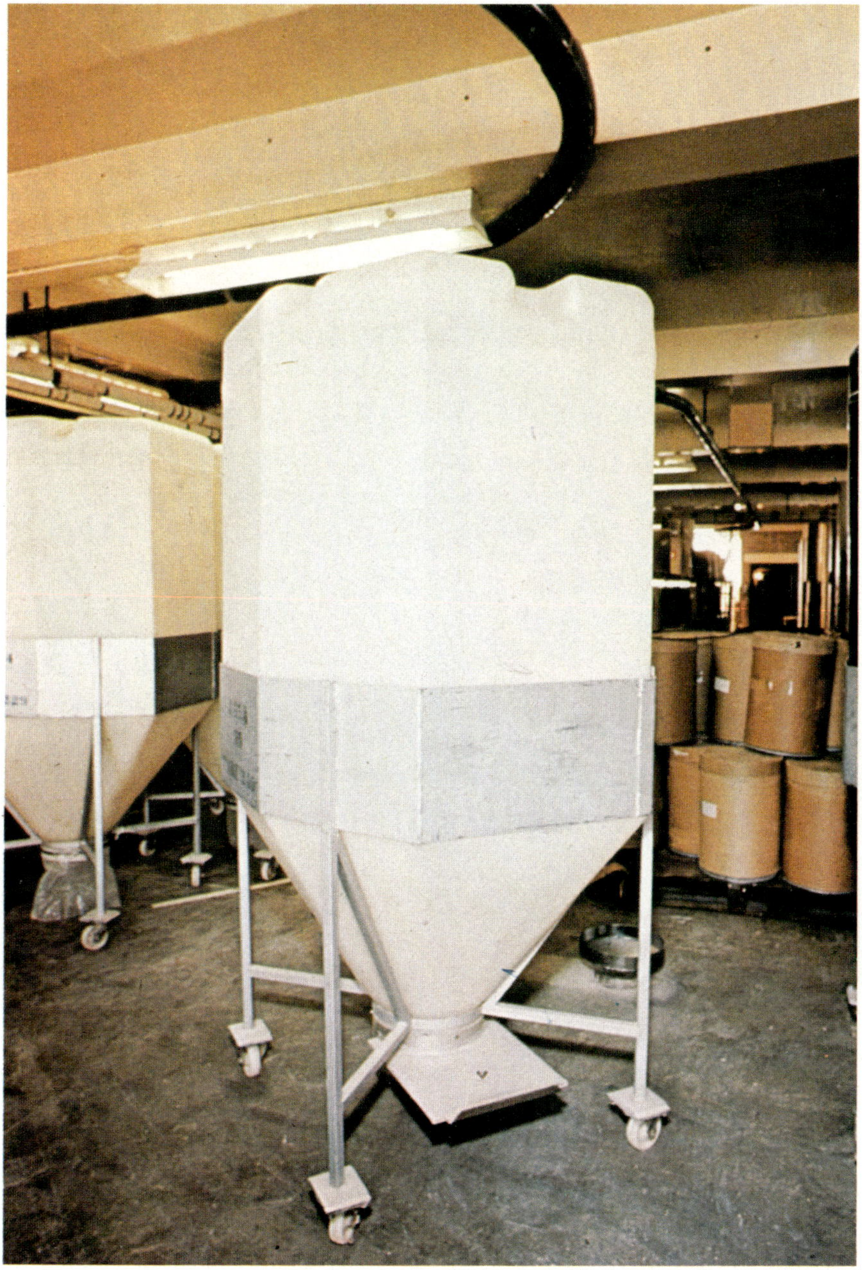

Fig. 7.7 – Bulk raw materials delivered and stored in plastic silos on wheeled metal stands to be dispensed through a hopper to the mixing floor below. This obviates such foreign body sources as wood, paper, string, nails, and wire.

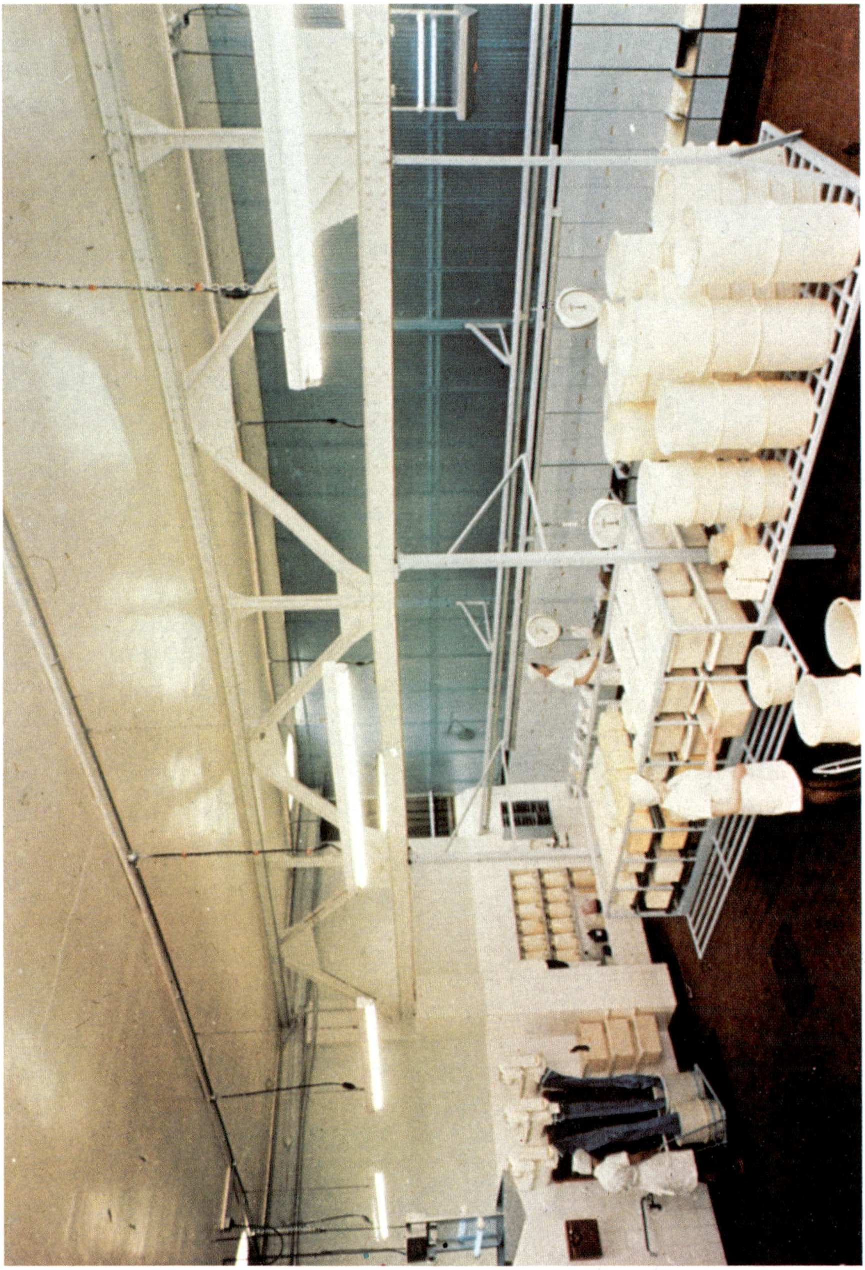

Fig. 7.8 – A clean modern raw materials dispensary in an old factory. The weighed ingredients are stored in clean containers off the floor. Individual small ingredients dispensers can be seen along the far wall.

Electrical hazards

The cleaning of a machine often involves the use of high-pressure hoses, steam lances, and much water, the floors and machinery frequently becoming wet during the process. It is often the case that the guard can only be interlocked by electrical means. It is vitally important that the electrical limit switches and associated cabling which are exposed to wet or steam are adequately protected. (BS 5420: 1977 describes the degree of protection available). In a factory where the Electricity (Factories Act) Special Regulations 1908 and 1944 apply, Regulation 27 requires that adequate protection and special precautions be taken to prevent danger.

One of the principles of industrial health is the removal or replacement of toxic substances. This principle can be applied to the use of lethal voltages in guard interlocks. Voltages at which the interlocks work should, whenever possible, be to the extra low voltage standard defined in BS 5304: 1975, that is:

> **extra low voltage.** A voltage normally not exceeding 50V between conductors and not exceeding 30V ac or 50V dc between any conductor and earth.

Where this is not possible, other precautions which adequately prevent danger in the conditions prevailing must be used.

Reference has been made to wet conditions, but it must not be overlooked that Regulation 27 applies equally to other conditions which may give rise to danger. There may be a danger of fire from the product, and in these circumstances adequate precautions should be taken with the interlocking to ensure that any risk from electrical sources is removed. This could be by substituting pneumatic interlocking for electrical interlocking, or the use of a key exchange system in which the electrical components are housed in a safe area and the machine guards are mechanically interlocked.

Design factors

The food industry embraces such an enormous field of operations and different types of machines, that it is impossible to deal in this paper with all types of guarding. However, the following factors should be considered in designing a machine which is safe to work upon and can be safely cleaned.

The best standard of safety is obtained by eliminating the hazard rather than by adding a guard. This is not always possible, and it is when the hazard cannot be eliminated that we should turn our attention to methods of guarding.

The first object of a guard is that it should prevent injury and it should not in itself, or in combination with some other part of the machine, present a hazard. The guard should also, as far as is possible, not interfere with production, although the Courts have held that safety must take precedence over production. So far as food machinery is concerned, guarding should not interfere with the cleaning of the machine, but the standard of machinery guarding should still be that required of it by law. To achieve this standard, guards which require to be removed or displaced for cleaning should be efficiently interlocked by one of the methods outlined in BS 5304: 1975.

There is no requirement within factory safety legislation for any particular type of material to be used for guards. Factory occupiers and machinery makers are free to use whatever type of material they wish provided that the guard is of substantial construction as required by Section 16 of the Factories Act 1961. From the hygiene point of view, stainless steel probably offers the best results. Because of cleaning difficulties, mesh or expanded metal are unlikely to be suitable for guards in close proximity to the food being produced. Guards which allow the operator to see the process would be easier to clean if made from a perforated sheet, the perforations of which should be of a size which prevents finger access to dangerous parts. Plastic-dipped mesh appears to be easier to clean than ordinary uncoated mesh, but if it is to remain hygienic and easy to clean the plastic covering must be kept intact. Hence the material presents a possible maintenence problem. Plastics materials which do not shatter offer a high standard of mechanical integrity, but in some circumstances quickly become obscured and may be damaged by steam cleaning.

Guarding materials must be chosen by each machine user to suit his needs, bearing in mind that the materials must prevent access, be strong enough an a long-term basis, and be capable of being maintained in a clean condition. It is also becoming the practice in some parts of the industry to design a guard to produce the maximum attentuation of noise produced by the machine and its product. This is a logical development as it can obviate the need for a second look at the problem later, and it can save costs. It is obvious that the materials used must not encourage micro-organic growth, or have toxic qualities. Very thick plastics sheeting is being evaluated by one large group to provide both guarding and noise reduction, the sheeting thickness being in excess of 10 mm. in many instances permanently attached guards have been fastened direct to the machine framework, forming a contact surface in which residues can lodge and create a growing medium for bacteria. In most cases there is no need for this, as guards can be mounted on spacers or be cut back locally to minimize the areas of contact, though with this arrangement it is essential to ensure that the spaces between the guard and machine frame are insufficient to allow finger access to dangerous parts.

Access from below

On some machines, access to dangerous parts can be obtained from beneath the bed of the machine, and the easiest way to prevent such access is to underdraw with a solid or perforated metal sheet, care being taken to ensure that finger access to dangerous parts is not possible through the perforations. However, there are problems with machines which manufacture or pack an edible product: parts of the product inevitably fall through the machine and need to be removed. This may well entail the removal of the underdrawing material with subsequent failure to replace it. In practice, a better system of guarding in these circumstances is to bring the sides of the machine down to within 150 mm of the floor and to place trays beneath the machine to catch the residues. Access to local drive mechanisms can be prevented by local enclosure guarding round the drive units. In one large company where a flume was provided to remove apple residues, the machine sides were arranged to slope towards the flume gulley, a spray pipe being fitted to enable the residues to be washed into the gulley. This arrangement appears to have added to the efficiency of the waste removal from the machine.

Other considerations

When manufacturing a guard the maker should bear in mind that it will need to be cleaned, and this may involve an employee in a handling operation. He should, therefore, ensure that the weight of the section to be handled will not cause injury. Care should also be taken to ensure that the guard edges have been smoothed so that they will not cut a person wiping the edges. Stiffening along the edges of guards should not form traps from which residues are difficult to remove.

Finally, it should be borne in mind that the enclosure of a machine by solid guards will affect the air flow and cooling, and unwanted temperature rises may occur. If this is a possibility, arrangements should be made to ensure adequate ventilation in a safe manner.

APPENDIX

HEALTH AND SAFETY AT WORK ACT 1974

Section 6 (part)

'(1) It shall be the duty of any person who designs, manufactures, imports or supplies any article for use at work –

(a) to ensure, so far as is reasonably practicable, that the article is so designed and constructed as to be safe and without risks to health when properly used . . . .'

FACTORIES ACT 1961

Section 17 (part)

'(1) In the case of any machine in a factory which is a machine intended to be driven by mechanical power –

(a) every set-screw, bolt or key on any revolving shaft, spindle, wheel or pinion should be so sunk, encased or otherwise effectively guarded as to prevent danger: and

(b) all spur and other toothed or friction gearing, which does not require frequent adjustment while in motion, shall be completely encased unless it is so situated as to be as safe as it would be if completely encased.

(2) Any person who sells or lets on hire, or as agent of the seller or hirer causes or procures to be sold or let on hire, for use in a factory in the United Kingdom any machine intended to be driven by mechanical power which does not comply with the requirements of this section shall be guilty of an offence and liable to a fine not exceeding two hundred pounds.'

DISCUSSION

H. Gilchrist (Alfa-Laval Company): What procedure could a manufacturer follow if he disagreed with a local H. M. Inspector's recommendations? Secondly, what are the guidelines generally laid down for proceeding with a prosecution?

Mr Daniels: If a firm doesn't like the advice given by the local H. M. Inspector you have the right as any citizen has, to go higher than the local Inspector; and the new system that has come out now means that you have bigger areas, so what you have the right to do is to go to that chap's Area Director and to say to him 'Look, I don't agree with this standard; can we have somebody else come over to discuss at your level', and you would find that you would get a discussion. If you aren't happy with the type of advice you've been getting technically then you have the right to get hold of what is called the Field Consultant Group, and if you don't know where the Consultant Group is and you can't find it from any other source you can always get on to the Factory Inspector's Head Office and they will tell you where the Field Consultant Group's Office is, and you can talk to them. If you don't get any satisfaction from them, you can come to Head Office. If it's a food machine, a packaging machine, I still deal with packaging machinery, bottling beer, and that kind of thing. The food machinery and food processing machinery have gone to our office which is now in Chelmsford or Hitchin, and you can get in touch with either of those two and you can sort it out.

So far as the prosecution side is concerned that's a little bit more difficult to answer. What the department normally does is to advise the company that in the opinion of the department they are in breach of the Act. They usually go along and the inspector says to them 'Look, I think that one needs guarding', and they say 'Yes, OK we agree it needs guarding' or 'We don't agree it needs guarding', and if the firm does nothing about it, and they don't correct the defect, then the inspector is placed in the position where *he* has to do something about it. Now he may decide to prosecute straight away or may decide to go to see the company's managing director or chairman and say 'Look if you don't do something we will have to take action', and it's done in this sort of way. If the company have obviously done nothing and they have been told on a number of occasions to do something, the inspector is forced to prosecute. I would say that inspectors do not prosecute just for the fun of it. It means a lot of work for them, and they try to avoid it as far as they can. They try to settle the problems amicably as far as they can between the company and themselves.

Mr Roger Coulthard (Baker Perkins Ltd.): You start off by saying that there isn't necessarily a conflict between hygiene and safety, and later on you mention the specific 6-inch ground clearance. That conflicts a little with something we mentioned in our paper; we said that what we try to do is to reach the centre line of the plant from either side of the machine with the brush held at 30° to the horizontal, the idea being to make cleaning an easy job. This obviously means that the width of the plant and the height from the ground are related to one another, and the height is not a fixed 6″. The idea is obviously to keep the cleanability quite constant. Have you any comments on that because as soon as you relate the height to the width say on a 1 to 2 m wide plant, you've got the same problem.

Mr Daniels: Yes, I think that when I said 6 inches I had in mind things like packaging machines which is usually fairly narrow; but if you've got a machine outside of the figures, if 6 inches is a figure that doesn't allow you to clean properly underneath, then I think it wants to be looked at as an independent and separate item. What we're aiming at is something that prevents you coming into contact with the parts that are likely to inflict injury, and I think you have to take into account the circumstances and the situation prevalent with the particular piece of plant you've got. Now, we had one particular machine in East Anglia where it was difficult to get 6 inches of space. We sloped – we started off with about 18 inches to 2 feet above the ground and sloped the panels inwards. This meant that the water that had been washed through the machine was now running down a sloping plate, and it went into a gulley underneath the machine so that the residues were taken away through a flume and there was no problem.

Mr Coulthard: How do you clean the inside?

Mr Daniels: There were pipes on them for washing the residues away. They were dealing with apples – something that did wash away. If you've got other materials that don't wash away then you may have problems. I think that it's difficult at a meeting of this nature to give an answer to all problems. I would suggest that Baker Perkins get in touch with us at head office and we would talk to them about their problem. That applies to any other company that has a similar sort of problem, and I think you would find that we would be quite ready and willing and able to look at the situation. We know your company very well indeed. We would be prepared to look at the situation, and I hope come up with an answer which is satisfactory to you and the customer who has the machine. One way we have tried in the past is to put trays under the machine where you can pull the whole tray out. OK, it's not perfect, but there are ways of overcoming this problem – sometimes expensive.

Mr Charles Rand (Associated Biscuits Ltd.): To assist cleaning staff gain easy access to machinery, hygiene officers are often very keen to see quick-release screws and butterfly-nuts fitted to various items of food machinery. Have you any comments relative to those hygiene aids in relation to safety?

Mr Daniels: Well, as I said earlier on, you have to take care of things like overrun on the machine. Now we as an inspectorate don't mind what sort of fastenings are on a machine provided that when you've released them you can't get access to the dangerous part before it has come to rest. If you wanted to fit quick-release devices we would not object provided that the guard is interlocked and access to dangerous parts cannot be gained before that part comes to rest. That's the criterion. If you have a bolted guard I would say that that's a guard which is not easily cleanable. Now we say to the company that has the machine, 'Which bits do you want to clean, which bits do you want to remove the guard from'; and if they say it is x, y, z we say 'Right, we'll interlock x, y, z', and having got it interlocked and having got it time delayed (you couldn't do a time delay with a quick-release device) – but having got it arranged so that a brake or some other device stops the motion of that dangerous part before the cleaning personnel can come into contact with it, we don't mind. We don't care what sort of fasteners you have on it if the machine is dead before anyone can come into contact with the part that is liable to inflict injury.

Mr L. G. Heighton (Geo. Bassetts): Having seen the experience we have had with the factory inspectorate at our own factory and seen the standards that were quite rightly required, and having had the opportunity of looking around a razor blade factory, I was quite frankly horrified. Do the standards vary a great deal from factory to factory or area to area?

Mr Daniels: They should not vary. The requirements in all factories are the same, but you may get a different inspector who has had perhaps a different experience from another one, and he may have found that your particular sort of machines were absolutely dangerous – and they may well be dangerous; but the razor blade machines which look dangerous might not be. I don't know – I don't deal with razor blade machinery, but the standards are the same, irrespective. The law is the same.

CHAPTER 7

Plant Design to Minimize Non-microbial Contamination

J. N. **Robson** and G. **Barnes**, Marks & Spencer Ltd.

INTRODUCTION

This paper is concerned with what are generally described as foreign bodies, including foreign odours and flavours, and we will concentrate on those which are likely to have originated in the plant itself, and might therefore be due to poor plant design.

The food processing plant is made up of four basic components:

1. Factory lay-out, structure, fittings, and perimeter.
2. Equipment.
3. Personnel.
4. Handling of foodstuffs from raw material to the final finished product.

Each part can contribute to the foreign body problem, and it is often as a result of a combination of factors that contamination occurs.

Firstly, some facts : in 1977 our company received 13 477 customer complaints of foreign bodies in foods. This was a marked increase over the previous year, even allowing for the greater number of units sold. Of this total, 6289 or 47%, were in categories that could have been due, in whole or in part, to defects in machinery or its design. These complaint types are set out in the table below.

	Foreign body type	Number	Percentage of total foreign body complaints
1.	Dirt	1303	9.7
2.	Metal (detectable)	966	7.2
3.	Plastic/rubber	963	7.1
4.	Oil/grease	762	5.6
5.	String	587	4.4
6.	Wood	571	4.2
7.	Fibres	525	3.9
8.	Glass	257	1.9
9.	Bristles	202	1.5
10.	Metal (non-detectable)	153	1.1

In addition there were 1166 (8.7%) complaints due to insects, and a proportion of these were undoubtably derived from poor factory and machinery design.

These figures are facts. What follows is conjecture.

Marks and Spencer represents about 2% of the food trade of the UK. If their experience is reasonably representative of the whole, then foreign body complaints on foods sold throughout the UK in 1977 should have been of the order of 700 000. Since experience shows that only between 10% and 20% of the actual foreign body complaints find their way back to the company, then it is possible that the actual number of incidents nationally could be of the order of 3 to 4 million. Perhaps the food industry should be thankful that only 13 000 foreign body complaints were received by Public Health Departments during 1976 (the last year of published figures).

Now, if poor plant and factory design is responsible for a third or a half of this figure, then this today is a massive and urgent subject, especially when many highly emotive foreign body incidents are 'unseen' by the consumer and hence are not the subject of complaints, such as contamination due to rodents, S.P.I. (stored product insects) etc.

Table 1 lists the proportions of each category of foreign body within some of the principal product groups of the food industry.

TABLE 1

Percentages of foreign bodies found in some food product groups

Bread	%	Cake	%
Foreign dough	13.7	Human hair	9.9
Dirt	13.1	Dirt/black marks	9.8
Oil/grease	8.7	Stones	9.4
Metal	7.3	Plastic/rubber	7.9
Dirty dough	7.0	Insects	7.6
Oven blacks	6.6	Metal	5.4
String	5.5	Stalks, thorns	5.4
Stones	4.7	Wood	5.1
Plastic/rubber	4.4	Oven blacks	4.3
Insects	4.2	Fibres	3.9
Fibres	2.8	Oil/grease	3.5
Wood	2.5	Bristles	2.7
Stalks, thorns	2.0	Paper/card	2.3
Human hair	2.0	String	1.8
Paper/card	2.0	Foreign dough	1.8
Glass	1.4	Dirty dough	1.8
Bristles	1.2	Glass	1.2
Cigarettes/matches	0.2	Cigarettes/matches	0.6
Other foreign bodies	10.7	Other foreign bodies	15.6

Table 1 (*continued*)

Dairy

	%
Insects	14.2
Plastic/rubber	13.7
Hair	10.8
Metal	8.4
Stalks, thorns	7.5
Dirt	7.2
Wood	6.6
Stones	6.1
Oil/grease	3.0
Glass	2.1
Fibres	1.9
Bristles	0.6
String	0.5
Oven blacks	0.2
Paper/card	0.2
Cigarettes/matches	0.1
Other foreign bodies	16.9

Delicatessen

	%
Insects	18.3
Plastic/rubber	11.2
Metal	10.9
Hair	9.3
Wood	6.3
Dirt	5.7
Stones	4.4
Bones	4.4
Fibres	3.0
String	2.1
Stalks, thorns	2.1
Glass	1.9
Oil/grease	1.9
Cigarettes/matches	0.5
Bristles	0.3
Paper	0.3
Other foreign bodies	17.4

Meat pies

	%
Plastic/rubber	13.0
Metal	11.8
Bones	8.1
Hair	7.6
Insects	6.9
Stones	6.9
Dirt	4.8
Fibres	3.7
Wood	3.6
Oil/grease	3.3
Oven blacks	2.9
String	2.4
Bristles	2.2
Glass	1.9
Paper/card	0.9
Stalks, thorns	0.8
Cigarettes/matches	0.4
Other foreign bodies	18.8

Biscuits

	%
String	14.8
Dirt	14.6
Fibres	13.1
Hair	12.2
Oil/grease	12.1
Oven blacks	5.3
Paper/card	3.8
Metal	3.1
Plastic/rubber	2.8
Insects	2.7
Stones	2.4
Wood	1.8
Bristles	1.6
Stalks, thorns	0.4
Glass	0.4
Cigarettes/matches	0.2
Other foreign bodies	8.7

Table 1 (*continued*)

Savoury snacks	%	Confectionery	%
String	14.3	Dirt	13.0
Metal	11.8	Metal	11.0
Fibres	8.6	Stones	8.0
Dirt	8.0	Wood	7.7
Wood	6.2	Hair	7.0
Plastic/rubber	6.2	Plastic/rubber	7.0
Insects	6.1	Insects	6.1
Oil/grease	5.8	Oil/grease	5.4
Hair	3.3	Bristles	2.9
Bristles	2.4	Fibres	2.9
Stones	1.3	String	2.7
Paper/card	1.3	Paper/card	2.6
Glass	1.2	Stalks, thorns	1.0
Stalks, thorns	0.9	Oven blacks	1.0
Cigarettes/matches	0.8	Glass	0.8
Oven blacks	0.4	Cigarettes/matches	0.5
Other foreign bodies	21.4	Other foreign bodies	20.4

Table 2 shows the total percentage breakdown of foreign body complaints due to all causes.

TABLE 2

Foreign body complaints due to all causes

(Marks and Spencer annual figures for 1977)

	%		%
Dirt	9.7	Fibres	3.9
Insects	8.7	Foreign dough	3.8
Metal	8.3	Oven blacks	3.1
Plastic	7.1	Stalks, thorns	2.5
Human hair	6.3	Glass	1.9
Oil/grease	5.6	Dirty dough	1.9
Stones	5.6	Paper	1.6
Bones	4.9	Bristles	1.5
String	4.4	Cigarettes/matches	0.3
Wood	4.2	Others	14.7

Plan of paper

This paper has been constructed from the accumulated, practical experience of this problem over the last 25 years. There are two alternative approaches to the examination of the subject:

a) To take each category of complaint and determine the causes and remedy.
b) To study those principles of factory design which avoid potential contamination sources.

It is proposed to take the latter approach, and it is hoped that this choice will be justified as it progresses.

Many of the points made will be obvious and already well-known. There will be little that is new or dramatic in this paper. So much of this topic stems from straightforward commonsense.

FACTORY LAY-OUT

In designing a lay-out for a new factory, certain pitfalls must be avoided to minimize foreign body contamination. It must subsequently be remembered that no lay-out is permanently ideal, owing to unforeseen later changes in patterns of production. With such changes often come the wholesale replacement of equipment and modifications to structure. Certain compromises to lay-out may then have to be accepted; but, in doing so, the following points should not be overlooked as they may well lead to product contamination.

a) Lack of space for the storage of raw materials and packaging can result in these items being kept in production areas. Similarly, lack of space for separate de-boxing and re-palletizing of raw materials should not be ignored. In both cases, contamination can arise from wire, string, staples, glass, wood, paper, card, etc. The need for adequate space for thorough raw material screening cannot be over-emphasized, as experience shows that a high proportion of foreign bodies come in with raw materials. When materials are by their nature dirty (vegetables being a good example), primary cleaning must be physically contained to prevent the spread of contaminants.
b) Congestion, especially in areas of open food production, makes cleaning and maintenance difficult to achieve without putting food products and other equipment at risk. The hazards are greater if these activities take place during production time.
c) Inadequate space for the separate storage of finished products may again necessitate the use of production areas for this purpose. In some factories there is also the practice of storing finished, but unwrapped, product in uncovered containers: such goods must be at risk, as are materials that have to be 'conditioned', (for example, doughs, fats, wafers, or trays of pre-prepared fillings.

Even more dangerous is the storage of finished goods next to incoming raw materials. Dirt and cross-infestation are obvious hazards; odour tainting is another, a good example being where finished goods share the same storage area as cleaning or maintenance materials.

d) Insufficient space for maintenance operations will result in many problems. Work benches in open production areas should never be permitted. Fitters forced to work in cramped, dirty conditions will find it difficult to conform to the required hygiene standards when working in production areas.

   Lack of storage space for temporarily disused equipment often results in it being kept in production areas. Such equipment is frequently infested because it is not being cleaned before and during storage.

e) If equipment cleaning centres are located too far from production areas, there will be temptation to neglect cleaning schedules. An equal temptation will be for cleaning materials, including concentrated detergents, to be kept in production areas. The quantities of foodstuffs tainted by detergents should not be under-estimated. See Fig. 7.1.

f) The location of amenities is important. If they are too far from production areas, obvious hazards arise, for example cigarette smoking behind production machinery, or the consumption of food in unauthorized parts of the factory site. If it is too far to the canteen or rest-room, why not provide properly equipped smoking/snack rooms adjacent to production areas?

g) Short and direct routes for waste removal are essential. It cannot be desirable to have waste trailed through open production rooms, especially in view of the insanitary condition of much equipment used for waste collection.

h) The siting of the returned-goods area can be crucial. Such goods are often infested, and/or in a state of decomposition. They must, therefore, be isolated from all raw material and production areas.

i) Certain aspects of perimeter control must not be forgotten, examples being:

   i) Elimination, or at least control, of weed growth.
   ii) Adequate surface drainage to avoid ponding.
   iii) The provision of a surface which can be easily cleaned.
   iv) The correct siting and construction of waste-collecting areas.
   v) Good housekeeping controls in perimeter buildings.
   vi) The correct siting and control of such operations as effluent treatment, incineration etc.
   vii) Control (or possibly elimination) of stocks of surplus equipment, wood, empty containers and similar items often kept because 'it might come in useful'. See Fig. 7.2.

All the above points will influence the attraction of pests to the perimeter and probably into the factory.

FACTORY STRUCTURE

Contaminant sources associated with the actual structure and its fittings are countless. Some problems which are frequently encountered are as follows.

Overhead fittings

One certain way of reducing many foreign matter complaints is to reduce overhead equipment to the minimum. In conventional buildings it is not uncommon to see ceilings covered in a network of ducting, pipework, lights, cable trays, heaters, public address systems etc. The problems are obvious:

i) Maintenance work overhead, causing direct contamination to product or contamination of equipment, and, subsequently, of product. Many complaints of metal arise in this way. Factory standards demand that this work takes place out of production hours and only then after production lines are covered. In practice this requirement is often ignored or cannot be met, owing to emergencies.
ii) Difficulty in cleaning, especially in bakeries, where dust from powdered raw materials settles on overheads, causes subsequent mouse or insect activity which in turn endangers production lines.
iii) Sparrow problems are aggravated by overhead structures which provide easy roosting. Droppings on equipment and raw materials are unpleasant, and the source of many complaints.

For new factories and factory extensions these problems can be remedied by providing a separate service floor which will house much of the ducting, pipe work, compressors etc. Feeds to production equipment are direct, and lighting and duct openings can be flush. The result is a clear ceiling which is easy to clean, and the removal of many activities, which could cause contamination, to the separate service area. Further, it does not restrict maintenance work to outside production hours. This system is also flexible and allows direct feed to be maintained after production line layout changes. See Figs. 7.3 and 7.4.

In more conventional designs, common problems can be avoided by:

i) Ensuring that the finish to pipe insulation is of the necessary quality to resist damage and corrosion and to endure frequent cleaning. Aluminium sheaths are to be recommended.
ii) Providing drainage collection for chronic condensation points.
iii) Using metalwork capable or suitably treated to withstand corrosion.

Production areas can also be fed from side or cellar service areas; the benefits are similar, namely, keeping the production area to a minimum amount of fittings and equipment and reducing all operations likely to cause contamination. Cost benefits are also apparent through reduced total cleaning costs. It must, however be remembered that those separate service areas must be easily accessible for cleaning, maintenance, and pest control.

Equally, efforts should be made to eliminate or open-up many of the small voids and ducts found in the fabric, as these have been often associated with heavy infestation.

Open planning

The number of partition walls required is worthy of consideration. They should be kept to the minimum and used only to isolate operations which otherwise lead to the spread of contaminants. Too many separate rooms will result in a 'nooks and crannies' situation which only complicates inspection, control, and the achievement of uniform standards.

Finishes – Walls and ceilings

Internal finishes to the structure should be selected for minimum maintenance. This reduces the need to employ contractors whose labour is often difficult to discipline to food factory standards. Painting must be a controlled exercise if tainting of finished product, raw materials, and packaging is to be avoided. Such was the concern at the large quantities of foodstuffs being rejected through this type of tainting that four years ago a joint Marks and Spencer–ICI code of practice for *Food Factory Painting* was published. This document is avilable from ICI Paints Division.

In existing factories areas of painted surface can be reduced by using;

i) Plastic-faced boarding for underlining ceilings.
ii) Sheet plastic for wall cladding.

In both cases manufacturers must be given full details of the environment in which these materials are to be used. Fire authorities must also be consulted to ensure that these materials are acceptable.

When underdrawing ceilings the insulation factor should not be ignored. Condensation occurring under the outer membrane may result in the gradual disintegration of the underdrawing material. This process may be further aggravated by a corrosive atmosphere.

Recent legislation for fresh meat and poultry plants and the proposed EEC directive for meat product establishments require that walls are impervious up to a specific height. It is then arguable that the extra expense of similarly treating the remainder of the walls is worthwhile, long-term. However, it must be emphasized that whatever wall finish is selected its protection is essential. In areas of high traffic, crash rails or plinths should be installed. No wall surface will withstand repeated impact from trolleys, pallet trucks etc. If wall damage occurs the product contamination risks are:

i) Pieces of plaster, paintwork or tile.
ii) Cockroach infestation behind loosened tiles or cladding.

The need for 'permanent' construction of partitioning should also be questioned, as there are many benefits to be derived from the use of prefabricated sectional walls namely:

i) Easy and speedy erection and dismantling, which minimizes hazards to production.
ii) Salvage potential which is not the case with conventional brick construction.

In looking for convenient partitioning, double-faced stud construction should be avoided as the voids which are formed give easy harbourage for infestation. Glass must never be built into partitions.

Protection is required for doors and door-frames to avoid wood splintering on impact from trolleys carrying foodstuffs from one department to another.

Finishes – Floors

Floor design is worth considerable thought and high initial investment. The disruption caused by defective floors may be very costly; piecemeal repair is difficult to achieve. .Many floor defects arise from poor planning and preparation, not from the actual finishing material. The use of epoxy resin floors needs to be approached with caution as the odour risks associated with this type of material are high. Floorings which do not use high-odour materials should be used.

Drainage

Correct floor drainage is important in the control of insect infestation and odours. Covered channels present major cleaning problems when compared with appropriately sited gullies or open wall junction channels. The latter provide the advantage of preventing any equipment or materials being sited tightly against walls.

Similarly, it is unnecessary and undesirable for equipment to drain directly on to the floor.This spreads dirt into inaccessible areas and is uncomfortable for operatives. Motorway-type drains should never be used, because of lack of access for shoulder cleaning.

Water cleaning systems are very much restricted in dry production areas such as in bakeries because of lack of drainage. This precludes the use of high-pressure systems for areas of high and tenacious soiling, and leaves as the only alternative, inefficient manual methods, which demand a greater level of supervision. This situation needs more attention from the manufacturers of 'dry cleaning equipment'.

Ventilation

The problems associated with the lack of adequate ventilation are:

i) Corrosion, perished plaster, peeling paintwork, and insect or mite attraction to mould growth. Wherever possible, steam or heat sources should be tackled by extraction at source, as ceiling or wall ventilators are not adequate.

ii) Personnel discomfort. Undoubtedly this contributes to many of the complaints of hair in products (6%). In excessively warm and humid conditions headcoverings will not be worn properly, and other manifestations of poor discipline will result.

Pest proofing

Proofing against pest entry is a fundamental necessity. Where possible, effective ventilation systems should overcome the necessity for openable windows. Where windows have to be proofed, it should be remembered that the proofing has to be removed periodically, for cleaning. Doorways are more difficult to flyproof but can be tackled effectively by:

i) Self-closing mechanisms.
ii) Overlapping heavy-duty plastic strips.
iii) Double door construction incorporating a lobby containing either an electrical trapping device or an insecticide vapourizer.

The last system is probably the most efficient and therefore worth installing at busy entry points. The need for rodent proofing is straightforward to establish when dealing with mice and brown rats, but in areas where ship rats are encountered, proofing will be necessary throughout the entire height of the structure because of the climbing ability of this rodent. All engineering work which entails pipework through outer walls must be inspected on completion for satisfactory proofing.

PRODUCTION MACHINERY AND RELATED EQUIPMENT

Siting

There are no easy rules of thumb for the siting of equipment except that sufficient space must be left to allow access to *all* external and internal surfaces, and the easy removal of strippable parts. Failure to make these provisions will hinder inspection, cleaning and maintenance.

It is not always possible to locate machinery clear of the floor, but where equipment has hollow bases, as is the case with some dough mixers, every effort should be made to give access to the area in which debris collects. Fermenting dough is highly attractive to insects. See Fig. 7.5.

Construction

Metal—In the construction of machinery every effort is needed to reduce the amount of direct contamination from metal, which in Table 2 represents 8% of all complaints. This figure is alarming as all the contaminated product had been screened by electronic metal detectors. On the other hand it may be considered that this figure is not surprising since nearly all machinery now used in food processing is metal.

However, it can be calculated that if the metal detectors are working at 95% efficiency (and Marks and Spencer surveys suggest that this figure is correct), some 5 million metal–contaminated products are being produced annually in the UK.

What machinery improvements can be suggested to reduce this figure?

a) A major contribution would be the reduction of metal fastenings to the absolute minimum. Fastenings have to be removed frequently during cleaning and maintenance, and many become lost. Inspections of machinery reveal considerable numbers of missing nuts, bolts, split-pins and washers.
b) Nondetachable fastenings and/or shakeproof fittings must become standard for food equipment. The increased cost of the machinery would be negligible, especially when compared with the cost of contamination.
c) There should be a reduction to a minimum of machine parts, moving or not, sited over exposed product. If this cannot be avoided, catch trays, possibly magnetic, should be fitted.

Wood—Over the years there has, thankfully, been a reduction in the amount of wood used in food machinery construction. However, examples of its use still occur. In confectionery production, chocolate and starch moulders still incorporate much wood, the consequence being difficulty in controlling S.P.I. in chocolate moulders and wood contamination from starch moulding frames.

Nowadays wood is most frequently used for temporary construction, repairs, or production 'aids' such as prodders, dip-sticks, and stirrers. Discipline must overcome these practices.

Paint—Painted surfaces on machinery should be reduced. Certainly no food contact surface, or surfaces above exposed food products, should be painted. See Fig. 7.6.

Seals—More efficient oil seals must be developed in the future. In the meantime, protection trays should be fitted to any piece of equipment liable to oil loss. Oil and grease contamination could be further reduced by more careful sitings of motors and the increased use of self-lubricating bearings.

Gaskets—Care must be taken to avoid infestation (S.P.I.) and disintegration of gaskets.

Conveyors—Complaints regarding biscuits indicate a high incidence of string, most of which comes from fraying cutting webs, conveyor belts, and scrap return webs. Apart from the discipline of routine trimming, automatic tracking devices would reduce wear to belts.

Plastics—Plastics used for machinery or equipment, especially holding bins, cause problems if the correct grades are not used. Fragments of plastic in product can be as damaging as metal, and static attraction can cause cleaning problems. The use of welding solvents for plastic pipelines may, if not used properly, lead to taint risks.

Free-flow surfaces—Free-flow surfaces should be built into all transfer systems. Many S.P.I. infestations have occurred where surfaces do not clear themselves. Additionally, where sticking is encountered in transfer systems and clearance is effected by hitting with a hammer, metal, wood, and paint chips are contaminant risks.

Access—It should now be standard procedure to provide access to all areas of suspected product build-up. An examination of a typical flour line, from silo to mixer, will show many potential traps to which there is no access. In providing access for cleaning or inspection the removal of panels must be made easy and not the subject of major engineering. This is true of all machinery stripping for for routine purposes, subject, of course, to personnel safety considerations.

Lidding—Lids of hoppers and vessels are often ill-fitting, difficult to remove, and badly designed, especially when there is a need for pipework or stirrer shafts to pass through the lid.

Waterproofing—Improved waterproofing, particularly of electrical gear, would allow the greater use of high-pressure water cleaning systems.

OPERATIONAL SYSTEMS

Raw material handling

If it is true that many foreign bodies are associated with raw materials, it follows that correct screening procedures must be practised. In addition to the appropriate use of specific pieces of screening equipment, other commonsense points need to be remembered:

a) More use of bulk handling systems to avoid the problems associated with bags (string, paper), cans (metal swarf), bottles, wooden boxes etc. See Fig. 7.7.

b) The application of mechanical sieving and filtration to as many raw materials as possible. Sieves for powders should not be constructed of stainless steel wire. Although this material is durable, it tends not to be magnetic and therefore, if sieves break up, there is wholesale contamination which will not be magnetically detectable. The recommended material is 22 S.W.G. high tensile steel.

   Sieve sizes must be appropriate for the raw materials, for example, white flour can be sieved through an 850 micron sieve, which will remove adult and larval S.P.I. However, 2000-plus micron sizes are often used which will not remove such contamination. By-pass systems must be fitted with sieves.

It must never be accepted that post-sieving equipment is free from trouble. Again, S.P.I. activity has been found in worm elevators from centrifugal sieves and in post-entoleter pipework. Similar ironies have been found with other raw material cleaning equipment, such as fruit-washing machines which, because of poor design, are difficult to maintain free from fruit fly infestation.

c) The opening of cans has caused major problems of swarf contamination. Punching openers should be used – not those based on a cutting action. After can-opening operations, magnets become a necessity in subsequent handling equipment. There is a good case for the greater use of magnets in many food handling systems: the Marks and Spencers survey shows that approximately 80% of all metal contamination is ferrous.

d) Manual systems for raw materials inspection must incorporate the following features:

   i) Suitable conveyor colours to provide contrast.
   ii) Correct belt speed to facilitate satisfactory inspection.
   iii) Correct product depth.
   iv) Correct lighting levels.
   v) Easy methods, such as vacuum pencils, for removing contaminants.

e) Having screened raw materials, it is only sensible to ensure that they are not subject to further contamination and are dispensed in properly-controlled areas. Transfer systems based on bins, trays, etc. must be protected by adequate lids. Similar protection must be afforded to 'scrap' or re-work materials. See Fig. 7.8.

f) The hazards due to odours and foreign bodies derived from incoming packaging materials (including cans, bottles, and plastic containers) must be dealt with by appropriate accommodation and quality inspection techniques. Goldenberg and Matheson† refer to financial losses due to packaging materials, while Table 2 shows the high level of plastic foreign bodies found in dairy and delicatessen products.

Metal detection

The correct application of metal detectors is obviously impottant. Considering their value in detecting contamination and their cost, it is surprising how often they are misused. It is not rare to find them switched off during production. The following points are important if full value is to be gained from this equipment:

i) Detectors should be sited in-line so that product cannot be removed before scanning.

ii) Detectors should be equipped with automatic rejection systems, fail-safe devices, memory systems, and automatic head balancing. Conveyor rollers must be constructed to minimize metal pick-up.

†Goldenberg, N. and Matheson, H. R., *Chem. Ind.* 5 July 1975, 551.

iii) Siting of the units is important to avoid electrical or magnetic interference from other equipment.
iv) A basic stock of spare parts must be kept, especially spare circuit boards.
v) Sensible operating sensitivities will ensure consistent performance, and avoid problems of excessive spurious rejection.

However valuable metal detectors may be, they must be regarded as the last line of defence and should in no way minimize efforts to avoid initial contamination.

Cleaning routines
Good cleaning systems will naturally reduce much potential contamination, and the following points should be borne in mind:

The installation of ring mains for vacuum-cleaning systems, and variable-pressure water/detergent systems. These should be designed to reach to all parts of production machinery and those areas of the structure requiring routine cleaning.
b) The elimination of compressed air cleaning which can create and spread contamination.
c) The creation of central dispensing points for detergents and sterilants to prevent contamination from concentrated cleaning materials in production areas. Such central points help to ensure that cleaning/sterilizing solutions are made up to the correct concentrations.
d) Hand equipment needs careful control, as many complaints arise from the poor conditions of mops, wooden-handled brushes, and frayed cloths.

Engineering maintenance practice
Many foreign bodies arise from undisciplined engineering maintenance. This is especially evident with 'Monday production'. This work needs to be clearly and precisely scheduled, and thorough post-inspection is vital to obviate loose small parts, excessive lubricants, and the use of non-approved materials such as string, wire, wood. Mechanics should be provided with adequate facilities for the accommodation of their gear while working in production areas. These should ideally include tool trolleys, magnetic trays, and blankets, and (where appropriate) mobile partitions.

PERSONNEL ATTITUDES

This paper has been concerned with statistics, observations, facts, and technical information, but the picture is incomplete without a reference to the part played by the management and operatives who are running the plant. As with so many other aspects of food production the price one has to pay for safe, clean food is constant vigilance at all levels, and it is imperative that this vigilant attitude is impressed on all workers from the day they start on the production line.

The simple maxim that one should only produce for others the food that one would be prepared to eat oneself cannot be repeated too frequently and is a good starting point for putting this message over, particularly to unskilled operatives. Staff training in the general principles of hygienic food production is a 'must' for any well-run food factory, and such training must include detailed reference to foreign bodies of all kinds and their prevention in food products.

The management and line supervisors have a very special responsibility in this. They must institute properly drawn-up practical operational routines and ensure that these are carefully followed by staff attuned to the dangers and problems of foreign matter. Management must also be observed by staff *at all levels* to be personally concerned with the cleanliness of the plant *at all times.* If a departmental manager ignores a piece of loose string or wire on a single occasion it will be taken for granted that it is a matter of little importance, and all workers in the department will respond accordingly.

It is interesting how an old and badly- designed plant can be kept clean and relatively free from foreign matter by careful attention and vigilance. It is equally significant that modern, well-equipped factories can rapidly deteriorate and cause hazards to the food product if they are not operated and maintained correctly. The difference between these two extremes is the attitude of mind of the people working in the factory. Without proper guidance this attitude can prejudice the care and thought that went into the original design of a safe and hygienic food production unit.

DISCUSSION

Mr Ridgway (Baker Perkins Ltd.): I think we all have a very great regard for Marks and Spencer, and I wonder from their central type of position whether they could tell some of the engineers in the service industry what proportion of costs relating to turnover the industry is prepared to spend annually. In other words what are people spending in the endeavour to get hygienic conditions? How much do we spend in a normal factory for interstation removal for cleaning, for materials and so on? Nowhere today have we had a feel of the size of the monetary problem, and I think it is very inportant that we do because that then places a very great emphasis, I think, on the limits to which people are prepared to go. If Mr Robson could answer that I would be very grateful.

Mr Robson: I am sorry, Mr Chairman, I can't answer it. I don't have this sort of information. Obviously we could provide part of the answer. For instance, taking the one example we questioned today we could give you an approximate estimation of the cost of infestation control. I would, however, be able to supply him with data on this matter from a completely different point of view. I could, supply him with data as to the cost to the food industry of not doing it – and that is astronomical. But that is another topic, Mr Chairman, for another day. Some of that information we do have available.

CHAPTER 8

General Philosophy of Hygienic Operation and Quality Standards

I. von Bockelmann, Lund University

INTRODUCTION

Hygienic food is understood all over the world to be that which is safe for consumption. Governments specify for different food items the highest acceptable counts of microbes and sometimes the greatest amount of specific contaminants or additives which may be present. In certain countries even processing equipment and production areas are subjects of specific regulations. Further, each lecturer on industrial hygiene has his own way to interpret hygiene, estimate safety, and recommend working routines and product control methods in order to meet government requirements.

Microbiological standards for foods are normally very modest but not always logical. The quality of available raw material and the effect of accepted, normal processing methods in many cases determine the microbiological quality of a food commodity, no matter how good are the working conditions. As an example, in spite of the fact that bacterial spores in raw milk are known to survive the pasteurization process, there are in Sweden now proposed regulations limiting the highest acceptable counts of *B. cereus* in some pasteurized dairy products, but no limits for the spore counts of raw milk.

Legal requirements for food quality normally include no information about *how* this quality is to be obtained. It is left to the food manufacturer to work out details for hygienic operation and to establish a product standard which must meet the legal requirements, but which must also consider processing methods as well as several quality characters necessary for economical production of successfully competing goods for the market. It was claimed by a well-known German food scientist, some months ago, that a person qualified to work on food industry hygiene should have full academic training in human medicine, animal husbandry, food chemistry, and microbiology. To this list should also be added food technology and engineering!

A chemical or microbiological analysis of food may be complicated, but so far as food standards are concerned, standard methods are available. For the food processing industry it is, however, not sufficient to have a figure for antibiotic residues or lipolytic changes or psychrotrophic micro-organisms in a product. The manager must also be capable of interpreting the results, and – in due time – he must know why the quality characteristics are as they are and what the possible consequences for his production and marketing may be. If laboratory results are not evaluated and used to keep quality under control, a manager may sooner or later encounter serious problems and trouble-shooting may turn out a very expensive way to restore quality and reputation. That is probably one good reason why a food hygienist should be more than just a well-trained laboratory technician. On the other hand, nothing is more expensive than a highly-specialized pure scientist on a factory floor, since his task is not only to analyse but to provide practical solutions. He may cause a lot of problems, simply because he knows too much about too little. In a food process it is usually not enough to make one step perfect. Food processing is much like a chain, and the weakest link determines the strength of the whole chain. Making one link very strong does not necessarily strengthen the whole chain at all.

A good food hygienist should be able to help during the layout of the factory and the process line, set up adequate and relevant control programmes for process and product, interpret results, negotiate with manufacturers of machinery, detergents, packaging material, etc, set up routines for collection, transport, storage, and control of raw material – all in order to ensure a process which with optimum use of money, energy, and labour is hygienic enough.

WHAT IS HYGIENIC OPERATION?

Hygienic operation is often superficially exaggerated. We all recognise 'rules' like: Workmen in the food industry should wear protective clothes and head covering. Floors, walls and ceilings should be easy to clean. Machinery should be kept spotless and shining, inside and out. Washrooms should be equipped with bacteriostatic, or at least liquid, soap, single-use towels, etc.

This is all very well. It probably has a psychological effect. But this should not be mistaken for hygienic operation.

If food is processed open and touched by hands, all the rules in the world are nothing but written lines in a drama where the performance is made by the staff and the success is entirely dependent on their personalities.

People handling food in open processes should be handpicked – carefully chosen with a personal hygiene level clearly above the average of 'normal' beings. Such people are quite able to maintain hygiene even in a rather indifferent environment. If, in such food processing, one has all the external elegance available and a very sophisticated hygiene programme, but *one* member of the staff, who *once* 'forgets' about toilet hygiene, his or her fingerprints could spoil your production – no matter how carefully the rest of the staff is working. Incidentally, foot-operated door-locks would be of more help in a food factory washroom than a beautiful mirror: doorhandles touched by *one* dirty hand are likely to infect several well-washed hands!

Another detail in open handling is the risk of airborne infection. This is often overlooked in spite of the well-known fact that micro-organisms may be carried long distances in aerosols, which are easily produced during cleaning of yards, floors, and the outsides of machinery, not to mention water treatment.

Another point of importance in open food processing is the traffic of people in process areas. It is a common misconception that managers, office, and laboratory staff are clean compared to people working in production areas. Because such persons are not obviously dirty they have less motivation to wash hands, change footwear, and 'keep their fingers off'. All visitors to production areas should be banned unless they agree to wash their hands and cover themselves, including feet and heads, with protective dress. If laboratory staff are to take samples in production areas they should be very well trained and tested to make sure that they understand the very different degrees of cleanliness appropriate in a lab and in production.

As between the raw material area and the process area, staff, facilities and even air should be kept strictly separated.

In a closed process the function of the equipment, the cleaning efficiency, and the control of process parameters are most important for hygienic operation. Cleaning is often looked upon as a necessary evil, and there is a tendency to trust automation rather than common sense. Food manufacturers are quick to ask for flexibility in process equipment, but it should be clearly understood that flexibility increases complication in installations intended for circulation cleaning. Every connection between different processing or packaging units means, when it comes to automatic cleaning, a number of valves. Assuming that a component like a pump or a valve or a measuring device has an average running time without malfunction or service of one year, with 400 components, on average, malfunction will occur at least once every day. In a large factory you may meet single valve batteries of 100 units or more.

Further, there is often a space problem which forces the installation of automatic valves in a position where they cannot even theoretically be sufficiently drained and can hardly be inspected.

Cleaning must be considered as a process, and the product of cleaning should be clean equipment. Inadequate cleaning may be due to mechanical malfunction , the wrong type or concentration of detergent, the wrong time and temperature during cleaning, or the wrong water quality with regard to detergents used, or to several of these in combination. Inadequate cleaning should be discovered on process control and never be allowed to cause loss of product through poor hygienic quality.

Inadequate cleaning, however, has many other economic consequences, beside the contamination risk. Poor product shelf life, malfunction and corrosion of equipment, over-consumption of detergents and water, expensive wastewater treatment, and energy losses are just a few examples.

SAFETY OF FOOD

If we assume that the choice and training of staff, installation, and maintenance of equipment, processing, and cleaning are all done to the best of all knowledge – would then industrially processed food be *absolutely* safe? Of course not!

Raw material may be heavily contaminated with chemicals and micro-organisms not wanted or not allowed in food sold for consumption.

During storage and processing food may become contaminated by heavy metals like nickel in very small concentrations, impossible to analyse but enough to give rise to allergy in some sensitive consumers.

There may be a considerable time between factory product control and food consumption during which growth and toxin formation or contamination could occur.

For most food-borne infections the minimum infection dose is high – 10^5 to 10^7 – and for intoxication often this number of microbes per gram of food is necessary. With reasonable care during processing and distribution food-borne illness caused by micro-organisms should never occur. Nevertheless, there is a trend towards increasing frequency of such illness, seen by some investigators as parallel to increasing industrialization in food handling.

KNOW-HOW, STANDARDS, AND CONTROL

In spite of the fact that 'cleaning' is hardly recognized as a science and is often subject to very broad generalizations, a great deal of scattered information is available which a food manufacturer could make use of to find the optimal cleaning for his system.

To start with, specify the required food quality. At which temperature and for how long should it be possible to keep the product before consumption? It is then possible to state which types of contamination are to be avoided.

The next step would be to consider the choice of equipment from a cleaning point of view. If sterility is needed it must be heat-resistant; if highly alkaline detergents are necessary it must be alkali-resistant, and so on. It is necessary to calculate investments and running costs for different cleaning systems, considering the safety in cleaning and disinfection or sterilization they can give.

Finally, raw material quality must be specified (and paid for) as well as packaging systems.

All steps in the operation must be considered, and their influence on the quality should be carefully studied. If a whole system is clean but one valve is leaking, the product quality is endangered. If the main raw material is well-controlled but one minor constituent is handled inadequately, food spoilage is to be expected.

The control of a food operation includes not only product but also process control. Process control is necessary in order to avoid malfunction due to inadequate cleaning and also to keep running costs low. Not only a test of the over-all results, such as a rinse test or control of first-processed product, but also a regular inspection of components is recommended. Dead ends in pipe lines pressure and temperature control devices, pumps, air-blow valves and product valves are known to cause problems in circulation cleaning as well as, especially, the functioning of spray balls in tanks.

If, during inspection, visible impurities are recognized, there is no point in a microbiological control of this. Such residues may be sterilized but they still represent a risk for the function of equipment and for the product quality. In such case the cleaning process has to be changed – by a change of detergents, by a temperature rise, or by improving the mechanical cleaning effect.

Microbiological control methods must be relevant and informative – a total count or coliform count is usually of very limited interest. Much better is a count of thermoduric bacteria or psychrotrophic organisms if such may multiply in the processed food.

It is very important to control water quality. Many food plants are cleaned adequately but recontaminated with chemicals and micro-organisms in the final rinse water.

Finally, food processing hygiene includes careful control of the handling of liquid and solid wastes within the factory and also in the immediate neighbourhood. Considerable product volumes are lost in rinse water, and ways to reduce losses and recover product must be considered.

Hygiene is as important as other process parameters, and the desired hygiene level should be established for each process as well as pressure, temperature, etc, if the process is to be optimized.

Adequate hygiene means not only safe production but also sound economy. It is the author's belief that food manufacturers will in future realize this, and that they should never have to fear a public health inspector since his legal demands are so modest compared to what the manager finds necessary and is able to maintain.

CHAPTER 9

Hygienic Handling and the Influence of Raw Material Condition

E. D. Hulland, Londreco Ltd.

INTRODUCTION

The primary objective of food manufacturers is to prepare and market food products of good quality which are both safe to eat from the public health aspect and which will have a reasonable shelf life under the anticipated conditions of distribution and storage. Furthermore, it is essential that the operations are carried out as efficiently as possible with the minimum of loss if the manufacturer is to remain in business; the protection of a good reputation is also important in a highly competitive market. These aims can only be achieved by purchasing good quality raw materials and processing them in well-designed hygienic plant and equipment, and by the use of good manufacturing practices.

By far the greatest part of any food manufacturer's expenditure concerns the purchase of raw materials, and it is not surprizing, therefore, that a considerable amount of time and effort is spent in obtaining good quality materials of suitable bacteriological specification. The problems, however, of ensuring that large bulk deliveries of materials are of good bacteriological condition throughout are considerable, and just one batch of heavily contaminated material passing through poorly designed equipment can give rise to serious product infection which may persist throughout the production run. Furthermore, unexpected types of infection may occur in materials occasionally, and it is important that the microbiologist responsible for their examination is aware of the products in which they are to be used and chooses the tests he will make accordingly. The presence of one type of infection in raw material does not necessarily condemn it, but it may indicate that some form of selection may have to be exercised on its use. For example, sugar contaminated with heat-resistant thermophilic spores would be unsuitable for use in low-acid canned foods, but it would be quite satisfactory for use in acid products such as soft drinks and jam, in which non-acid-tolerant organisms could not develop and would therefore be insignificant. This situation occurs mainly with manufactured or 'preserved' materials such as sugar, starches, flour, and some canned products; with fresh materials heavily contaminated samples usually contain a wide variety of organisms.

Because the death of bacteria, whether it be caused by heat, chemicals, or preservatives, generally proceeds in a logarithmic manner, it follows that the heavier the initial infection the longer it will take to destroy or inactivate the organisms; or to put it another way there is a possibility that the scheduled process or preservative system in operation in the factory will be overloaded resulting in spoilage of the finished product. It is therefore very important that the total number of organisms passing into the final product mix is restricted to a reasonably low level.

Assuming that the plant and equipment have been thoroughly cleaned initially, then excessively high numbers of micro-organisms can only result from the use of heavily contaminated raw materials, the use of poorly designed equipment, or the use of poor, unhygienic manufacturing methods. In all cases the contamination will originate from the raw materials passing through the plant, and the more heavily contaminated they are, the more critical will become the other two factors.

This paper will now discuss just some of the major raw materials used in the food industry and examine a few specific instances which illustrate how their microbiological condition can influence the manufacturing plant and consequently the final product.

The microbial contamination of raw materials entering a food processing plant depends partly on their origin and partly on the methods of handling and preparation they have already received. Thus the influence of fresh materials on plant hygiene is related directly to the efficiency of the trimming and cleaning operations and the standard of handling to which they have been subjected. However, the need to transport some materials over long distances and to store seasonal crops over a twelve-month period necessitates the use of some form of preservation (canning, dehydration, cold storage, etc.) which may further modify their bacteriological condition. It is therefore convenient to distinguish between fresh materials and those which have been subjected to some form of preservation or have had their flora modified to some extent by processes such as refining.

FRESH MATERIALS

Because the soil is an enormous reservoir for bacterial spores, vegetables – particularly root crops and dwarf growing plants such as many herbs – usually carry large numbers of micro-organisms after harvesting. The situation is made considerably worse in a wet growing season – especially if conditions are wet during harvesting when infected soil adheres firmly to the vegetables. Fresh peas, because of the method of their harvesting when the entire plant is pulled from the soil and passed through a vining machine, are particularly prone to carry a heavy bacterial contamination. Tomatoes are another crop which can suffer heavy bacterial contamination as a result of summer showers splashing soil over the fruit. It is clear, therefore, that considerable attention must be paid to the cleaning and washing operations if an unacceptable level of contamination in the plant and spoilage of the product is to be avoided.

Mercer et al (1958) carried out extensive investigations into the contamination on tomatoes entering American canneries. Analysis of tomato field soils showed average counts in excess of 50 millions per gram of heat resistant, acid tolerant spores capable of growing in tomato products; the higher the organic content of the soil, the higher the spore count. They found that in a wet season as much as 8 lb of soil per ton of fruit could be found adhering to the tomatoes arriving at the cannery. If this soil and debris is allowed to accumulate in the washers, then the sterility of the final product is affected. In many washing operations studied, the tomatoes leaving the soak tank or flume were found to carry a heavier bacterial contamination than when sampled before washing. The presence of a final spray wash with warm water (50°C) at the end of the belt after leaving the washers was found to be very effective in reducing contamination. They were also able to demonstrate the importance of careful handling before and during the washing operations, when it was found that damaged tomatoes carried seven times the bacterial load of those with unbroken skins. This was attributed to the organisms penetrating the tissues of the tomato, making it virtually impossible to remove them by normal washing methods.

The use of recirculated water is not recommended for washing vegetables because of the danger of a rapid build-up of micro-organisms in the system. Chlorination of recirculated water would be largely ineffective because the free chlorine would be rapidly absorbed and neutralized by the accumulated organic content of the water. Even if this were not the case, the benefit of chlorination would be limited, since these spores often exhibit considerable chlorine resistance.

The advent of machine harvesting of tomatoes in America in the early 1960s increased the problem considerably. Thus Mercer (1967) reviewing the situation stated that machine-harvested tomatoes could carry 10 to 200 times the spore load of hand picked fruit, and on average 37.5 lb of soil per ton of tomatoes, of which 4.1lb was present as a difficult-to-remove smear. He recommended in-field washing stations to clean the fruit immediately after harvesting and before the soil smears had time to harden. Factory washing at a later stage could remove only 50% of the soil present as a smear. Krochta and Bellows (1974) investigated the effects of machine-harvesting tomatoes and state that up to 30% of the fruit delivered to packers may be damaged. The exudate resulting from broken skins encouraged the formation of soil smears and also increased insect problems. They found that soil with a moisture content in the range 20 to 40% easily formed smears which were difficult to remove, and recommended the use of detergents in cleaning operations. In attempts to reduce the water usage in cleaning operations they experimented with foam cleaning and oil-water emulsions.

The situation described for tomatoes applies equally to other vegetables, the differences being the degree of difficulty in removing the contaminating soil and micro-organisms. Hersom and Hulland (1969) mention an outbreak of spoilage in canned carrots in which the vegetables from one particular farm were found to be heavily infected with a thermophilic organism, while Cameron (1938) reports a similar case concerning asparagus. Failure to remove the contamination and prevent its build-up in the washers, results in the infection being carried further forward with the raw material until the entire production line may become contaminated.

Perhaps one of the most difficult materials to deal with is the mushroom, although it represents a special case in that it is grown commercially in compost produced by microbial fermentation. Natural composts are usually prepared from straw and horse manure with a little powdered gypsum, and are allowed to ferment in stacks until an homogenous friable mixture results. The process takes 10 to 14 days, and in the early stages temperatures up to 70°C are attained and, although the stack is turned over every 2 to 3 days to encourage aerobic fermentation, it is inevitable that there will be periods when the centre of the stack is under anaerobic conditions. This may lead to the rapid growth of the very heat-resistant thermophilic anaerobe *Clostridium thermosaccharolyticum;* indeed most mushrooms will carry some spores of this organism, but occasionally crops will be very heavily contaminated. The author can recall an instance some years ago when an increase of twenty minutes on the normal process time at a temperature of 118°C failed to inactivate such an infection in a canned speciality pack, samples subjected to routine incubation tests blowing within twenty four hours. Because they float on water, are difficult to wet, and the fact that compost may become stuck in the gills, mushrooms are very difficult to wash adequately. However, the use of a wetting agent in the water and vigorous spray rinsing will remove much of the contamination.

In addition to spoilage organisms, soil contamination may also introduce food-poisoning bacteria into the plant, including the heat-resistant and very toxic mesophilic anaerobe, *Clostridium botulinum.* This organism is widely distributed in nature, having been isolated from virgin and cultivated soils in America, Europe, Russia, India, and other parts of the world. Seven antigenically -distinct types of *C. botulinum,* designated A, B, C, D, E, F, and G, are now recognized. Types A and B produce heat-resistant spores, whilst types E and F are noted for their ability to grow and produce toxin down to temperatures as low as 4°C. Types C and D are associated mainly with botulism in cattle. *Clostridium perfringens* is another food-poisoning organism which may be present in soil in the form of spores.

Mesophilic clostridia, including the two food-poisoning organisms just mentioned, are often associated with meat, but if the carcases have been prepared under strict hygienic conditions the level of contamination is usually very low. The incidence of mesophilic clostridium spores in fresh meat has been investigated by Steinkraus and Ayres (1964) and by Greenberg et al (1966). Contamination was found to be low, the latter workers reporting the higher figures averaging 2.8 putrefactive anaerobes per gram of meat. No spores of *C. botulinum* were found by Steinkraus and Ayres, and Greenberg and colleagues obtained only one isolate from 2358 samples of meat. Roberts and Ingram (1976) found two spores of *C. botulinum* per kilogram of pork. Normally most of the bacterial contamination of meat occurs after slaughter during the dressing and handling operations, the chief sources being the hide, gut, implements used, and the personnel. Immediately after dressing it is important to cool the carcases right through to the centre of the meat as quickly as possible. This is achieved in refrigerated chill rooms when currents of cold air are passed over the carcases by forced circulation. Initially this air is humidified to prevent undue moisture loss due to the temperature difference between the meat and the circulating air. During the cooling the surface connective tissues undergo changes which will prevent excessive moisture loss during subsequent chill storage. While the surface of the carcase remains at chill temperatures, −2°C to 7°C, the growth of psychrophilic bacteria such as Achromobacter, Flavobacterium, and Pseudomonas will continue until the moisture content of the surface falls sufficiently to restrict their growth. If the carcase is removed from the chill store into the atmosphere of a food factory where higher ambient temperatures and humidities prevail, condensation will occur on the surface of the meat. This condition is known as 'sweating' and encourages microbial growth. If the meat surface remains sufficiently moist for any reason, then the psychrophilic organisms will grow to produce colonies which coalesce to form a film of bacterial slime. The time for this to occur is a function of temperature, average figures being in the region of ten days at 0°C and three days at 5°C. If meat with high counts of these psychrophilic organisms is used for the preparation of comminuted meat products such as beefburgers, heavy contamination will build up in the equipment and product. Freezing the product and holding it at a temperature of −10°C will inhibit the growth of the psychrophilic organisms, but some of their enzymes which will have accumulated in the product may continue to cause quality deterioration at temperatures approaching −30°C (Sulzbacher & Gaddis, 1968). It is interesting to note that beef prepared from cattle in tropical countries will be contaminated with fewer psychrophilic organisms capable of growth at chill temperatures (−1.5°C), and will therefore tend to keep better than beef prepared from cattle reared in temperate climates. This is because most of the contaminating micro-organisms originate from the soil, via the hide, and are adapted to grow at the prevailing soil temperatures which are, of course, much higher in the tropics.

DRY MATERIALS

Moisture is essential for the growth of micro-organisms, and the bacterial cell consists of about four-fifths by weight of water. Many organisms are damaged by drying in air, and different species vary widely in their ability to survive drying under natural conditions. Most pathogens die rapidly, but *Staphylococcus aureus* may survive for several months. Bacterial spores survive drying very well, and those of *Bacillis anthracis* have been known to survive in a viable state for over sixty years. More delicate non-sporing organisms will survive for several years if they are freeze-dried.

A considerable proportion of peas grown for canning are dried and then canned at a later date as 'processed' peas after being rehydrated, whilst 'baked' beans are pea beans which have been dried for storage and distribution before canning. After the dried vegetables have been subjected to a series of screening and sorting operations they are washed in cold water and then enter a soaking tank for reconstitution, or they may be fed direct into a hot-water blancher where reconstitution and blanching occur simultaneously. The water in the bottom of rotary blanchers is usually maintained at a temperature of 80 to 85°C, too high for bacterial growth; but as the inner reel revolves the internal surface of the shell becomes wetted and soiled with organic debris, and a temperature gradient is established. The spores of thermophilic 'flat-sour' organisms such as *Bacillus stearothermophilus* will germinate and multiply very rapidly under these conditions and, particularly in the case of peas, may lead to an overloading of the thermal process with the consequent danger of flat-sour spoilage occurring, especially in packs exported to tropical climates. Continuous tubular blanchers do not suffer from this problem to the same extent, particularly if the water is run to waste; recirculated water should be treated and chlorinated before re-use.

Thermophilic and mesophilic spores can be particularly troublesome in canneries, being well adapted for growth in heated equipment such as mixers, blanchers, and fillers. Other dry materials such as sugar, starch, and milk powder may contribute a heavy contamination of heat-resistant spores to the plant and final product.

An incident comes to mind which occurred some years ago of an intermediate product which contained, among other materials, both starch and milk powder. The ingredients were mixed together in water which was then heated to 80°C and pumped up to a header tank as a thin liquid. From here it was fed by gravity into the final product mix as required. The problem always occurred from about 3 p.m. onwards and was manifested by separation of the final product after processing. All the production up to this time each day was satisfactory. Checks showed that the pH of this intermediate product was much lower during the afternoons, and it continued to fall until production ended for the day. Further investigations revealed large numbers of thermophilic flat-souring organisms growing in the foam head on the liquid, the liquid itself being too hot to support their growth. The variation in the level of the liquid in the tank also aggravated the situation. Each evening the clean-down and disinfection procedure meant that the contamination had to build up from the ingredients again the following morning. The introduction of an extra clean-down of the tank at lunchtime and an hourly check on the pH value of the intermediate product eliminated any further trouble. The infection was thought to originate mainly from the milk powder.

Allen et al (1946) have shown that crude beet sugar may be heavily contaminated with thermophilic organisms, many of which presumably survive in the finished product. It is possible, however, to purchase certain grades of sugar which contain only a low level of bacterial contamination.

Herbs and spices may carry very heavy bacterial loads, particularly spores, and the contamination they contribute to the plant and product is far out of proportion to their quantities. The contamination of spices can be reduced considerably by heating the dry spice in shallow trays, but excessive heating destroys the spice flavour. More recently such materials have often been treated by fumigation with ethylene or propylene oxides. Thus curry powder containing over fifty million organisms per gram has been treated with ethylene oxide in a vacuum chamber to reduce the contamination to less than five hundred per gram. Care should be exercised in the use of fumigation, however, since Wesley et al (1965) demonstrated that chlorohydrins could be produced by the interaction of ethylene oxide or propylene oxide with traces of chloride usually present in the food. The presence of chlorohydrins could constitute a toxic hazard.

FROZEN RAW MATERIALS

At low temperatures some species of bacteria die rapidly, but the majority survive well. The process of freezing kills a proportion of the bacterial cells, but if the freezing is carried out quickly, as indeed it is in the food industry, then the number of cells dying is kept to a minimum. Lowering the temperature of food to −10°C inhibits the growth of all micro-organisms, although as we have seen earlier, some bacterial enzymes may still be acting slowly at much lower temperatures. As for the survival of bacteria at low temperatures (below 0°C), this generally increases as the temperature falls. Thus *Staphylococcus aureus,* a common food-poisoning orgsnism, will remain viable for longer periods at −20°C than it will at −10°C; indeed, a convenient method of preserving bacteria in culture collections is to store them under liquid nitrogen at −196°C when they will remain viable for several years.

Deep-frozen raw materials will, therefore,contain much the same type and degree of contamination as their fresh counterparts, and if thawed before use should be treated in the same manner as the fresh article. So far as I am aware, there is no evidence to substantiate a popularly held belief that deep-frozen food when thawed will spoil *more* rapidly or support more vigorous bacterial growth than fresh food. Indeed what evidence there is suggests thar the lag phase (the period of adaptation before logarithmic growth occurs) may be lengthened.

Compared with fresh foods there are inherent dangers in the handling of frozen foods. If we consider deep-frozen meat, perhaps one of the most common frozen raw materials, we find that, on thawing, the surface becomes very wet and sticky. Although this in itself does not lead to an increase in bacterial growth, it does mean that the meat surface will readily pick-up extraneous dirt and infect-tion during handling and preparation. To improve the hygiene of meat handling and, simultaneously, to save on the time required for thawing, meat can be prepared direct from the frozen state by cutting up on a band saw and then feed-ing into powerful bowl choppers or mincing machines. Careful control on the emerging product, however, is essential, particularly with regard to the temper-ature attained by the meat. For example, it is possible to cut whole frozen oxtails into lengths on a band saw and then feed them through a double mincing process (with the aid of added cold water) to produce a fine puree. Such a pro-cedure, however, is likely to achieve temperatures of up to 40°C in the final puree. If this is fed into large tanks or mobiles it is likely that the centre will remain warm and anaerobic for several hours – ideal conditions for the rapid growth of mesophilic anaerobes such as Clostridia including the food-poisoning species *C. botulinum* and *C. perfringens.* Although originally present in low numbers clostridia may rapidly come to dominate the original psychrophilic flora under these conditions. It is important, therefore, not to prepare such purees too far in advance of production and, if a hold-up in production appears likely, the puree should be filled into shallow trays and cooled rapidly.

CANNED RAW MATERIALS

Since most canned foods receive a thermal process sufficient to reduce the number of spores of *Clostridium botulinum,* the most heat-resistant food-poisoning organism, by a factor of 10^{12}, and to destroy or inactivate all but a few of the very heat-resistant spoilage organisms, it might be concluded that the amount of bacterial contamination contributed by these materials to the equip-ment and product would be very small. In the majority of cases this is certainly true, but the severity of the heat process given to canned foods depends to a large extent on the pH value of the pack, which in turn governs the types of organisms capable of growing in the product and spoiling it. Thus canned tomato puree, a major raw material in this category, has a pH value ranging from 4.1 to 4.4 and would normally only suffer spoilage by yeasts, lactobacilli, or moulds – all acid-tolerant, non-heat-resistant organisms. During its preparation tomato puree receives virtually little more than a pasteurization and hot fill treatment As we have seen earlier, tomatoes are likely to be contaminated with heat-resistant spores from the soil which are able to survive this level of heat treatment, and it is not unusual for thermophilic spores of *Clostridium thermosaccharo-lyticum* and *Bacillus coagulans* to be found in considerable numbers in some purees. They are unable to develop in the puree itself, but if this is mixed with other ingredients of a non-acid nature which raise the pH value, then rapid proliferation of the organisms will occur in heated equipment. I remember an instance concerning an acid product which was given an HTST process and then filled hot into preheated cans. The cans were held for a few minutes before being cooled and labelled. The spasmodic occurence of odd cans showing spoilage in the form of souring and off-flavour was traced to a heavy contamination of *B. coagulans* which had developed in the drip which built up on the filler heads. Intermittently, part of this drip fell into a can causing spoilage. The source of the *B. coagulans* was traced to the tomato puree.

Canned fruit, because of its low pH value and hence low-heat process, may also contain viable spores. In this case the most troublesome organism is perhaps the mould *Byssochlamys fulva* and the closely related *B. nivea.* The spores of these moulds possess quite exceptional heat resistance (for moulds); Gillespy and Thorpe (1962) state that they survive 10 minutes at 87.7°C, while Michener et al (1966) found that they could survive ten minutes at 92.2°C in grape juice. They can cause a complete disintegration of fruit due to the breakdown of pectinous material. The spores are likely to survive the canning process for fruit, particularly so in the case of the large 5 kg cans produced for manufacturing purposes. However, this does not always produce a complete breakdown of the fruit, so that even if each can is inspected on opening, it is possible for one infected can to contaminate a production batch. If the fruit is held in a balance tank the infection may spread over several batches. A case occurred some years ago of an instant fruit dessert which was required to set through the formation of a pectin gel. The pectin in the product had been destroyed by the pectolytic enzyme produced by the mould, with the result that no set was obtained when the pack was opened and mixed.

CROSS-CONTAMINATION

The possibility of cross-infection occurring between the raw materials and intermediate or final products, which have received some treatment to reduce their contamination, is an ever-present problem. Ideally, production lines should be so designed to ensure that the materials flow in a straight line and that the raw material is as far removed from the final product as possible. Care should be taken to avoid the build-up of intermediate products so that the materials flow smoothly at a constant rate along the line. If the accumulation of intermediate product is unavoidable, then special care is necessary to ensure that recontamination and build-up of infection do not occur at these stages. Problems may arise on occasions which are due partly to a false sense of security.

An incident occurred some time ago concerning the production of a certain beverage, the raw materials for which were stored in a separate building, adjacent to the one containing the production line but separated from it by a yard some 60 feet wide. A bridge connected the two buildings along which the raw material was transported. The first stage in the process involved extracting the raw material at a high temperature, the resulting liquor being cooled by heat-exchangers and then fed into a series of storage tanks connected by a manifold. From here the liquor received further processing before a final heat treatment prior to filling. An off-flavour occurred in the final product which was thought to be due to chemical contamination. However, this could not be demonstrated. Culturing the final product showed this to be sterile, but working back along the line examining samples at all points revealed a heavy growth of lactobacilli in the liquor storage tanks. These organisms are not heat-resistant and can grow well in the environment of the storage tanks, the liquor having a pH of 4.4 and a temperature of 20 to 25°C. No previous experience existed of microbial spoilage of this product, and the organism could grow only at this one stage in the production line. It was found later that contamination had occurred from the dust caused by handling the raw material, and that this had been carried through open windows across the yard and into the liquor tanks via the inspection covers which unwisely had been left open.

CONCLUSION

The subject of raw material contamination covers a very wide area, and although it has only been possible to mention and illustrate certain aspects, it is hoped that the importance of the raw material condition and its effect on the hygiene of manufacturing processes has been demonstrated.

To summarize, hygienically-designed and -operated plant and equipment will not produce a food quality final product if the raw material is microbiologically unsuitable. Conversely, good quality raw materials may become heavily contaminated if processed in unhygienically-designed and -operated equipment. To achieve our desired aim, all three – the raw material, the plant and the method of operation – must be hygienically sound.

REFERENCES

Allen, L. A., Cooper, A. H., Cairns, A., and Maxwell, M. C. C. (1946) *Proc. Soc. Appl. Bact.,* **1**, 5.

Cameron, E. J. (1938) *Food Res.,* **3**, 91.

Gillespy, T. G., and Thorpe, R. H. (1962) 'Survey of Byssochlamys fulva Ascospore infection on Strawberries for Canning'. Tech. Mem. No. 44. Fruit and Veg. Canning and Quick Freezing Res. Ass., Campden.

Greenberg, R. A., Tompkin, R. B., Bludel, B. O., Kittora, R. S., and Anellis, A. (1966). *Appl. Microbiol.,* **14**, 789.

Hersom, A. C., and Hulland, E. D. (1969) *Canned Foods* 6th ed. J and A Churchill.

Krochta, J. M., and Bellows, R. J. (1974) *Food Technology,* **28** (2), 34-37, 47.

Mercer, W. A., Rose, W. W., Butler, C. E., and Appleman, M. M. (1958). Nat. Canner's Ass. Inf. Letter No. 1666 (Convention issue) 56.

Mercer, W. A. (1967). Nat. Canners' Ass. Inf. Letter No. 2102 (Convention issue) 52.

Michener, H. D., King, A. D. Jr., and Ito, K. A. (1966) *Bact. Proc.,* A **15**, 3.
Roberts, T. A., and Ingram, M., (1976). Proc. 2nd Int. Symp. on Nitrates in Meat Products. Tinbergen, B. J., and Krol, B. (Ed.) Wageningen Centre for Agr. Pub and Doc.
Steinkraus, K. H. and Ayres, J. C. (1964) *J. Food Sci.,* **29**, 87.
Sulzbacher, W. L., and Gaddis, A. M. (1968) 'The Freezing Preservation of Foods'. 4th ed. AVI Westpoint, Conn.
Wesley, F., Rourke, B., and Darbyshire, O. (1965) *J. Food Sci.,* **30**, 1037.

DISCUSSION

Mr G Heighton (Geo. Basset & Co. Ltd.): Do you have any information as to how effective irradiation of raw material might be to sterilize it?

Mr Hulland; No, I haven't much information on irradiation except that it is a method which has been used for pretreating raw materials before use in other food materials. It certainly is coming – there is certainly more work being done in this area, and I think that it won't be long before it will be an accepted method of treating raw materials.

Mr John Lee (Distillers Co.): Mr Hulland mentioned the bacterial contamination of tomatoes from the field. How reliable is the Howard Mould Count to indicate the extent of bacterial contamination?

Mr Hulland: Well, it is really not a very reliable method at all if you look at it statistically. It's also not a very good idea, as a producer of tomato puree can easily get around that by picking the tomatoes before they are properly ripe, so although it is intended to increase the quality, in fact it could possibly have the reverse effect. Obviously the more ripe and soft the tomatoes are the better the flavour and the colour, but the more likely they are to have a high mould count because they are very easily broken during handling under adverse conditions.

Mr Lee: What alternative method of incoming quality control would you suggest for a user of canned tomato puree?

Mr Hulland: Well, certainly I would consider the spore count content if it's going into low-acid canned foods.

Mr Lee: You mean the mould spore?

Mr Hulland: No, I mean the bacterial spore. If it's going into a low-acid canned food where the bacterial spores are important.

Mr Lee: Something like baked beans?

Mr Hulland: Yes, *Clostridium thermosaccharolyticum* can be important in baked beans because they are normally within the pH range of the growth of that organism in the tomato puree.

Mr T. Lloyd (Walls Ice Cream): Dr Jarvis, Leatherhead Food RA, has in fact developed a new method for the examination of tomatoes to replace the Howard Mould Count. The textbooks say that the Howard Mould Count is a useful general index of the state of the tomato either as a processed or a partly-processed material. I was just wondering what your opinion was.

Mr Hulland: Well, it doesn't give any indication of the kind of process it has had at all – only the preprocess contamination. It does indicate – if it is a very high mould count, of course – that the hygienic conditions in the puree-producing plant were not good. But, as I say, by picking unripe tomatoes you can bring about a much lower count. Would Mr Thorpe like to comment on this interesting question.

Mr Thorpe (Campden Food RA): Yes, I think I would agree that if you are looking for low-acid canned products then the Howard Moult Count is not really going to be very much use to you, and it would be very much better to be looking for bacterial spores, particularly *Clostridium thermosaccharolyticum* which is the one most likely to cause you the most spoilage in that type of pack.

Mr M. J. Carpenter (Cadbury Ltd.): There is one point in Mr Hulland's paper on which I would like clarification. He said in the storage of meat at –30°C the micro-organisms present were inactive, nevertheless the meat deteriorated because of enzyme activity. Are these the *meat* enzymes or enzymes within the inactive micro-organisms which cause deterioration of the meat?

Mr Hulland: Many psychrophilic organisms found on meat release extracellular enzymes into the meat during growth, and meat with high bacterial counts may contain significant amounts of these extracellular microbial enzymes. Freezing the meat and holding it at –10°C will inhibit the psychrophilic organisms, but their extracellular enzymes may continue to be active at temperatures down to –30°C.

Sulzbacher and Gaddis in 'The Freezing Preservation of Foods' give an example of lipases released by a Pseudomonas culture which are able to act on fats at –29°C within two weeks.

CHAPTER 10

Bacteriology of Raw Materials, Handling, and Processing of Fish

W. **Hodgkiss**, Torry Research Station

INTRODUCTION

The bacteriology of marine fish intended for use as human food involves two main avenues of investigation. Firstly, studies of the commensal flora and the putrefactive flora which develop from it, and secondly, the detection of food-poisoning and indicator organisms. Within recent years comprehensive data on the microbiology of fishery products have been presented by colleagues at Torry Research Station [1,2,3,4]. The main features of this work as they relate to the subject of this Symposium follow.

In their natural environment marine fish carry numbers of commensal bacteria on the external surfaces, on the gills, and in the digestive tract. Most of the fish landed at UK ports are caught in temperate or sub-arctic waters, so their commensal bacterial flora consist mainly of psychrophilic organisms, that is, bacteria which have an optimum growth temperature of 20°C and are capable of moderate to rapid growth at temperatures of 0° to 10°C. The temperatures of growth of these and other micro-organisms are shown below:

Temperature of growth of Micro-organisms

	Optimum temperature °C	Range of growth °C
Psychrophiles	20	–4 to 28
Mesophiles	30 to 37	3.5 to 45
Thermophiles	55 to 60	37 to 65

The commensal organisms are prevented from invading the tissues of a healthy fish by the protective action of its surface tissues and by its natural defence mechanisms [5]. When the fish is killed these bacteria multiply rapidly. invade the tissues, and eventually cause putrefaction. The rate at which putrefaction proceeds depends upon the rate of growth of the causative bacteria, and this in turn is dependent upon a number of factors including an adequate supply of nutrients, moisture and suitable pH, temperature and gaseous environment,

As fish is in every way a suitable substrate for bacterial growth, temperature is the factor which can be controlled most effectively in order to restrict that growth and yet preserve the organoleptic qualities of the fish.

CHILLING

Chilling to near 0°C by the use of ice is the traditional method of short-term storage and has been used in basic studies of the bacteriology and biochemistry of fish spoilage [1,2,3,4,5,6,7,8]. Apart from slight seasonal variations, the commensal bacteria are fairly constant in total numbers and types of organisms, but once the fish is killed changes occur in these flora and changes continue to occur throughout the processes of evisceration, washing, icing, filleting, transportation etc. They continue until the fish is cooked and consumed. See Fig. 10.A. These changes may be summarized as follows. At chill temperatures (which may vary from 0° to 10°C) and under conditions of ideal storage, the growth of psychrophilic bacteria is quite rapid; during the first period of storage (3 to 4 days) the total numbers of bacteria increase but organoleptic changes in the fish are only slight. After 5 to 6 day's storage the total numbers of bacteria increase still further to millions per gram, the Gram-negative bacteria (*Pseudomonas, Moraxella, Acinetobacter*) multiplying more rapidly than the Gram-positive Micrococci, coryneforms). After 10 days' storage signs of putrefaction become evident, *Pseudomonas* species dominate the bacterial flora and after 14 to 16 days the product becomes unacceptable.

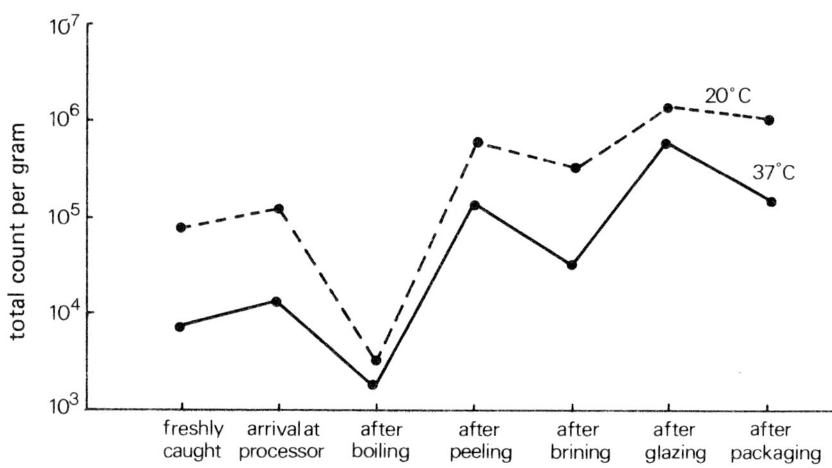

Fig. 10.A – Total viable counts on temperate shrimp during processing.

Tables 1 and 2 give an outline of bacteriological analyses of the marine environment, fish, and items with which it comes into contact. During processing additional bacterial contamination may get on to the fish if filleting boards, knives, conveyor belts, and containers are not cleaned efficiently; and, if the temperature of the fish is allowed to rise, bacterial multiplication is also increased. Efficient cleaning and the maintenance of low temperatures throughout processing are therefore essential for a good quality product by keeping the numbers of putrefactive bacteria at a minimum level.

Table 1

Psychrophilic bacteria: total viable counts from marine fish, its natural environment and the processing environment

Fish	*Numbers of viable bacteria at 20°C*
Surface of skin	4 000 to 150 000 per sq cm
Gills	5 000 to 64 000 per gram
Intestines	17 million to 417 million per gram
Sea water	
5 fathoms	390 to 1 200 per ml
40 fathoms	25 to 110 per ml
Sea muds	1 million to 31 million per gram
Ice	
Ice	440 per ml
Ice in trawler's bunker	106 000 to 12 500 000 per ml
	Bacteria per sq cm (20°C)
Wooden box, new	100
Wooden box, used once	3 000 000
Wooden box, used once, after washing	300 000
	Bacteria per sq cm (20°C)
Filleting bench	450 000 to 3 200 000
Filleting knife	219 000 to 265 000

Table 2

Psychrophilic bacteria on fish

Quantitative changes

Days in ice	*Fish surface* *Bacteria per sq cm fish surface (20° C)*
1	10 000 to 100 000
6	100 000 to 1 000 000
12	50 000 000
12	50 000 000
21 (inedible)	500 000 000

Qualitative changes in the bacterial flora of iced cod during chill storage

		Gutted, washed un-iced	*5 days in ice*	*12 days in ice*
			% of total isolates	
	Pseudomonas	9	29	67
Gram - ve	Moraxella Acinetobacter	51	49	22
	Flavobacterium Cytophaga	9	7	1
Gram + ve	Coryneform	20	14	5
	Micrococci	8	1	0
	Other organisms	3	0	5

FREEZING

Freezing to recommended cold storage temperatures stops all bacterial growth and kills 60 to 90% of the bacteria present. Gram-negative bacteria are more susceptible to freezing than Gram-positive forms, but as soon as the product is thawed they quickly resume growth and putrefaction proceeds as if uninterrupted. Efficient freezing, the use of correct cold storage procedures, and a controlled cold chain distribution ensure that bacteriological problems with frozen products are negligible.

SMOKING

The smoking process alters the bacterial flora of fish because of the combined action of salt, heat, and bacteriostatic substances derived from the smoke. The total numbers of bacteria are reduced and Gram-positive organisms dominate the flora immediately after smoking. The shelf-life of a smoked product depends upon the method of smoking; the greater the reduction in water activity, the greater the retardation in subsequent bacterial growth. Lightly cured products quickly develop a Gram-negative spoilage flora and in consequence have a relatively short shelf-life. In drier products the main spoilage agents are moulds derived from the sawdust or wood chips.

CONVENIENCE FOODS

In the production of convenience foods, the addition of batter, breadcrumbs, or sauces introduces additional bacterial flora (Table 3). Foods such as fish fingers produced under a system in which the bacterial flora are monitored and which are distributed frozen are bacteriologically acceptable. However, convenience foods intended for chill display cabinet distribution are susceptible to unusual spoilage changes. It should be understood that certain areas in chill display cabinets may reach temperatures several degrees above the specified level. For this reason shelf-life should be calculated upon storage at the maximum probable temperature of storage (10°C).

Table 3

Changes in bacterial flora in processing

Sample	Total viable count per gram at 20°C	at 37°C	*E coli/gram*
Frozen fish	534 000	14 000	3
Batter	482 000	36 000	0
Breadcrumbs	37 000	5 000	0
Enrobed fish stick:			
before cooking	2 100 000	19 200	5
after cooking	172 000	2 400	0
after freezing	401 000	32 000	5

INDICATOR AND FOOD-POISONING ORGANISMS

Marine fish caught in unpolluted waters are free from human enteric organisms and from *Staphylococcus aureus.* The significance of *S. aureus, E. coli,* coliforms, and enteric pathogens in foods is well documented and need not be stressed here. Cleanliness is important as a means of keeping the putrefactive organisms at low levels, and from the hygiene point of view adequate methods of sanitizing, such as the use of in-plant chlorination, are essential. In the cleaning process it is important to remove all traces of proteinaceous material such as fish debris and fish slime, for these not only become foci of bacterial growth but absorb and inactive sanitizing agents. In this context plant design and engineering play an important role. A plant which is difficult to clean because of inaccessible crevices and corners quickly becomes a reservoir of all types of bacteria. These accumulations of bacteria, either in the vegetative stage or in the resistant spore stage, can become a source of endless trouble and cross-contamination.

Although the commensal flora are mainly psychrophilic two important mesophilic organisms which cause food poisining are found on fish; these are *Clostridium botulinum* and *Vibrio parahaemolyticus.* Botulism is a form of food poisoning caused by the ingestion of toxin produced in the food by one or other of a group of spore-forming anaerobic bacteria classified as *C. botulinum.* The potential hazard in the food industry is well recognized, and the importance of it in fishery products has recently been reviewed. [9]. Before 1960 it was assumed that the botulism hazard in commercial food processing had been largely obviated. Botulism outbreaks were generally the result of inefficient home-processing or were due to the consumption of raw fermented products. The sudden increase in cases of botulism in the USA in 1963, when some of the outbreaks involved fishery products, led to a new awareness of the problem. At Torry Research Station considerable effort has been applied to this subject [10,11,12,13,14]. These investigations have established that the incidence of *C. botulinum* in the British marine environment and in fish landed here is very low indeed (Table 4). In fishery products the important serotypes are non-proteolytic types B, E, and F. as these are capable of producing toxin at chill temperatures. Toxin production is subject to the influence of many factors, most important of which are temperature, salt content of the substrate, and time. The botulinum toxins are destroyed by normal cooking processes, so the greatest potential hazard is hot-smoked products which are eaten without further cooking. Much of the recent work at TRS has been in studies of toxin production in smoked products and the influence of factors which can be controlled to obviate the hazard. This work has included extensive investigations in farmed rainbow trout [15,16,17]. As a result, recommendations have been made by the Department of Health and Social Security on rainbow trout products. The recommendations for the smoked product include efficient evisceration and washing (removal of the gills being advantageous), a minimum salt concentration, appropriate temperature control during storage and distribution, and a specified limit on shelf-life.

C. botulinum spores are found on the gills and in the intestines of fish, having been picked up from the environment, particularly from bottom deposits. Investigations during the botulinum work revealed that spores of *C. welchii* (perfringens) were present also on the gills and in the intestines, but heat-resistant strains were not detected [18]. *C. welchii* type food poisoning is rarely associated with fishery products.

Table 4

Distribution of *Clostridium botulinum* Type E

Source	Type of sample	No tested	*C. botulinum* Type E present
Shops in Britain	Vacuum packed fish	646	5
Skagerrak	White fish (intestines)	130	0
,,	,, ,, (whole)	130	0
North Sea	,, ,, (intestines)	96	0
,, ,,	Herring (intestines)	200	0
Norwegian Sea	,, (intestines)	22	3
,, ,,	,, (whole)	44	24
Britain	Rainbow trout (intestines)	700	45
,,	,, ,, (whole)	700	43
England and Wales	Shellfish	106	0
Skagerrak, Kattegat, and Sound	Bottom deposits	114	57
North Sea	,, ,,	171	1
Arctic fishing grounds	,, ,,	26	0
Britain	Shore samples	59	0

V. parahaemolyticus is a more recently defined hazard in seafoods [19,20], the first cases bring recognized as a specific bacterial gastro-enteritis in Japan in 1951. In that country the persistently high incidence of cases correlates not only with the extensive use of seafoods but with the consumption of them in the raw state. The causative organism is the subject of study by fishery and public health laboratories in many countries, and in consequence a number of publications exist. The most recent comprehensive review of the literature was presented by Cabassi and Mori [21]. *V. parahaemolyticus* is a Gram-negative, non-sporing rod which is unique in being the only food-poisoning organism of true marine origin. It grows rapidly at 37° and can grow over a wide range of sodium chloride concentrations (0.5 to 8.0%). It appears to prefer estuarine and coastal waters which are warmer than the open sea and contain more organic detritus. Its presence in UK waters was reported by Barrow and Miller [22], and a recent collaborative survey has shown that it is widely distributed in relatively small numbers in our coastal waters, sediments, and shellfish especially in southern and western areas [23]. In the UK cases of food poisoning caused by this organism have been reported not only in incoming airline passengers on international flights [23] but also in local outbreaks [24,25]. As the organism is quickly destroyed in the normal cooking process the main hazard is cross-contamination of cooked products with organisms from uncooked material [25]. Although reports state that the organism is susceptible to freezing, it has been isolated in the author's laboratory from imported shellfish [4]. The current increase in international trade in shellfish therefore could give rise to infection of processing premises with organisms from these frozen products. In turn estuarine and coastal waters could support growth of the organism during the warmer season of the year.

The production of a safe food of good eating quality involves bacteriological analyses. Whilst bacteriological standards were originally introduced to check the hygiene condition of drinking water and milk, their application has been extended to all types of foods, not only to assess safety of the product but also as a measure of quality [26]. In consequence all aspects of bacteriological standards have become the subject of debate, and the literature on them is extensive. In this country data on fishery products have been published [2,4,27] and the philosophical attitudes have also been expressed [28,29,30]. From the producer's point of view there is no doubt that bacteriological monitoring of the raw material and of samples taken throughout the processing line is most useful in maintaining high product quality.

Bacteriological analyses are expensive in materials and man-hours as well as being lengthy procedures. However, two new techniques in bacteriology, the spiral-plating method and electrical impedence measurement of estimating bacterial populations, now being tested on food materials, show promise of shortening the time involved and reducing the costs of materials [31,32].

To summarize, careful control of temperatures and attention to cleanliness and hygiene are the factors which are most effective in reducing the activities of spoilage bacteria. Food-poisoning organisms are rare in this raw material; these and any which gain access subsequently can be rendered innocuous by this same care and attention, and the reputation of fish as a safe food material thereby maintained.

ILLUSTRATIONS

Figs. 1 to 10 and 12 to 16 are electron micrographs of gold-palladium shadowed preparations. Fig. 11 is an electron micrograph of an ultra-thin section stained with lead oxide. Fig. 17 is a photomicrograph taken by means of phase optics.

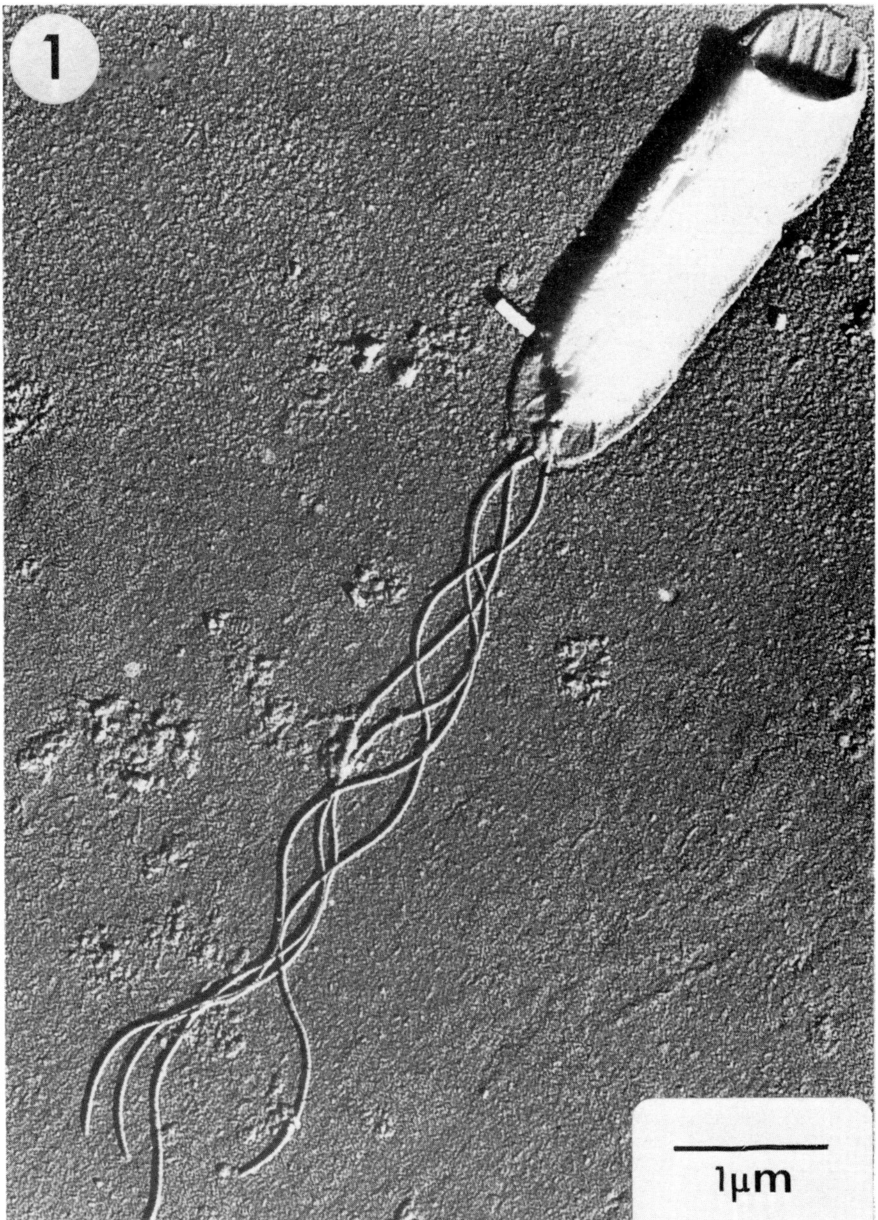

Fig. 10.1 – A cell of a *Pseudomonas* species showing polar flagella. The cells of pseudomonads are motile and possess from 1 to 16 polar flagella.

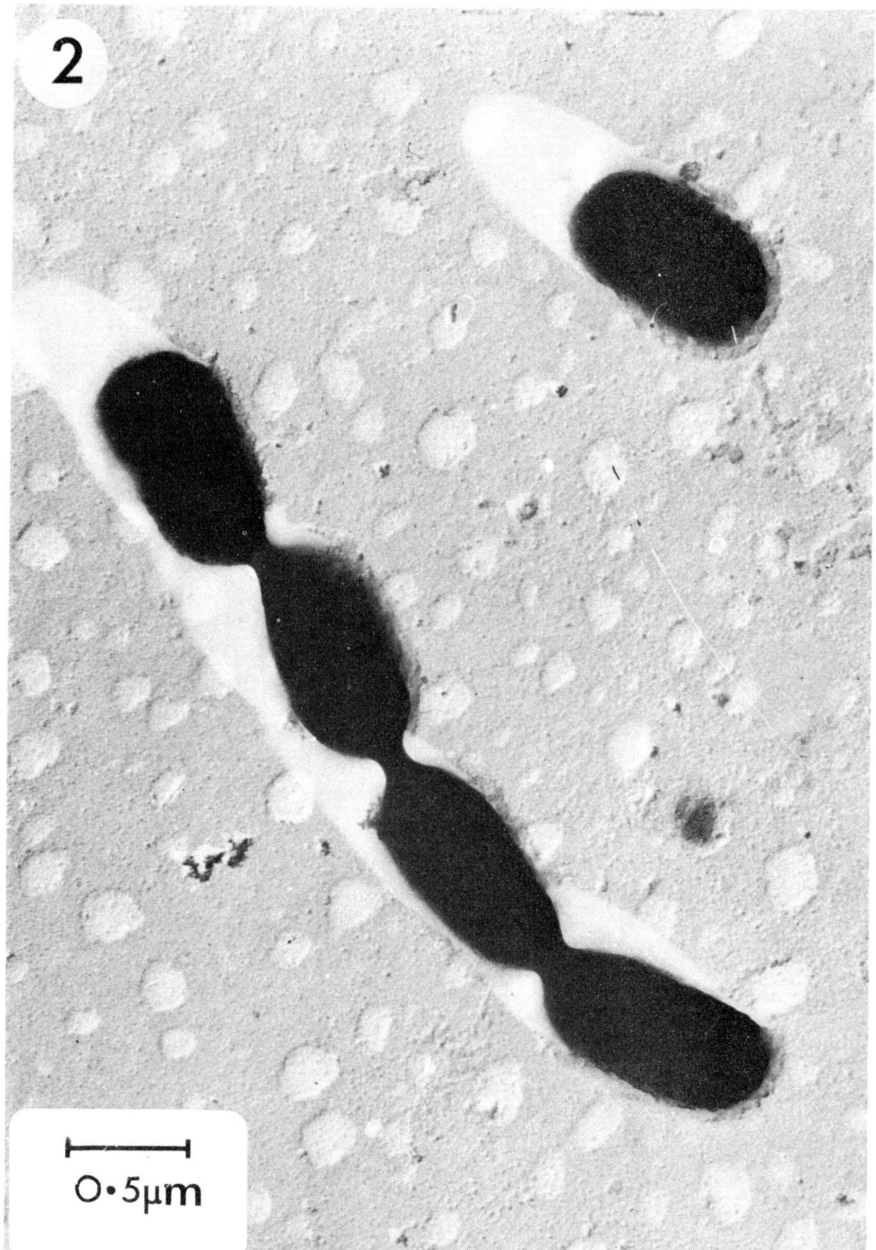

Fig. 10.2 – Illustration of the morphology of cells of the non-motile organisms of the *Moraxella-Acinetobacter* group.

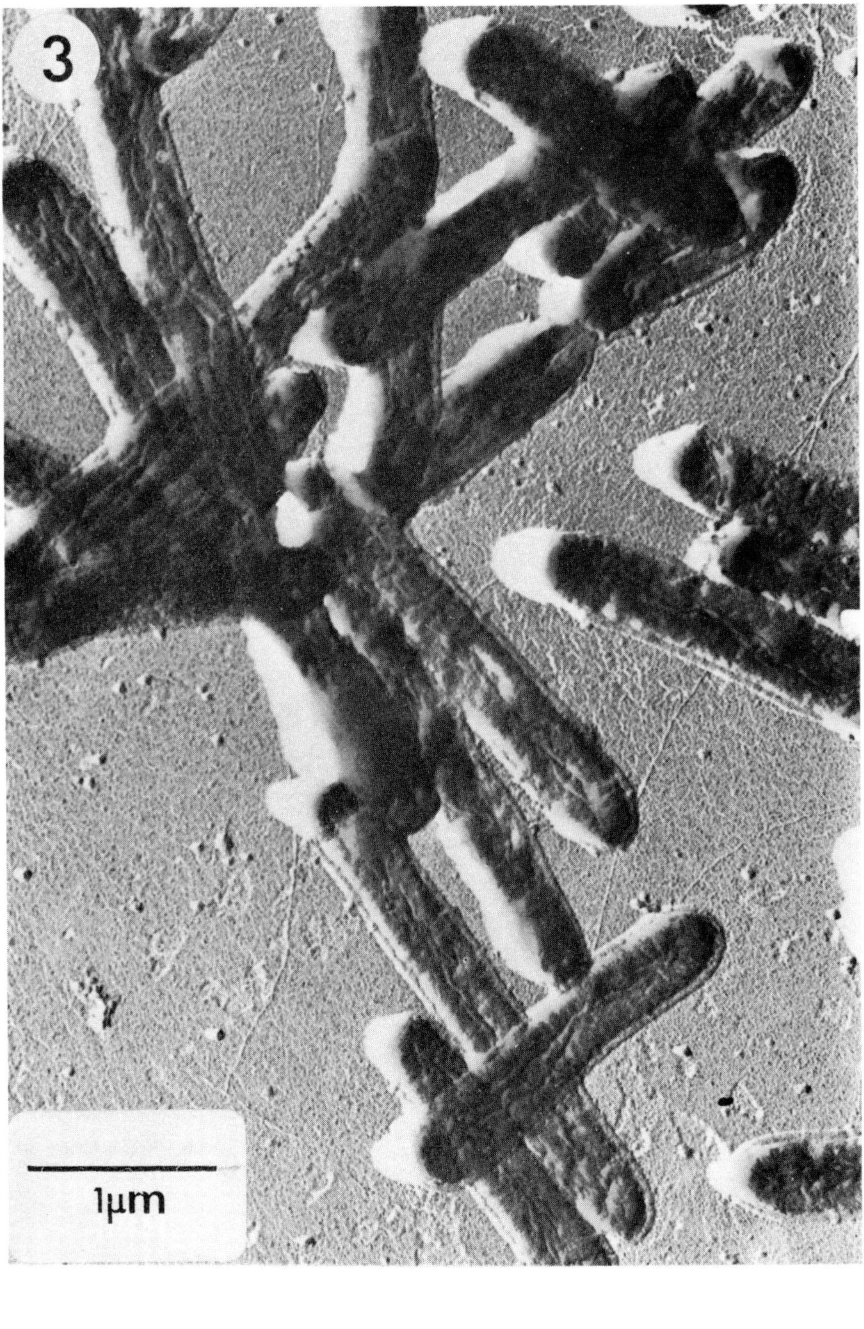

Fig. 10.3 – Cells from a culture of a *Cytophage* species: cells of *Flavobacetrium* species are similar in morphology.

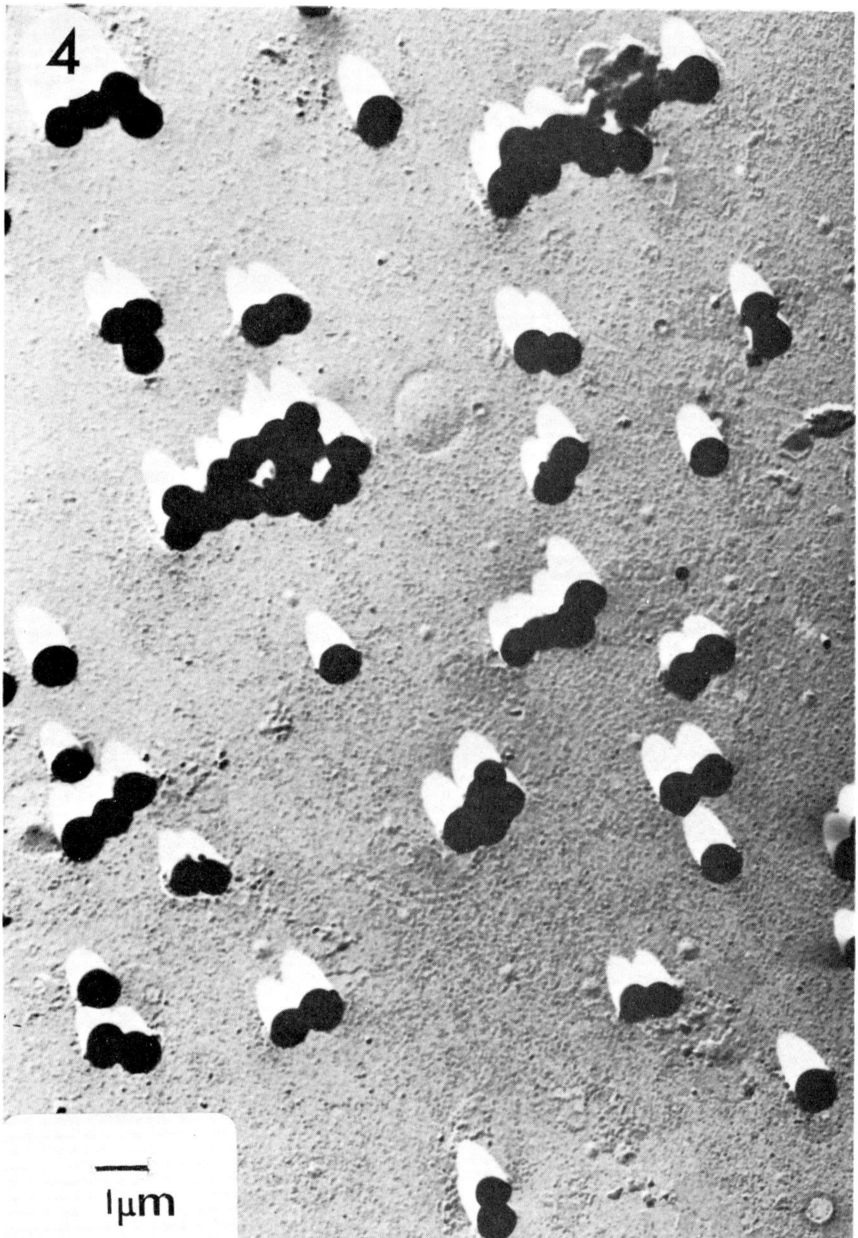

Fig. 10.4 – A *Micrococcus* species (*Staphylococcus aureus* is indistinguishable from this morphologically).

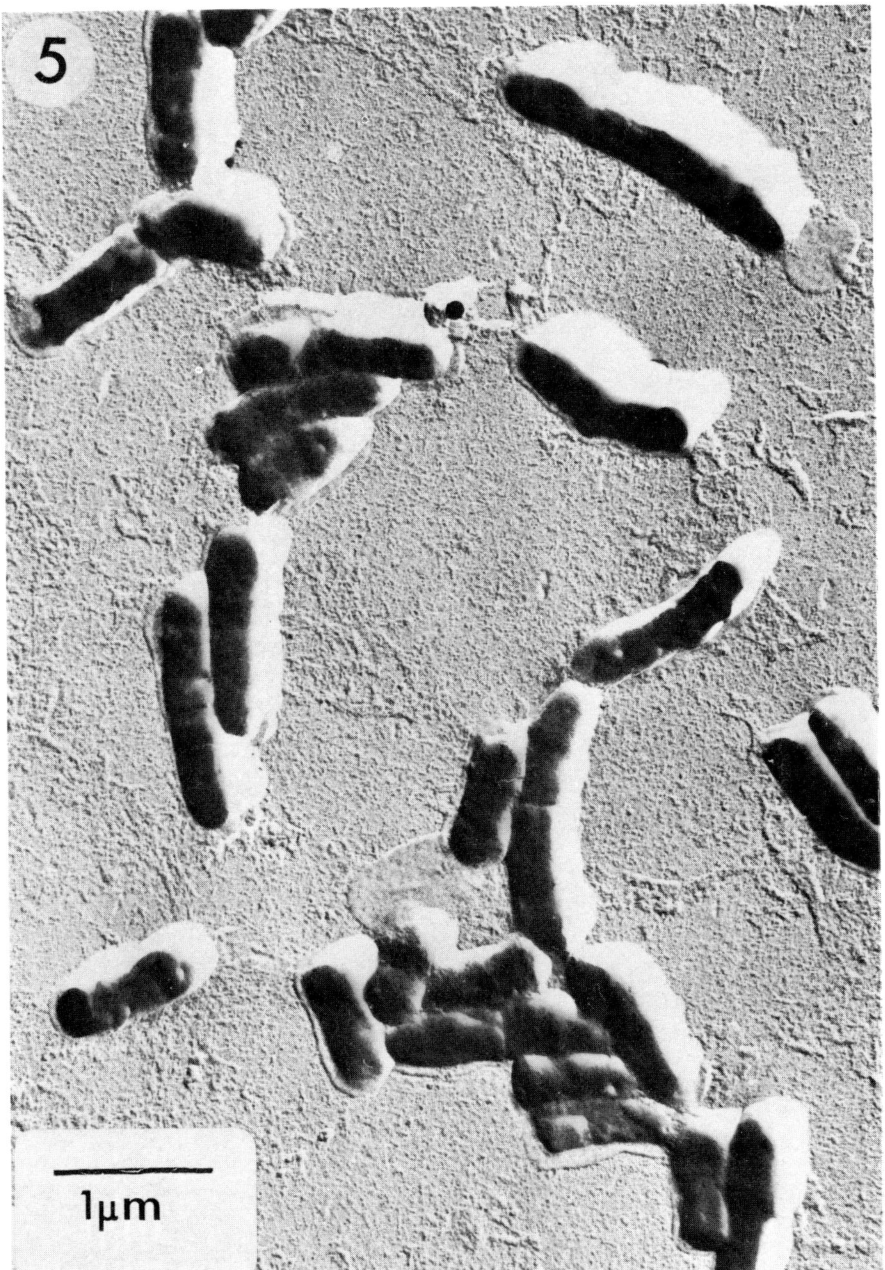

Fig. 10.5 – A coryneform organism.

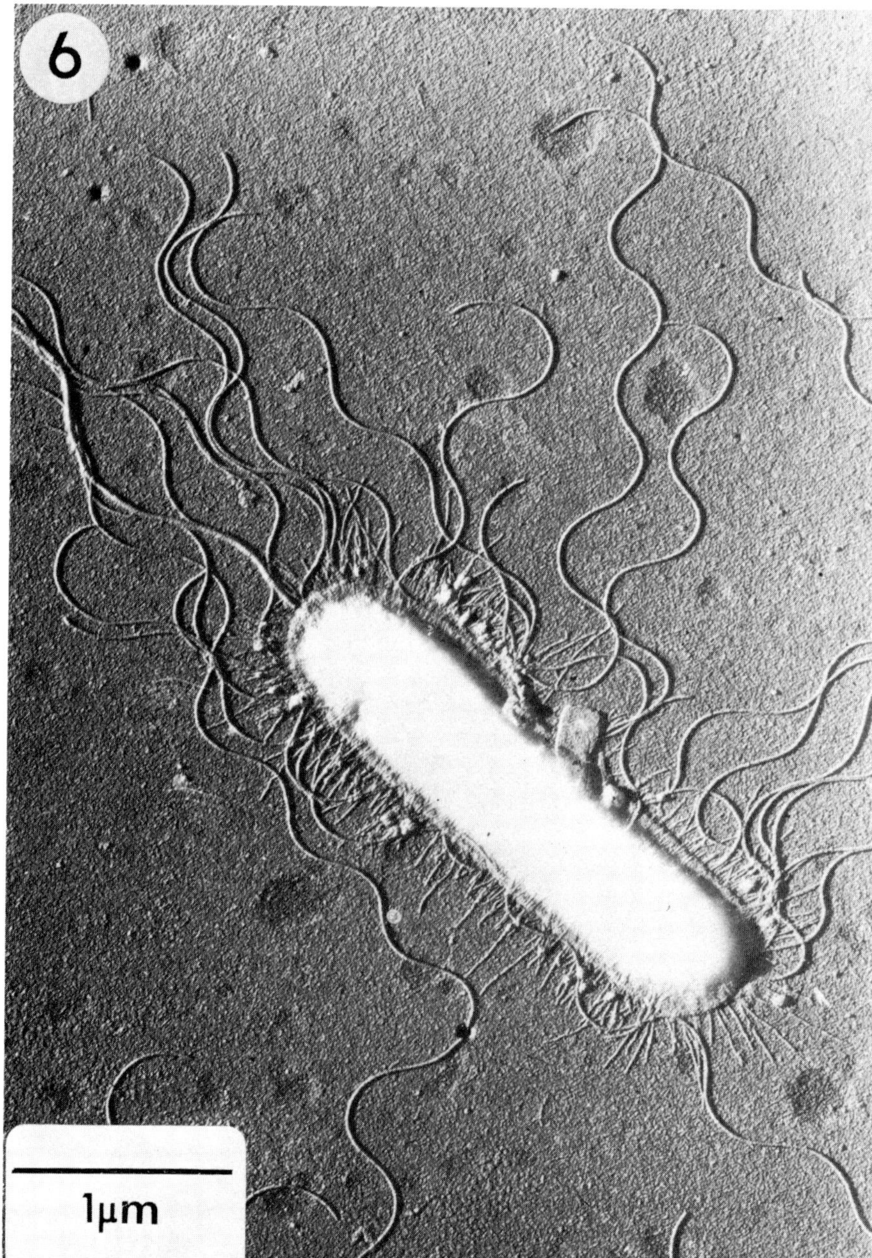

Fig. 10.6 – A cell of one of the many types of luminous bacteria found in the marine environment and frequently isolated from fish. The cells of this species, *Lucibacterium harveyii*, are similar in morphology to cells of *Vibrio parahaemolyticus* when grown at 20°C on solid culture medium (see Fig. 10.14).

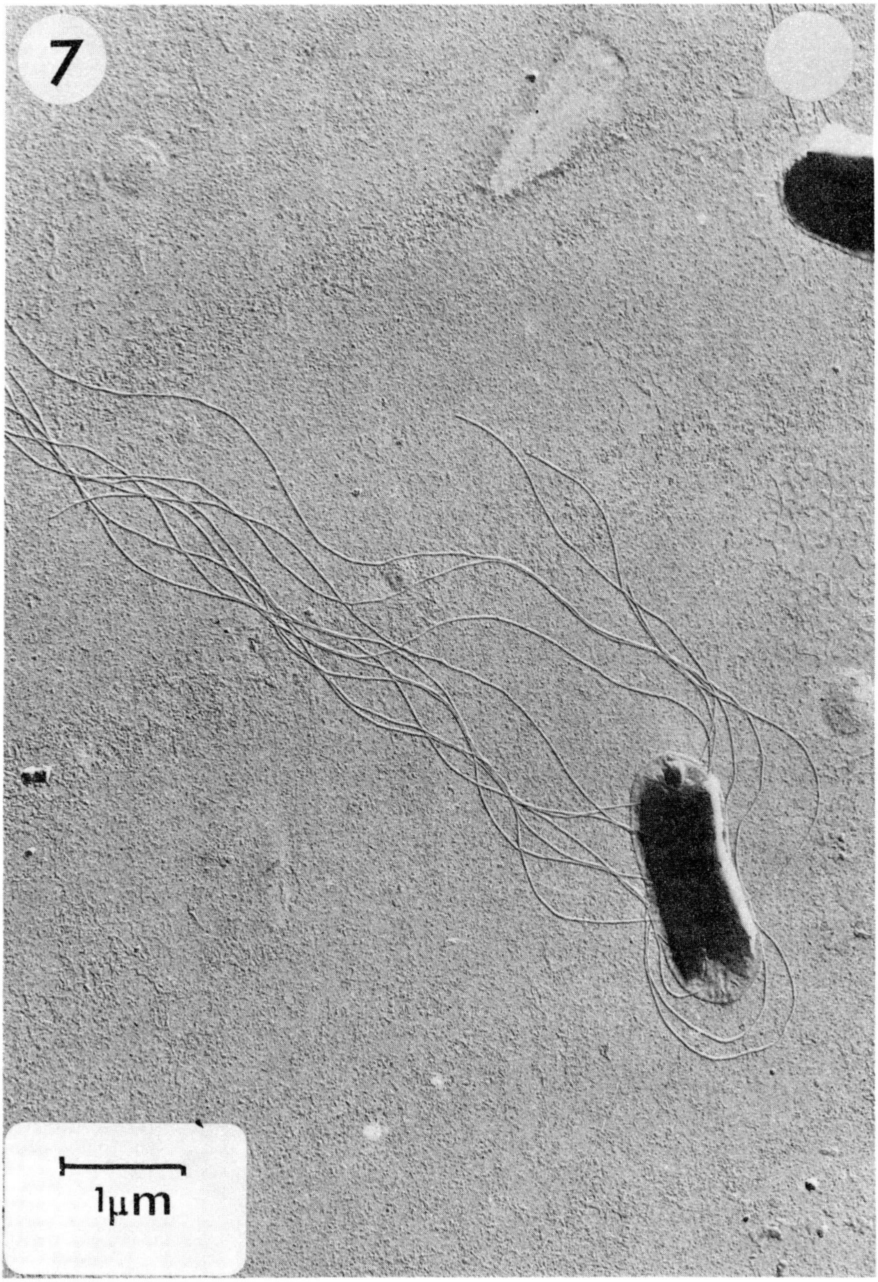

Fig. 10.7 – A coliform organism (peritrichous flagella).

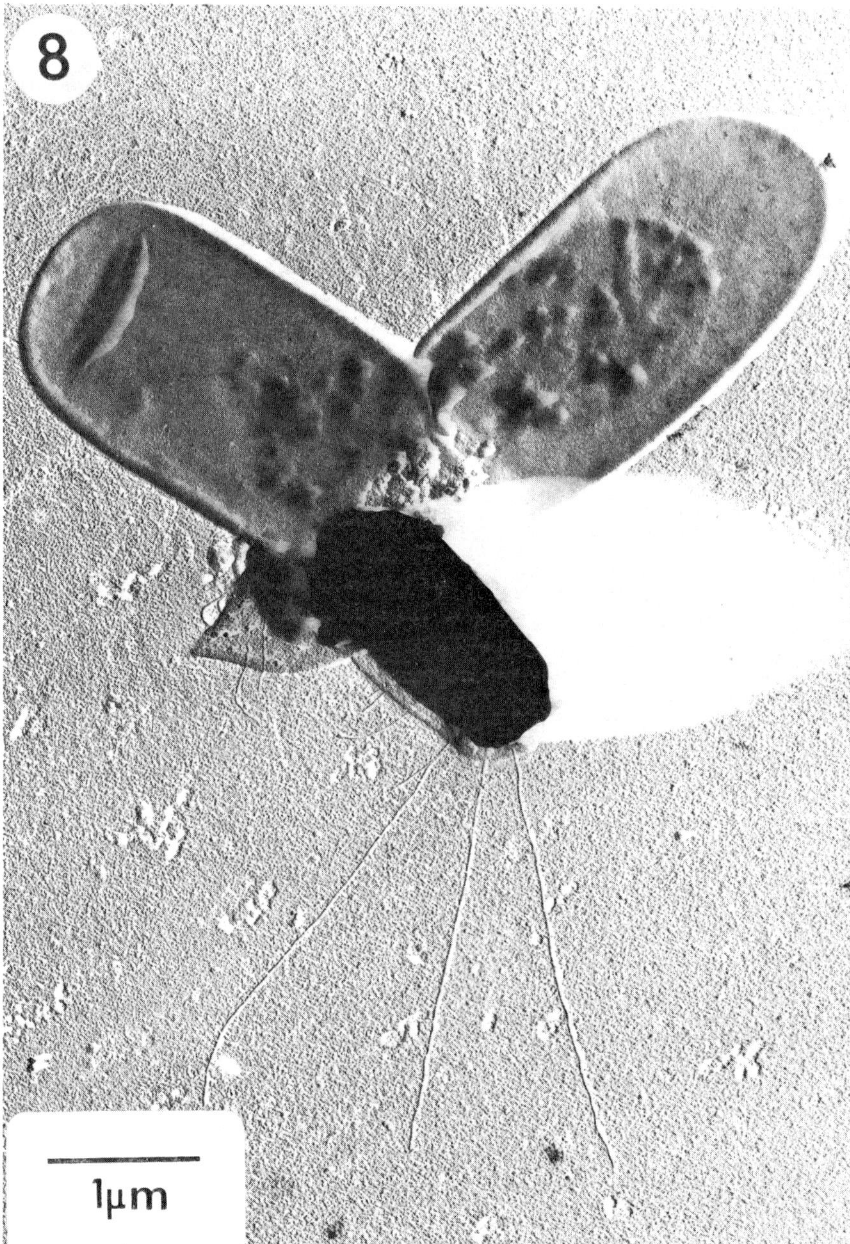

Fig. 10.8 – Resistant endospores are formed by organisms of the genera *Bacillus* (aerobes) and *Clostridium* (anaerobes). This micrograph illustrates the liberation of a spore from the remnants of the vegetative cell in *Bacillus cereus*, a food-poisoning organism.

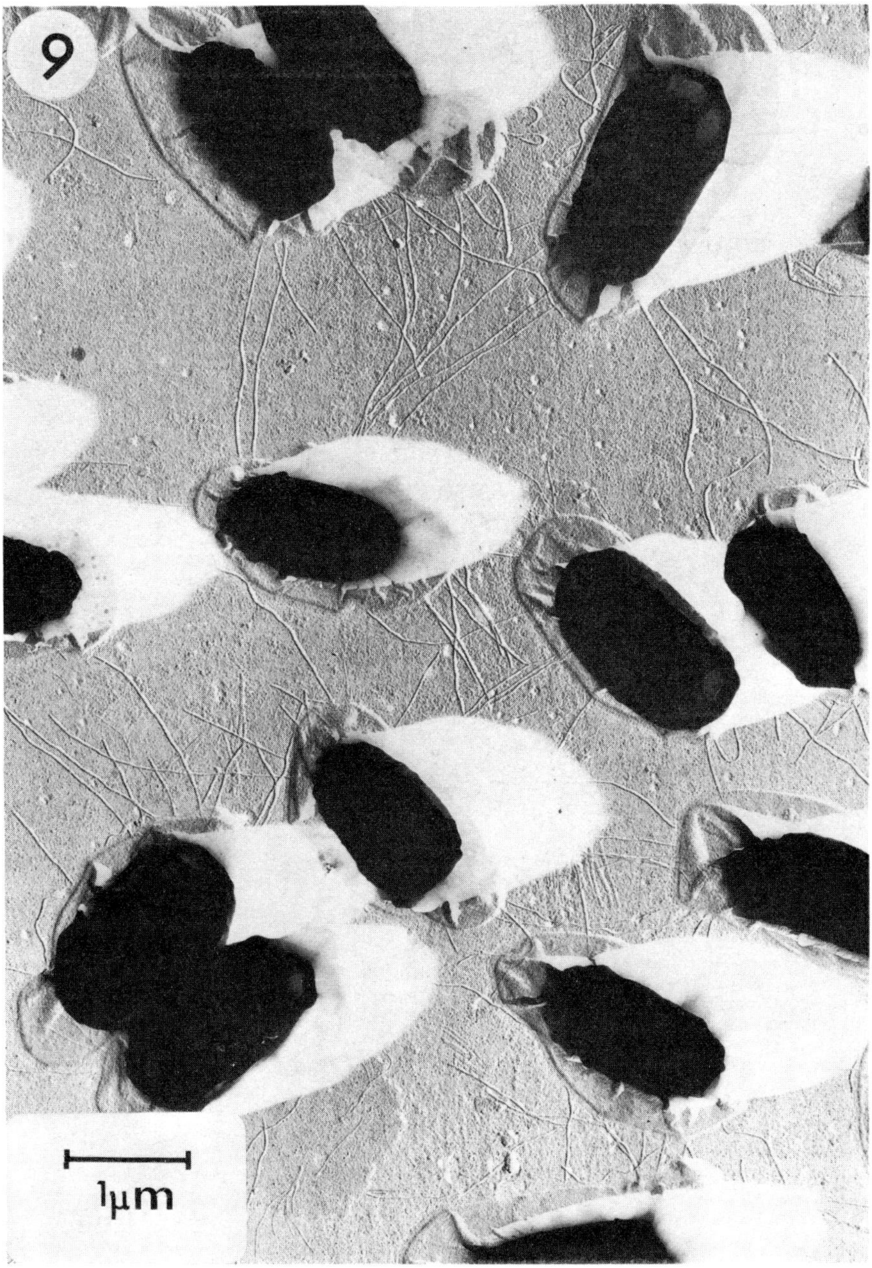

Fig. 10.9 – A group of spores of *Bacillus cereus*. Note the fine, filamentous appendages on the sac (exosporium) which envelopes the spore.

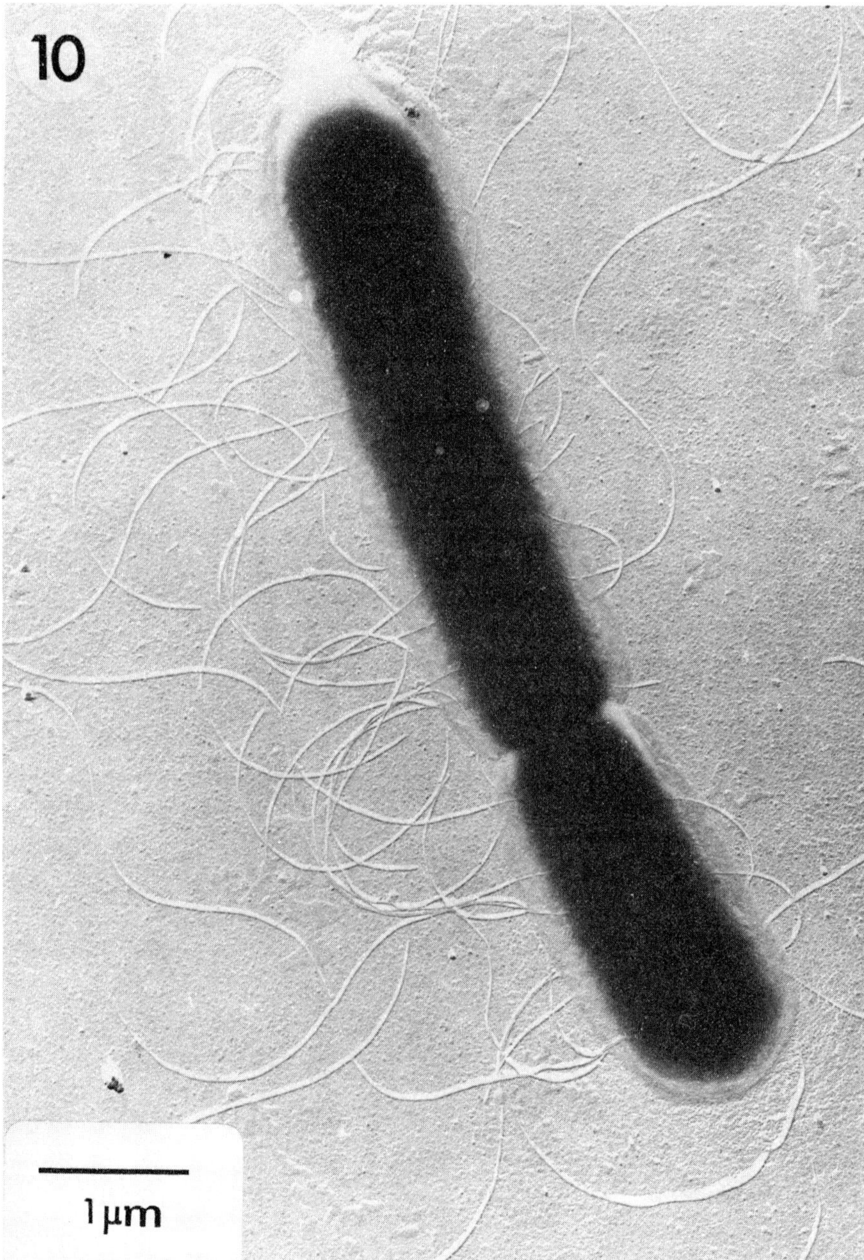

Fig. 10.10 – Vegetative cells of *Clostridium botulinum* Type E.

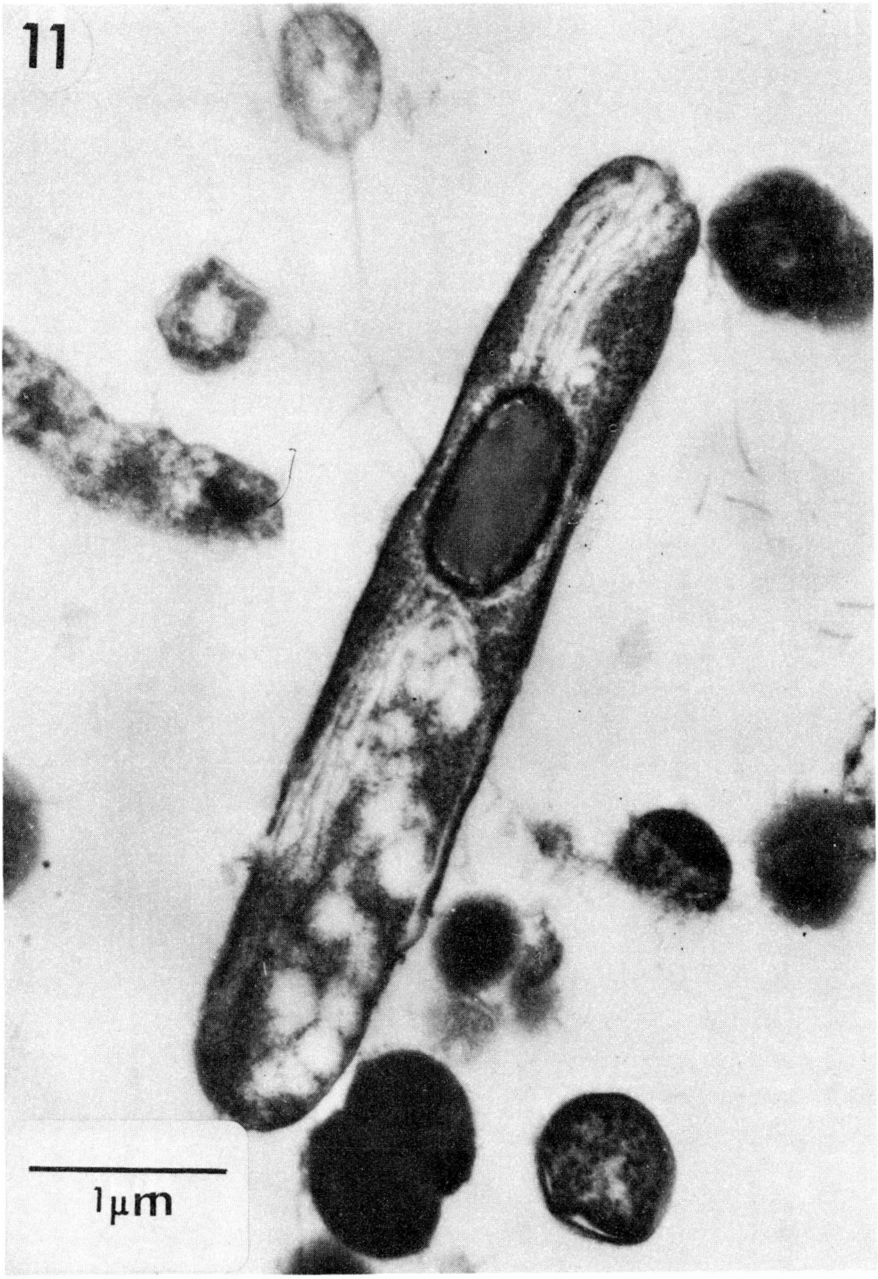

Fig. 10.11 – Ultra-thin section of a sporulating cell of a *Clostridium* species.

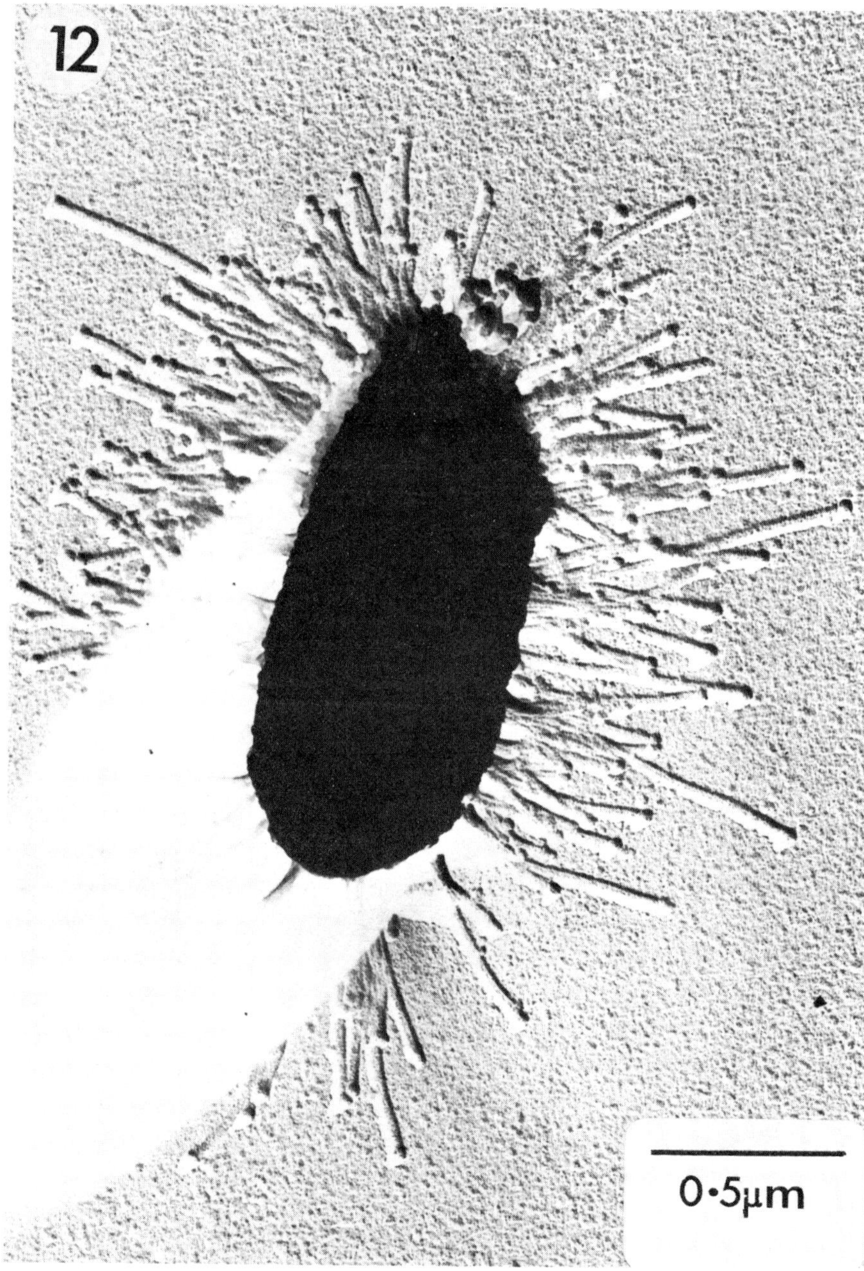

Fig. 10.12 – The spore of *Clostridium botulinum* Type E possesses many characteristic appendages.

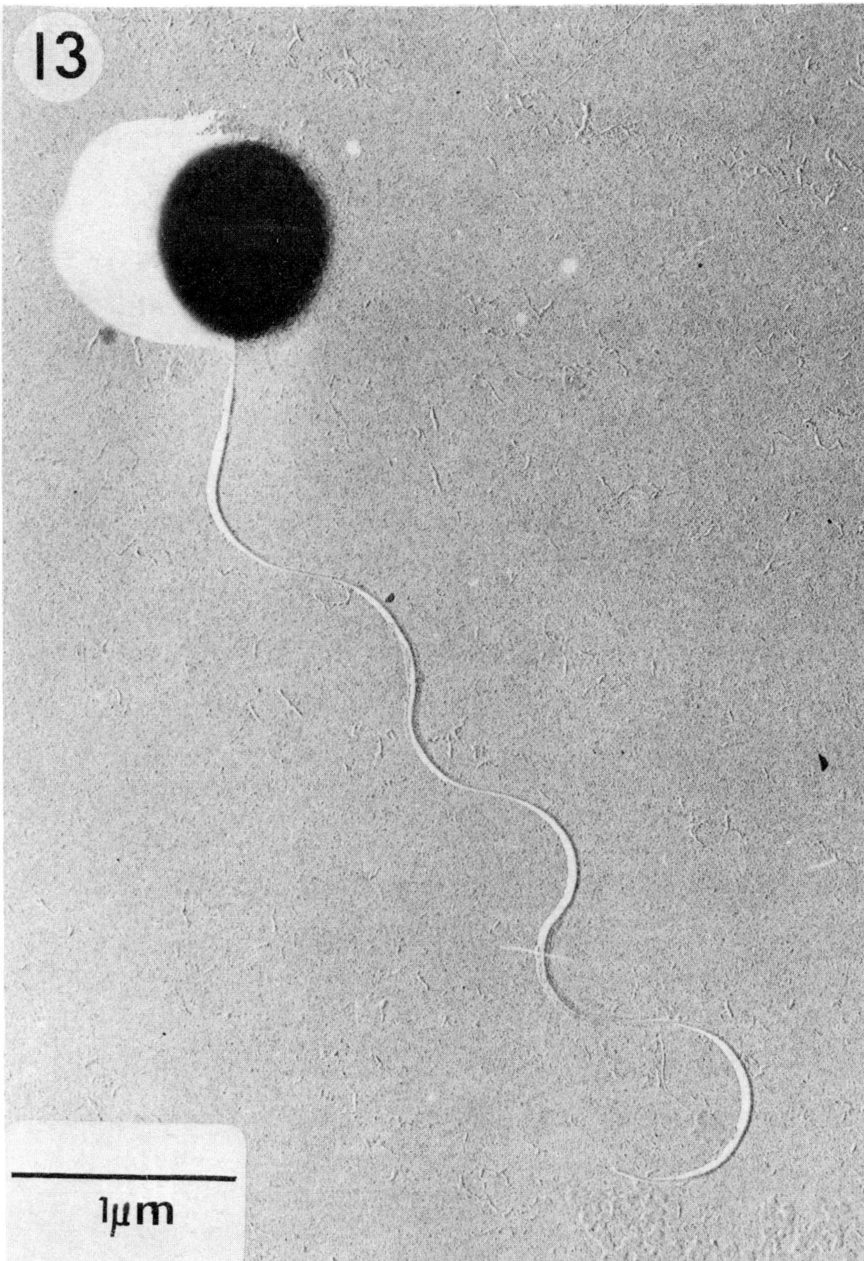

Fig. 10.13 – A cell of *Vibrio parahaemolyticus* from a culture grown at 30°C in liquid medium.

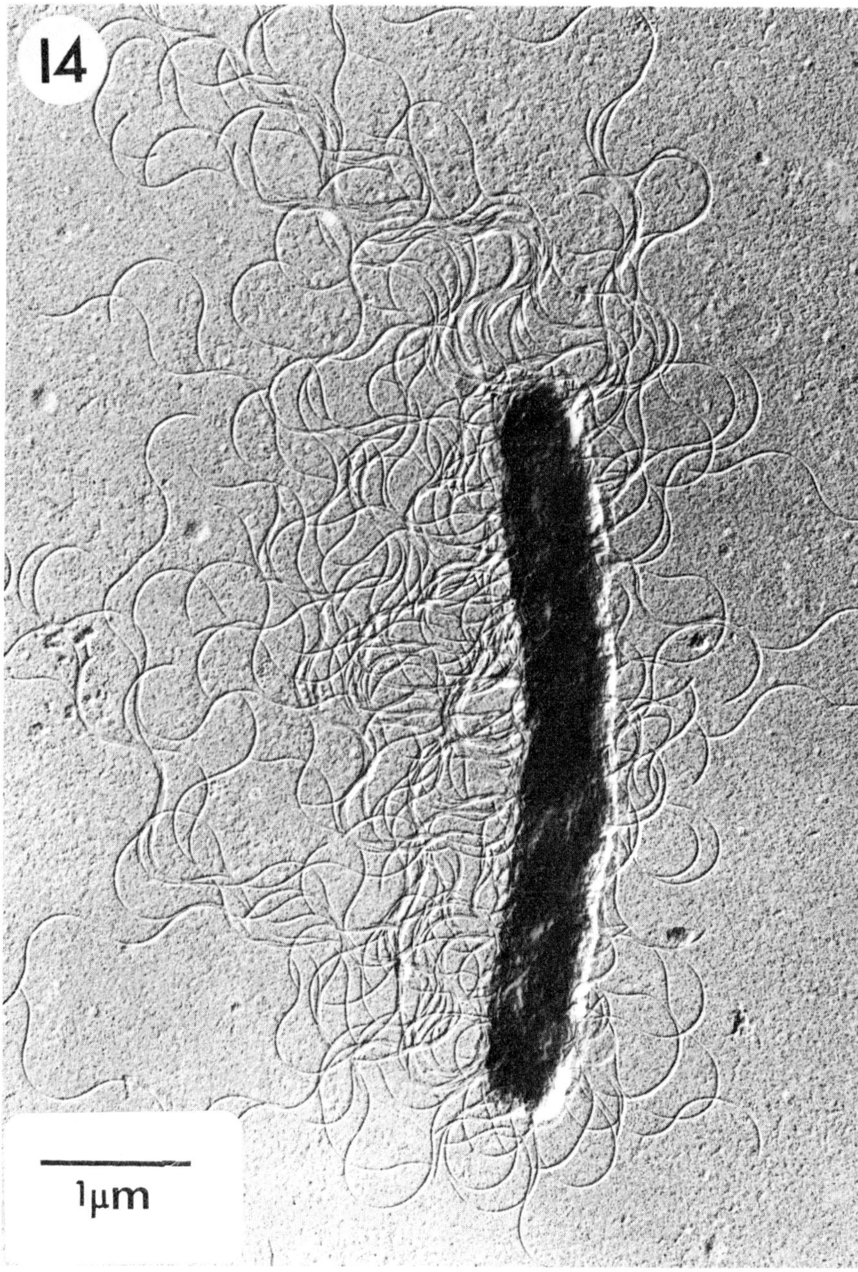

Fig. 10.14 – A cell from a culture of *V. parahaemolyticus* grown at 20°C on solid medium shows numerous peritrichous flagella.

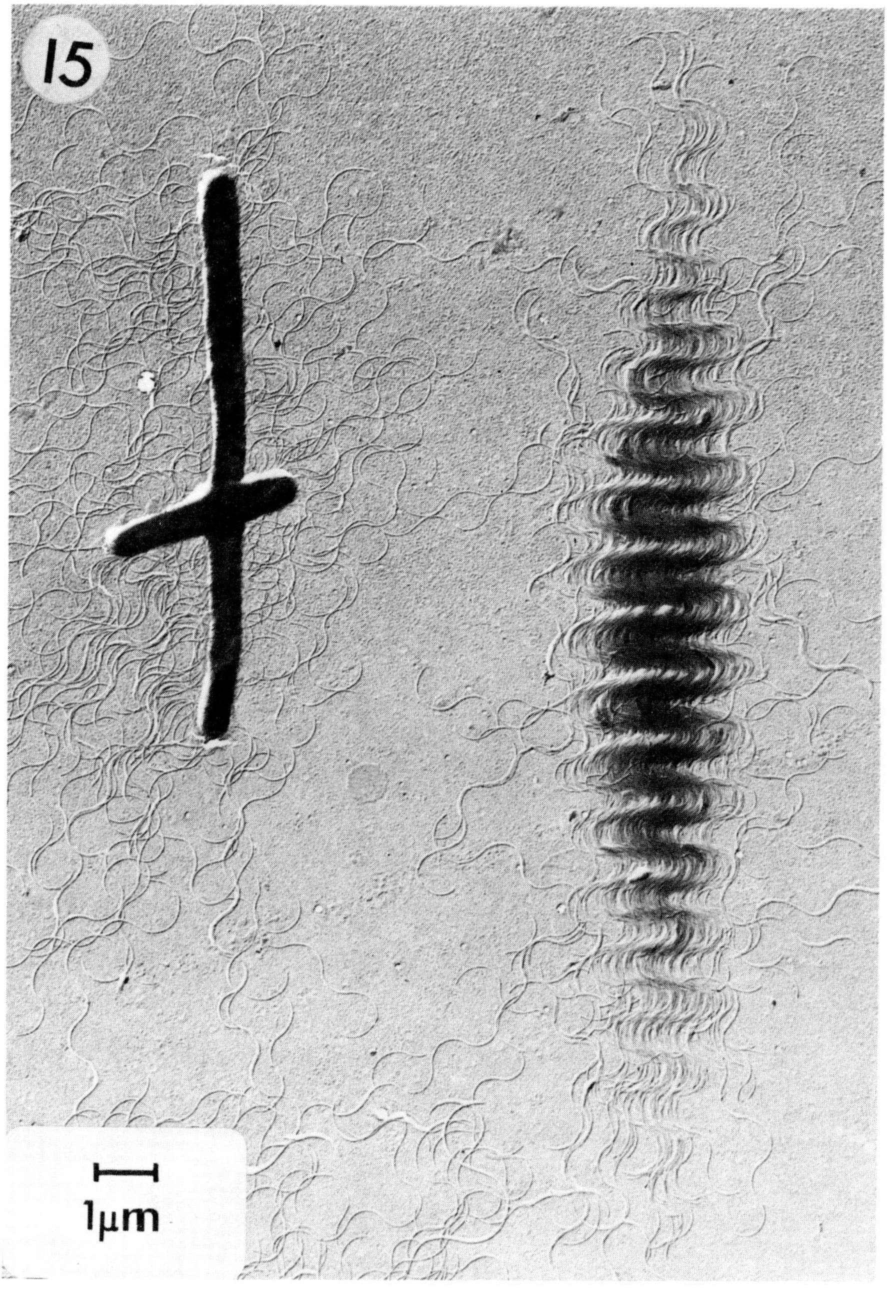

Fig. 10.15 – A preparation from the same culture (Fig. 10.14) showing a small aggregate of detached flagella (in 2.5% aqueous sodium chloride).

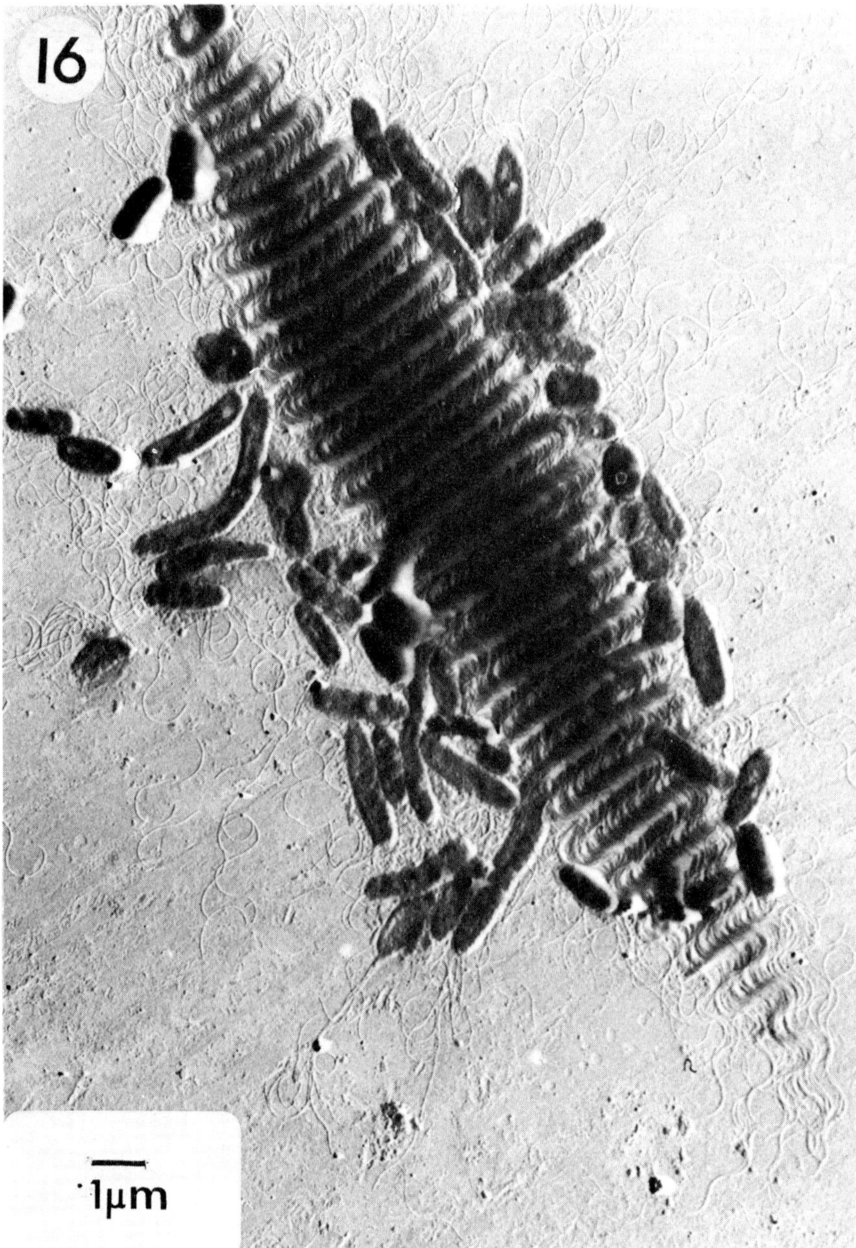

Fig. 10.16 and 10.17 – In one or two hours the flagella-bundles (fascicles) become large enough to be easily visible in the optical microscope.

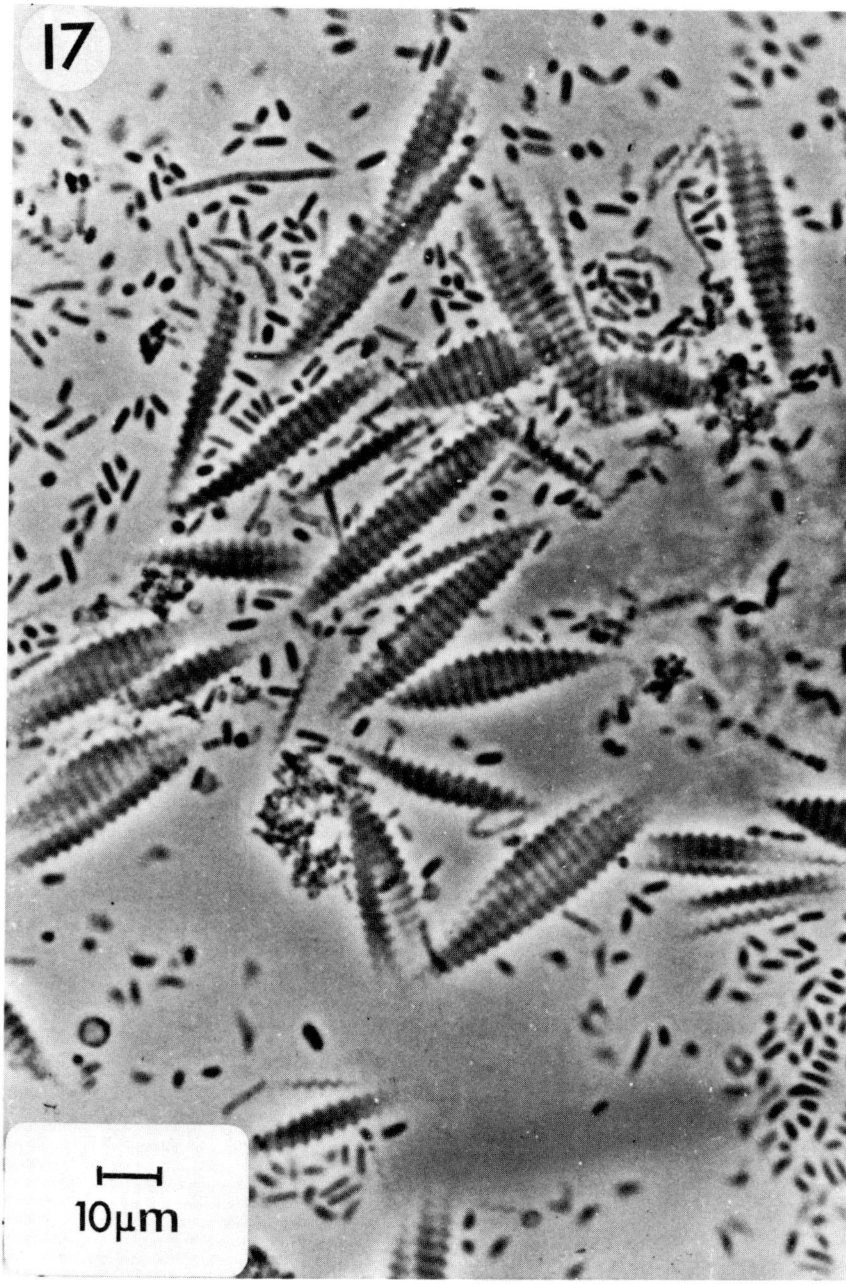

Fig. 10.17

DISCUSSION

Mr R. E. Welborn: Flesh such as beef and lamb needs to be inspected for disease. In what way is disease important or not important in caught fish?

Mr Hodgkiss: The inspection in this country is by Environmental Health Officers. At each port there is a Fishery Officer and an Environmental Health Officer, and and they have certain criteria for passing the fish. Most of these are very subjective. Torry Research Station has for a long time worked on the possibility of developing an objective test for the quality of the fish, but neither a quick chemical test nor a quick bacteriological test has been forthcoming†. By and large it is the experience of the Environmental Health Officer that is the main factor in this respect. With regard to the specific business of diseased fish, they are very rare. I was explaining to someone here at the meeting that we do get a lot of specimens of quite naturally occurring things that the processor couldn't do anything about – a malignant growth or a non-malignant growth occurs in fish just as in any other animal, and there are lots of parasites, of course, in fish. But one thing about it is that as soon as the fish becomes incapacitated in its natural environment it falls easy prey to the next bigger fish, so that you don't see many diseased fish landed.

Mr P. W. Thompson (APV Co. Ltd.): Would you expect to find any evidence of *C. botulinum* infection in fresh water fish?

Mr Hodgkiss: Yes, in the paper you will find that I have given some reference to this. My colleague, Mr Cann, has done most of the botulinum work and he has extended his work from the marine fish area to fresh-water fish over the last few years, particularly in trout farms, so I wonder if I could call upon him to answer your question.

Mr D. C. Cann (Torry Research Station): The incidence of *Cl. botulinum* in individual UK–farmed trout can vary from 0 to 100% according to the type and location of individual farms. In a survey of British trout farms an overall incidence of 9.4% was found. The incidence of the organism in wild, fresh-water fish could be expected to be of the same order.

REFERENCES

[1] Shewan, J. M. and Hobbs, G. *Prog. Indust. Microbiol.* 1967, **6**, 169.
[2] Shewan, J. M. *Chemy. Ind.* 1970, 193.
[3] Shewan, J. M. *Proc. Trop. Prod. Inst. Conf. Handl. Process. Mark. Trop. Fish.* 1977, 51.
[4] Cann, D. C. *ibid.* 1977, 377.
[5] Murray, C. K. and Fletcher, T. C. *J. Fish. Biol.* 1976, **9**, 329.

†An instrument, the Torry Fish Freshness Meter, is in use commercially for rapid determination of the 'equivalent days on ice' quality of fresh fish. It uses the change in a.c. impedance of the fish between two points on its surface as a measure of the loss of 'freshness', with which it correlates well – Ed.

[6] Herbert, R. A., Hendrie, M. S., Gibson, D. M. and Shewan, J. M. *J. appl. Bact.* 1971, **34**, 41.
[7] Herbert, R. A., Ellis, J. R. and Shewan, *J. M. J. Sci. Fd. Agric.* 1975, **26**, 1187.
[8] Herbert, R. A. and Shewan, J. M. *ibid.* 1976, **27**, 89.
[9] Hobbs, G. *Adv. Fd Res.* 1976, **22**, 135.
[10] Cann, D. C., Wilson, B. B., Hobbs, G., Shewan, J. M. and Johannsen, A. *J. appl. Bact.* 1965, **28**, 426.
[11] Cann, D. C., Wilson, B. B., Hobbs, G. and Shewan, J. M. *ibid.* 1965, **28**, 431.
[12] Cann, D. C., Wilson, B. B., Shewan, J. M. and Hobbs, G. *Nature (Lond.)* 1966, **211**, 205.
[13] Cann, D. C., Wilson, B. B. and Hobbs, G. *J. appl. Bact.* 1968, **31**, 511.
[14] Hobbs, G., Cann, D. C. and Wilson, B. B. *J. Fd Technol.* 1969, **4**, 185.
[15] Huss, H. H., Pederson, A. and Cann, D. C. *ibid.* 1974, **9**, 445.
[16] Huss, H. H., Pederson, A. and Cann, D. C. *ibid.* 1974, **9**, 451.
[17] Cann, D. C., Taylor, L. Y. and Hobbs, G. *J. appl. Bact.* 1975, **39**, 331.
[18] Hobbs, G., Cann, D. C., Wilson, B. B. and Shewan, J. M. *ibid.* 1965, **28**, 265.
[19] Hobbs, B. C. and Christian, J. M. B. (Eds.) *The Microbiological Safety of Foods* 1973, London, Academic Press.
[20] Barrow, G. I. *Postgrad. Med. J.* 1974, **50**, 612.
[21] Cabassi, E. and Mori, L. *Folia vet. lat.* 1976, **6**, 335.
[22] Barrow, G. I. and Miller, D. C. *Lancet* 1972, **i**, 485.
[23] Ayres, P. A. and Barrow, G. I. *J. Hyg. (Camb.)* 1978, **80**, 281.
[24] Peffers, A. S. R., Bailey, J., Barrow, G. I. and Hobbs, B. C. *Lancet* 1973, **i**, 143.
[25] Hooper, W. L., Barrow, G. I. and McNab, D. J. W. *Lancet* 1974, **i**, 1100.
[26] ICMSF (International Commission on Microbiological Specifications for Foods). *Microorganisms in Foods* 1974, Toronto, University of Toronto Press.
[27] Hobbs, G. *IFST Proc.* 1970, **3**, 98.
[28] Baird-Parker, A. C. *Postgrad. Med. J.* 1974, **50**, 644.
[29] Sparnon, R. B. *J. Assoc. Publ. Analysts* 1976, **14**, 87.
[30] Jarvis, B. *ibid.* 1976, **14**, 91.
[31] Jarvis, B., Lach, V. H. and Wood, J. M. *J. appl. Bact.* 1977, **43**, 149.
[32] Gibson, D. M., Hobbs, G., Christie, R. H. and Jason, A. C. *J. Phys. E.* 1978, **Vol. 11**, 560.

CHAPTER 11

CIP Technology, Detergents, and Sanitizers

T. C. Tamplin, APV Co. Ltd., Crawley

This chapter is divided into two main sections: Part 1 deals with the description and selection of CIP units, whilst Part 2 is more specifically orientated to cleaning and sanitization in the food industry, viewed from a chemical/microbiological standpoint.

Part 1. – CLEANING-IN-PLACE SYSTEMS

CIP systems have many forms. Originally it was customary to use detergents only once and then throw them away, but with the growth and complexity of plants and the number of circuits to be cleaned, the re-use of detergents was adopted.

It is not possible to describe and specify a system which will be optimum for all occasions, because there is no universal CIP system which can be specified for all applications.

There are two different basic techniques, single-use and re-use systems, which have evolved with time. The latest development is to use combined systems which incorporate the best characteristics of the single-use and re-use units. These are generally known as multi-use systems.

SINGLE-USE SYSTEMS

General

In single-use systems, the detergents are used for cleaning only once. This means that the detergent chemist has the facility to make a mixture of ingredients which have an activity which is good for a short time but might deteriorate or lose effectiveness if the material with this formulation was stored and packaged.

In general, single-use systems are small units which are normally placed adjacent to the equipment to be cleaned. On occasion, when a plant needs a number of CIP units, concentrated detergents can be distributed in small pipes to the various units. Thus if the units are situated near the equipment, the quantity of chemical and rinse water can be relatively small.

Certain circuits may be heavily polluted, and such circumstances may make a single-use system highly desirable. For instance, heat treatment circuits may contain such a high soil load that detergents cannot be re-used and therefore must be discharged to drain.

With some single-use systems, it is possible to recover detergent and rinse water from a previous cycle and use this for a pre-rinse cycle for the subsequent cleaning operation.

Description

Single use CIP systems are compact, preassembled units with a low capital cost. Installation is relatively simple. Fig. 11.1 shows a typical single-use system. The principal components of a single-use system, which are assembled on a frame, are:

One tank with level probes and pneumatically-controlled valves to inject steam, to admit water, and to regulate the circuit inclusive of discharge, overflow, and through-flow.

One centrifugal pump and control panel and programme cabinet with temperature-controller, solenoid valves, and pressure and temperature instruments.

One set of dosing pumps for caustic, acid, and additives.

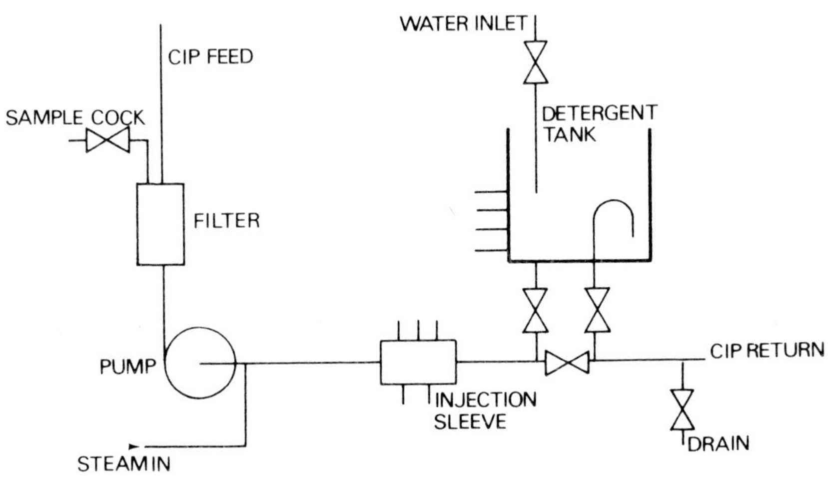

Fig. 11.1 – Typical single-use CIP system.

Fig. 11.2 shows a typical single-use system with limited recovery. Here an additional tank with high-level probe is mounted so that the wash and rinse water can be collected for the next pre-wash cycle.

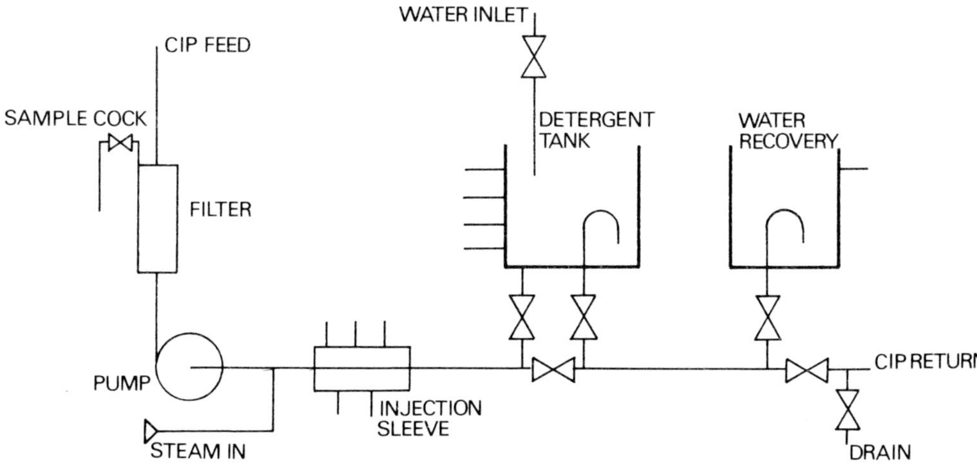

Fig. 11.2 – Single-use system with limited recovery.

The cleaning operation:

A typical cleaning sequence for a tank clean occupies a 20-minute programme which runs as follows:-

Three pre-rinses of 20 seconds with intervals of about 40 seconds each to remove the gross soil contamination. A CIP return pump discharges the water to drain. (If this pre-wash is derived from a rinse recovery tank, this can aid pre-washing efficiency).

Dosage of cleaning media and injection of steam to provide the preadjusted temperature direct into/the circuit. This circuit is maintained for about 10 to 12 minutes, after which the spent chemicals are discharged to drain or taken to the recovery tank.

Two intermediate rinses with cold water with an interval of 40 seconds each which either go to drain or to water recovery.

A further rinse and recirculation is established and may include the injection of acid to lower the pH value to 4.5 – 5. This cold circulation is continued for about 3 minutes and then discharged to drain.

Cleaning media vary, but a general technique would be to use:

An alkaline cleaning medium, concentration 0.2% – 0.5%.

A product containing emulsifying, surface-active and anti-foaming agents. Dose 0.08%, depending on the make.

A liquid chlorine sanitizing agent, concentration 50 – 100 ppm, depending on the make.

A food-grade acid product at a concentration of 0.08 – 0.1% to give pH 4 – 6, depending on the make.

RE-USE SYSTEMS

General

Re-use CIP systems are based on the principle that the detergents should be recovered and re-used as much as possible. Detergents are not polluted very much by cleaning pre-rinsed equipment, therefore the detergents can be re-used many times. Wastage of detergents can be caused by:

Operating plant manually instead of on the automatic mode.

Cleaning self-desludging centrifuges in the plant.

Excessive dosing of detergents into grossly contaminated solutions.

The concentration of detergents is important. Reasonable sequencing versatility enables the times and sequence of operations (alkaline/acid or acid/alkaline) to be varied, or to exclude one of the two on some occasions.

The tanks with the detergents are usually standing hot, which means that a big heat source is available. This might give a shorter cleaning time and demand less steam load on the boiler than when starting with cold detergents. The tanks may be heated by plate heat exchangers.

If cleaning detergent is lost for any reason – sometimes it is part of the programme – the loss is easily replaced by new detergents in a re-use system.

Re-use systems are equipped with a tank for each chemical.

If hot-water rinse is used, a hot-water tank or a bypass loop is necessary to save energy and water.

Description

Usually, the essential components of a CIP plant are caustic and acid tanks, fresh-water tank, return water tank (if required), a heating system, and CIP feed and return pumps. The piping layout of the CIP system is fixed in the plant and equipped with remote-controlled valves and measuring devices. A programme control unit ensures automatic sequencing of the predetermined cleaning operations. The cleaning liquid is conveyed from the CIP unit through the production plant and the appropriate circuits and machines to be cleaned. Careful attention to hygienic design and engineering is essential when the production plant is planned.

Fig. 11.3 shows the layout of a CIP plant for a typical re-use system. In this example, the cleaning liquid is heated by a coil. Two caustic detergent tanks are provided for the different concentrations; the lower concentration is used for cleaning the tanks and pipelines, the higher for cleaning the plate heat exchanger. The concentrations of caustic and acid are automatically adjusted by means of dosing pumps which feed corresponding amounts of detergent concentrate from containers into the tanks. Neutralization tanks with automatically-adjusted acid concentrations can be provided to neutralize effluents.

A typical dairy cleaning system may be required to work on the individual circuits about 15 to 20 times a day. Therefore it is sometimes advantageous to add extra CIP feed pumps and thus enable two CIP circuits to be cleaned simultaneously.

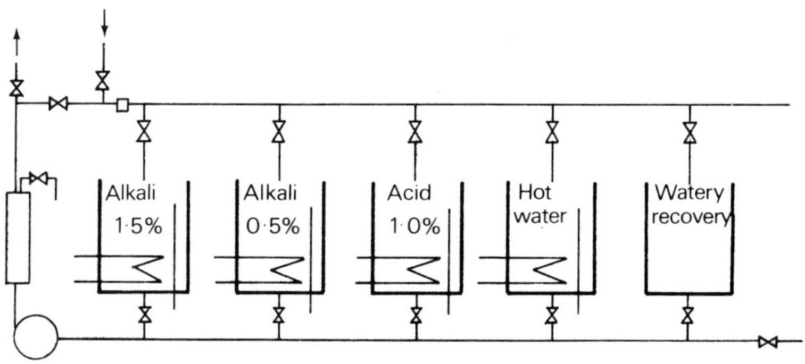

Fig. 11.3 – Typical re-use CIP system (simplified).

With this type of cleaning system, the tank capacity is defined by circuit volumes, temperature requirements, and desired cleaning programmes. The cleaning circuits in automated plants are switched on and off by valves remote-controlled from a central control console.

With the recirculation facility of the hot-water option and the use of a return water tank, the water consumption of a re-use system can be optimized.

The CIP unit would be designed to fill, empty, recirculate, heat, and dose contents automatically. The CIP sequences would generally be as follows: pre-rinsing, cleaning, intermediate rinsing, sanitizing, post-rinsing. These steps are discussed more fully in Table 3 of Part 2.

A typical programme for tank and pipeline cleaning with recovery of detergent and acid would be as follows:

	OPERATION	TIME (min)	TEMPERATURE
1.	Pre-rinse – softened cold water from recovery tank. Runs to drain. Burst rinsing may be advantageous on certain vessels.	3–5	ambient
2.	Detergent wash – 1% caustic base proprietary detergent purges out remaining rinse water to drain and is then diverted by a conductivity probe to detergent tank for circulation and recovery.	5–15	ambient to 93°C (200°F)

	TIME	TIME (min)	TEMPERATURE
3.	Intermediate water rinse – softened cold water from mains purges out remaining detergent to the detergent tank. When this is cleared, water is diverted to the water recovery tank.	3	ambient
4.	Acid wash – an appropriate acid solution (approx 0.5 – 1.0%) purges out remaining water to drain, then is diverted by conductivity probe to the acid tank for recirculation and recovery.	5–15	ambient to 93°C (200°F)
5.	Final water rinse – softened cold water from mains purges out remaining acid, and water is collected in the water recovery tank. When this is full the water diverts to drain.	3	ambient

The cleaning programme for pasteurizers as well as tanks and pipelines may include a final flushing with hot water at 90°C.

MULTI-USE SYSTEMS

General

Among recent developments are the combined systems termed multi-use because they combine features of both recovery and single-use systems.

Description

These units are designed for cleaning-in-place of tanks and pipelines. They work with automatically controlled programmes comprising different combinations of cleaning sequences in which water, caustic, acid, and highly-diluted acid solutions (acidified rinse) are circulated through the cleaning circuits for varying lengths of time at varying temperatures. Not all cleaning liquids are included in every cleaning programme.

Fig. 11.4 shows the simplified flow-diagram of a typical multi-use CIP system. This unit is modular and completely versatile in terms of CIP sequencing, chemical strength, and thermal performance. It comprises tanks for chemical and water recovery, with an associated single pump, recirculatory pipework, and heat exchanger all mounted on adjacent but integral sub-frames.

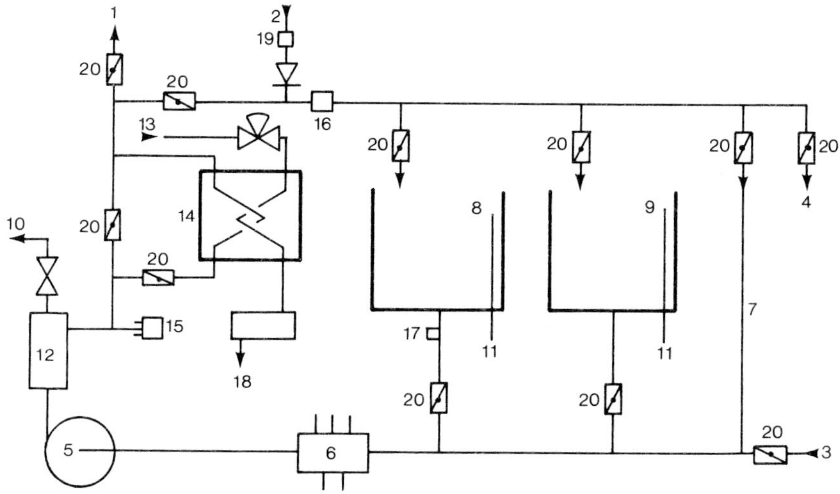

Fig. 11.4 – Typical multi-use CIP system (simplified).

1. CIP feed
2. CIP return
3. Water inlet
4. Drain
5. Puma pump
6. Injection sleeve
7. Recirculating loop
8. Detergent tank
9. Water recovery
10. Sample cock
11. Overflow
12. Filter
13. Steam in
14. 'Paraflow' heat exchanger
15. Temperature probe
16. Soluvisor
17. Conductivity probe
18. Condensate
19. No-flow probe
20. Butterfly valve

The plate heat exchanger is used to heat incoming water and the cleaning liquid to the desired temprerature. The inclusion of a heat exchanger allows flexibility of temperature control, full utilization of tank capacity, and versatile heating of water or other chemicals. It is common to fit a plate heat exchanger by-pass valve so that sterilant solutions do not have to pass through the plate pack.

The automatic mode of the system is shown in the following examples:

1. *Pre-rinse operations*

   Either from water recovery (usual) or mains supply.

   Variable periods available at various temperatures.

   Pre-rinse can be either directed to drain or diverted via recirculatory loop for a timed period and then sent to drain.

   If required, chemicals can be injected to aid pre-rinsing efficiency.

2. *Detergent recirculation*
   Recirculation can be established either via the detergent vessel or the by-pass loop.
   Recirculation times are variable, and chemical injection can either boost the strength or use any combination of chemicals as required.
   Recirculation can be achieved either via the plate heat exchanger or its by-pass loop. If a by-pass loop is installed, variable temperature programming allows for total detergent tank heating; or this can be limited to the recirculation loop and the main detergent vessel maintained at ambient or some other temperature.
   Chemicals can either be recovered or sent to drain.

3. *Intermediate rinse*
   This is variable but similar in principle to the pre-rinse except that chemicals would not normally be required at this stage.

4. *Acid recirculation (if necessary)*
   This is variable but similar in principle to the detergent facility. It may be used with or without an acid tank. In the latter case, the recirculatory loop is established on mains water either through the plate heat exchanger or via the plate heat exchanger by-pass loop.
   Acid is injected to a pre-set strength based on timing for a specific circuit volume.
   Recirculation time and temperature are both variable.

5. *Sterilant recirculation*
   This is similar to the acid injection sequence except that heating would not be required in normal circumstances.

6. *Hot-water sterilization*
   Recirculation loop is established on fresh water via the plate heat exchanger.
   Variable times and temperatures are available.
   The contents can be sent to either drain or water recovery.

7. *Final water rinse*
   Mains water is pumped through the CIP route and directed to water recovery.
   Both times and temperatures are variable.

APPLICATION OF CIP

CIP has largely replaced hand cleaning in many industries. The variable levels of automation which can be offered range from simple cam timers to fully-automated computer-controlled plant. The major factors to be taken into consideration in deciding which type of plant to provide are largely ones of finance and the geographical location of the installation. The following guidelines may aid selection, design, and installation of equipment.

Obviously it is imperative to follow the fundamentals of hygienic design, and in this context it is advisable to approach a reputable supplier of equipment, preferably on a consultative basis, and gain the benefit of his specialist advice and experience. Many companies offer specialist site survey facilities and provide confidential reports on the hygienic status of existing equipment etc. These design studies are sometimes referred to as 'hygiene audits'.

It is vitally important to obtain full consultative rapport with a reputable detergent supplier. It is futile to wait until bacteriological, scale or corrosion problems occur before obtaining advice. By that time both process plant and product brand name may be ruined. As with equipment, the cheapest product is not necessarily the best.

At the design/concept stage it must be recognized that the interrelationship between product routeing and control of process variables is closely allied to CIP. The closest possible collaboration is required between departments or companies involved in design, production control, quality control, maintenance, safety, etc. Similarly, it is important to discuss the impact of new equipment with trade union representatives.

The widespread use of CIP systems enabling plant to be cleaned and sanitized automatically has helped to minimize direct contact of personnel with potentially dangerous chemicals. Nevertheless, some involvement is always necessary, and commonsense safety precautions should be observed. Detergent and equipment suppliers will give advice on this subject.

A requirement in most liquid processing installations is the alternate filling, emptying, and cleaning of product storage tanks, sometimes involving more than one product. With such an arrangement, it is essential that products and cleaning solutions cannot mix owing to an error in the operation of valves or in making pipe connections. Fig. 11.5 shows one method of protection using a key piece system. Each key piece is arranged to fit only into a predetermined position to complete either a cleaning circuit or a product circuit but not both. This positively isolates cleaning fluid from the product flow. Sometimes, microswitches operated by associated manually-controlled cocks provide additional safeguards.

Some small cleaning systems may not justify full automation, or it may be decided to reduce the automated content of a system. In such cases the required circuits can be set manually by means of a flow-selector plate. Pipelines are brought to a backplate and the required connections are made by a U-bend inserted in the appropriate ports. If required, these can be supplied with microswitch logic interlocked to the CIP set.

Many fully automated systems have been developed in which the entire process and CIP operations are automatically controlled and electrical interlocks make an error in valve operation impossible. In these systems there is no manual intervention and systems are fully safeguarded.

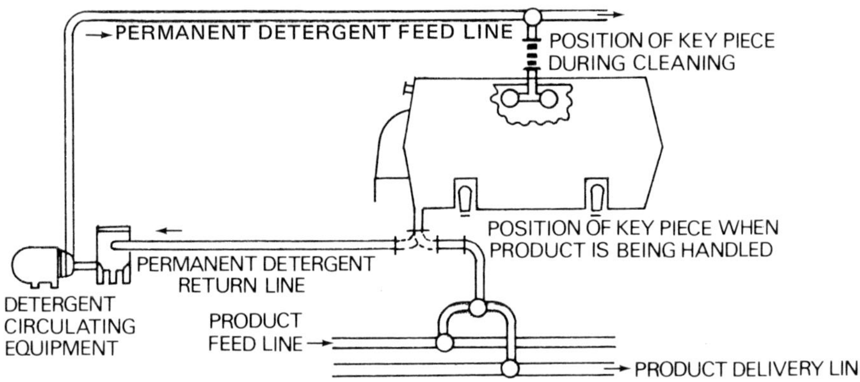

Fig. 11.5 – Protection method using a keypiece.

Within the context of automated product routeing and CIP it is possible to include facilities for product recovery, thus reducing product losses and minimising effluent factors.

The practical benefits of CIP include:

Cost saving

Optimum use of water, detergent, sterilant, and steam produces economy in operation.

Increased plant utilisation.

Tanks and pipelines can be cleaned as soon as they are empty and refilled immediately afterwards.

Minimum manual effort.

Manual operations can be reduced or eliminated according to requirement.

Greater safety

Personnel have no need to enter vessels. The risk of falls on slippery internal surfaces is eliminated.

Improved hygiene.

Cleaning schedules are adhered to exactly, and consistently satisfactory results are obtained. Thus product quality is improved.

This is by no means a complete list.

As in all commercial issues, the fundamental questions 'How much will it cost per unit operation?' and 'Which is the best practical solution for our requirements?' have to be asked. For example, a cheap, inefficient installation, wasteful in terms of water, chemicals, and heat may have attractive features when viewed as a capital plant item in isolation; but this initial view may require reappraisal when running costs (for example cost per clean) have to be examined in the light of increasing effluent, heating, and water charges, and the ever-rising cost of raw materials for detergent products.

To this must be added the important environmental considerations and the likelihood of legislation that will impose tighter controls on effluents.

The following guidelines may be of some assistance when considering a CIP installation.

SELECTION OF CIP UNITS

Single use

In these systems low-strength detergents are used only once for cleaning. It is possible to mix short-lived chemical mixtures which have no long-term stability but are effective for immediate cleaning.

Concentrated detergents can be metered to a number of CIP units.

Fresh detergents are used each time.

When positioned in close proximity to equipment to be cleaned, water and chemical quantities may be smaller than those for centrally placed re-use systems which may have to be located further away.

If soil loads are not excessive, chemical and rinse solutions can be recovered in additional equipment and used as the pre-rinse before the next cleaning circuit.

If a number of units are installed, each in close proximity to the corresponding equipment to be cleaned, less complex valve arrangements and fewer pipelines may be required. The engineering and installation of the pipework may thus be correspondingly easier.

A large central re-use system placed in the centre of the plant may give a more difficult layout and design problem. The optimum product flow through the plant may have to be modified by CIP requirements. Ideally, process equipment should not be positioned too far away from the central CIP system.

These small units are usually factory-made in batches and pre-tested.

With small units, the installation can be made in a few days. On the other hand, most re-use systems are usually tailor-made and need consequently more engineering and installation work.

Large re-use CIP systems may require special rooms for the installation, whilst the smaller units can be placed adjacent to the equipment to be cleaned.

If, through a failure in the system, infection occurs in a CIP re-use system, it can jeopardize the whole process plant. This, however, is a very unlikely occurrence.

Occasionally, process plants and production layouts require modification and expansion after a time. New products are introduced or higher production rates have to be handled. These operations may be facilitated if the CIP can be done from local CIP units. Usually, a further unit is easy to install.

The detergents for single-use systems are metered by volume each time, whilst in re-use systems it is common for the concentration to be controlled by conductivity meters which may give variable accuracy. Usually, the concentration is therefore checked chemically by laboratory staff.

As new detergents are metered for each cycle, the cleaning programme (concentrations and type of detergent mixtures) can be adjusted for each circuit depending on what kind of residues have to be removed.

Re-use CIP systems

These conventional systems are based on the principle that the detergents shall be recovered and re-used as much as possible in order to save money. Usually, detergents are not polluted very much, if pre-rinsing has been adequate, therefore the detergents can be re-used many times. However, the number of cleaning cycles before total discharge of tank contents depends upon several factors.

a) If air purge is used, between each cycle, more detergent can be recovered, but at the expense of increasing pollution within the detergent tank. That will have an influence on how often the detergent tanks have to be drained completely and replenished. It is usual for the tanks to be flushed out during the recharging operations.
b) If through intermixing or valve pulsing the losses of detergent are high, more water and detergents have to be added each day, but this will mean that solutions remain cleaner.
c) If a self-cleaning separator is connected to the cleaning process from time to time, the cleaning solution will be separated in it during the cleaning process, and the dirt particles will thus be eliminated from the detergent. Consequently, the cleaning solution will remain clean for quite a long time and can be used relatively longer.

With this type of system, the worst circuit, that is, the most heavily-soiled, decides the necessary cleaning concentration of the detergents. Apart from the concentration, it is possible to set the times and order of steps – alkaline/acid or acid/alkaline or alkali/sterilant, or exclude any one or more operations if required.

Normally, detergent tanks are standing hot, which means that a big heat source is available. This should give a shorter cleaning period and give less steam load on the boilers than when starting with cold detergents, as in the case of the single-use system.

If some cleaning detergent is lost to drain, for example in valve pulsing, this loss is easily replaced by new detergents in the re-use system. In a single-use system, the missing quantity is normally replaced by water, or a special programme step would need to be added. Conventional re-use systems need a tank for each new detergent, and if a hot-water rinse is used, a tank is needed for that as well.

Probably the best way of heating the tanks is by plate heat exchangers. Some systems do not commence with hot detergent direct, for instance after having had a cold rinse in the process tanks. In these systems, the detergents are stored cold and heating starts after the circuit is established. Without adequate precautions, thermal shock can collapse tanks.

Large re-use systems are normally situated in a special room with good ventilation.

It could be argued that a weak point of the re-use systems is the equipment used for the detection of the interface between detergent and water or vice versa. Here, different principles have been tried, but probably conductivity meters are the most common. Without adequate precautions, deposits can develop and cause progressive drift of the set point, giving rise to increased losses of detergent. Another possibility is to change over valves based on time, after having made preliminary tests with a conductivity meter. As long as the pump capacities are the same, this method can be employed.

With re-use systems it is easy to check detergent strengths, as laboratory staff can collect samples at any time. With single-use systems, difficulty is sometimes experienced in obtaining representative samples at the correct time during the cleaning sequence.

With a central CIP unit, potentially dangerous chemicals can be stored at one specific point with associated safety equipment. Access to the CIP area can be prohibited. Some food processors do not like concentrated chemicals in the process area.

Re-use systems have centralized drain gulleys and services, for example electrical/water/steam/air/drain connections. For each smaller single-use unit, independent service supplies are required in that area.

With adequate sizing of CIP vessels and mains, several CIP feed pumps can be fed from the same CIP plant, enabling instantaneous cleaning operations to be performed at the same time without excessive steam loadings.

Neutralization of detergent contents is of course possible to any desired pH before discharge to drain.

It is of course arguable whether a small and uncomplicated re-use CIP system placed close to the specific equipment to be cleaned, may not have certain economic attractions.

In many re-use systems there is a more than adequate measure of 'overkill' in the strength of the chemicals employed. Some users consider this an important factor to cater for sporadic processing problems yielding higher than usual soil loads.

Multi-use CIP systems

Recent investigations by various companies have led to the development of multi-use CIP systems which attempt to combine the optimum characteristics of the single-use and re-use systems.

In one system, local small standard units are placed close to the circuits to be cleaned, but they are fed with detergents from a centrally placed storage unit. After use in the local unit, the detergent is sent back again to the storage unit.

In this system, one can save some piping and complex valve arrangements. Pipes between storage and units must, however not be too small because of the time for filling and emptying which has to take place several times during a cleaning operation.

In other systems, similar principles apply.

In general, the facilities offered by these systems mean that:

Pre-rinse solutions may be heated, recirculated, and dosed with a selection of chemicals before discharge to drain.

Variable chemical compounds as in the single-use system may be prepared in any combination, to any concentration, for circulation at any temperature, for any period. A basic detergent strength is stored, a portion of which may be boosted for a specific cleaning duty and either recovered or discharged to drain.

Chemical sanitization or hot-water recirculation facilities are available within the same unit.

It is considered by many that these systems incorporate most of the attractive features hitherto claimed by advocates of the single-use and re-use philosophies.

SELECTION OF SPRAYBALLS OR ROTATING JETS

The following notes compare the two basic types.

Static spray distribution devices ('sprayballs')

Sprayballs are cheap, simple, and effective.
There are no moving parts, and maintenance is negligible.
They are nearly all made of AISI 316 stainless steel.
They are unaffected by temperature.
They are self-cleaning and self-draining.
They provide continuous coverage during the entire discharge period.
There is a negligible effect of single hole blockage.
Flow rates tend to be high.
Pressures are relatively low.
Radial flow is limited.
In some instances only irrigation is provided.

Rotating jets

Rotating jets have a long radial throw.
They have a lower flow rate than the sprayballs.
They have higher impingement factors which can enable lower detergent strengths to be used.

In some devices (single planar), nozzle blockage could be serious.
Reliability is variable, and the maintenance on some models is complex.
Rotating jets contact the soil intermittently at each jet sweep.
They are not always considered to be self-cleaning and self-draining.
They are usually much more expensive than sprayballs.
Some devices do not tolerate high temperatures.

In conclusion it must be added that whichever CIP system is decided upon, and whatever spray distribution devices are installed, the whole will be doomed to failure unless adequate staff training is arranged and a planned maintenance procedure adopted, whether this be by a negotiated service contract or by the user's own internal resources.

PART 2.

CLEANING AND DISINFECTION: A CHEMICAL/MICROBIOLOGICAL APPROACH

INTRODUCTION

This section dicusses the philosophy of cleaning from a chemical/microbiological viewpoint and illustrates some of the considerations which should be borne in mind when selecting detergents and sterilizing agents. Examples are taken largely from the dairy industry.

ASSESSING THE PLANT HYGIENE PROBLEM

Most plant which has held and processed food or has been used in the manufacture of food products will become soiled and require cleaning. Several factors affect efficient soil removal and choice of cleaning agents:

What is the soil?
How much is there?
In what condition is it?
What are the materials of construction of the equipment? Hence,
What chemicals can be employed?
What is the cleaning method: manual? CIP? or specialized techniques?
What is the water hardness?
Is a combined detergent-sterilizer to be used?
What standards of cleanliness and sanitation are required?

TYPICAL SOILS

As a general guide, soil characteristics may be summarized as in Table 1.
Table 2 gives the characteristics of the common soil 'milkstone'.

Table 1

SOIL CHARACTERISTICS

Component on surface	Solubility	Ease of removal	Change on heating
Sugar	Water soluble	Easy	Caramelization: more difficult to clean
Fat	Water insoluble, alkali soluble	Difficult	Polymerization: more difficult to clean
Protein	Water insoluble, alkali soluble, slightly acid soluble	Very difficult	Denaturation: much more difficult to clean
Mineral salts	Water solubility is variable, but most are acid soluble	Easy to difficult	Generally easy to clean

Table 2

COMPOSITION OF WHOLE MILK AND MILKSTONE

Whole milk (%)		Milkstone (%)		
Water	87	Water		2.7
Milk fat	3.9	Fat		10
Lactose	5.0	Protein		20
Casein	2.5	Ash		50
Albumin and globulin	0.7	(Calcium oxide	28	
Minerals	0.9	Phosphorus pentoxide	22	
		Plus magnesium, iron		
	100.0	and sodium salts)		

The figures for milkstone can vary widely.

Many soil films can harden and set as they dry, making subsequent removal extremely difficult. These deposits can harbour micro-organisms which multiply and can subsequently be released into the process stream, along with flakes of scale, by turbulence or thermal cracking.

FUNDAMENTALS OF THE CLEANING PROCESS

Soil removal mechanisms aim to achieve a hygienic, clean surface.

Defining a 'clean surface'

General appearance

A clean surface is a surface, free from residual film or soil, that will not contaminate food products in contact with it, and which will comply with the following requirements.

Contamination will not be visible under good lighting conditions with the surface wet or dry.

No objectionable odour will be apparent.

The surface will not give a greasy or rough feeling to clean fingers when they are rubbed on the surface.

A new, white paper tissue wiped several times over the surface will show no discolouration.

The surface will show no sign of excessive water break while water is draining from it.

Confirmatory tests

If desired, the following confirmatory tests may be applied to the surface under examination.

No sign of fluorescence shall be detectable when the surface is inspected with long wave (340 – 380 nm) ultraviolet light radiation.

After sanitizing, the surface shall not cause serious reinfection of the product coming into contact with it.

Principles employed to yield a 'clean surface'

The basic steps in a typical cleaning process are set out in Table 3 (overleaf).

The soil removal mechanisms have four basic stages:

1. Intimate contact of the detergent with the soil, employing wetting and penetrating properties.
2. Displacement of soil: by saponifying fat, peptizing proteins, and dissolving mineral salts.
3. Dispersing the soil by deflocculation and/or emulsification.
4. Preventing re-deposition of the dispersed soil by providing good rinsing properties.

Table 3

TYPICAL CLEANING PROCESS

Operation	Function
Pre-rinse	Rinsing with water to remove gross, loose soil.
Cleaning	Removal of all residual soil by a suitable detergent.
Inter-rinse	The removal and rinsing away of all detergent and soil from plant items.
Sanitizing	The destruction of most micro-organisms by the application of chemicals with or without heat.
Post-rinse	Removal with water (of a suitable bacteriological quality) of sterilant chemicals from the system.

Water quality and hardness factors

A good-quality potable water supply is essential. To avoid water scale deposition detergent formulations must be selected for the specific water hardness existing on site. In nearly all cases, detergent costs will increase in proportion to the mineral salt content, because expensive detergent ingredients will be required to combat water hardness.

The water hardness is a very important factor in detergent formulations and must be known before detailed detergent recommendations can be given. The

water should comply with the prescribed standards of the World Health Organization International Drinking Water Requirements (WHO 1963). Water hardness may be explained as follows.
Water contains many cations, anions, and dissolved/suspended matter which can affect the pH range. Water, falling as rain, absorbs carbon dioxide from the air, thus making a weak solution of carbonic acid (1)†.
On contact with certain calciferous rocks, the water dissolves acid-soluble components to form calcium and magnesium bicarbonates (2).
The level of these dissolved salts is a measure of the water hardness. For general guidance, the United States Geological Survey Classification of Water Hardness is shown in Table 4.

Table 4

U.S. GEOLOGICAL SURVEY CLASSIFICATION OF WATER HARDNESS

Hardness	Total calcium + magnesium ions expressed as ppm. $CaCO_3$
Soft	0 – 60
Moderately hard	60 – 120
Hard	120 – 180
Very hard	Over 180

Soft water is preferred for cleaning processes involving alkaline detergents. It gives greater detergent economy and more efficient detergent action, and it prevents scale formation.
Water hardness is divided into two types – temporary and permanent.

Temporary hardness
Temporary hardness is due to the presence of calcium and magnesium bicarbonates. Temporary hardness can be removed by boiling, although heat is only one method of decomposing bicarbonates into insoluble carbonate salts. Some alkalis precipitate hardness constituents from water, unless other additives are present.

†Chemical formulae and equations are given in Appendix 2; the (number) refers to the corresponding expression therein.

Typical of carbonate scale is the 'fur' on the inside of kettles. This mineral scale accumulates on boiler tubes, evaporator surfaces, and heat exchanger plates, reducing overall heat transfer and providing an excellent key for other soil deposit ions, such as milkstone (3).

Not only does this hard film support underlying bacterial growth; but favourable conditions are established for crevice corrosion attack on stainless steel or other metals.

Permanent hardness

Permanent hardness is due to the presence of calcium and magnesium sulphates. Conversion to carbonates cannot be achieved by heating (as with temporary hardness), but addition of materials such as sodium carbonate (a common constituent of detergents) will precipitate insoluble carbonate deposits (4,5).

Suggested standards of water quality

The above factors affect cleaning efficiency and influence cleaning economy. The following desirable limits act as a guide to water quality for cleaning purposes.

The water should be good quality, potable mains water of acceptable bacteriological standards. The water should also comply with the brief chemical specifications below:

Total hardness	–	50 ppm expressed as $CaCO_3$
Chloride (as NaCl)	–	50 ppm
Chlorine (elementary)	–	1 ppm
pH	–	6.5 – 7.5
Iron (as Fe)	–	1 ppm
Manganese (as Mn)	–	0.5 ppm
Suspended solids	–	Substantially free

DETERGENTS

Most detergents are available as either solids or liquids. Powder formulations can usually be prepared to give any desired property. With liquid detergents, however, the ability of raw materials to blend and remain stable at high concentrations must be considered.

Many chemical sterilizing agents are available, and these may be used as terminal sanitizers, following a separate detergent recirculation, or they may be blended with appropriate detergent compounds to provide balanced products, which clean and sanitize simultaneously during a single period of recirculation. These combined detergent-sanitizers are mainly used for manual cleaning operations or CIP where soil loads are very light. See Table 5.

Table 5

CHEMICAL STERILIZING AGENTS

Chemical sterilizing agent	Active agent
Chlorinated trisodium orthophosphate	Chlorine
Dichlorodimethyl hydantoin	Chlorine
Sodium dichloro-isocyanurate	Chlorine
Sodium hypochlorite	Chlorine
Cetyl trimethyl ammonium bromide	Quaternary ammonium compound
Benzalkonium chloride	Quaternary ammonium compound
Iodophors	Iodine

Sanitizing and sterilization techniques are dealt with in greater detail later.

Detergent ingredients and factors affecting formulation

When formulating detergent compounds, a number of ingredients may be added to widen and extend the desirable characteristics of the end product. The main characteristics required for an effective cleaning solution are listed below and defined in Appendix 1.

Organic dissolving power.
Wetting power.
Dispersing and suspending power.
Rinsing power.
Sequestering power.
Bactericidal power.
Buffering action.

Relative properties of detergent ingredients

Regrettably, there is no single chemical substance that possesses all of these desirable detergent properties. This is shown in Table 6.

Table 6

RELATIVE PROPERTIES OF DETERGENT INGREDIENTS

(5 represents an optimum property)

Type	Detergent component	Organic dissolving	Wetting	Dispersing, suspending	Rinsing	Sequestering	Chelating	Bactericidal
Alkali	Sodium hydroxide	5	1	1	1	0	0	5
	Sodium carbonate	2	1	1	1	0	0	1
	Sodium metasilicate	3	3	4	3	0	0	2
	Trisodium phosphate	2	2	4	3	0	0	2
Surfactants	Anionic	0	5	5	5	0	0	0
	Non ionic	0	5	5	5	0	0	0
Sequestering & chelating agents	EDTA	0	0	0	0	5	5	0
	Sodium tripolyphosphate	2	1	3	2	3	0	0
Sterilants	Chlorine	0	0	0	0	0	0	5
	Quaternary ammonium compounds	0	4	4	4	0	0	5

The detergent raw materials may be outlined as follows:

Alkalis.
Phosphates.
Acids.
Sequestrants.
Surfactants.
Other minor groups such as suspending agents, anti-foaming agents, and inhibitors.

Alkalis

The inorganic alkalis most widely used are:

Sodium hydroxide (caustic soda).
Sodium orthosilicate.

Sodium metasilicate.
Trisodium phosphate.
Sodium carbonate (soda ash, soda crystals).
Sodium hydrogen carbonate (sodium bicarbonate).

These raw materials contribute the desired degrees of alkalinity, buffering, and rinsing power to the final formulation. Therefore, if high alkalinity is required, sodium hydroxide or sodium orthosilicate will form a large proportion of the mixture. These materials should be handled with care because they can cause severe burns on the skin. In use, caustic alkalis are gradually converted to carbonates. In the absence of sufficient suspending or sequestering agent this will eventually cause scale or bloom to appear on equipment and utensils.

Sodium orthosilicate, sodium metasilicate, and trisodium phosphate are very effective for removing heavy soil. They also possess good buffering and rinsing properties.

Because of their low alkalinity, sodium carbonate and sodium hydrogen carbonate are used in detergent solutions which come into contact with the skin.

Phosphates

Phosphates are usually divided into two groups: the orthophosphates and the poly-phosphates.

The most important member of the orthophosphate group is trisodium phosphate (TSP); other less alkaline members are monosodium dihydrogen phosphate and disodium hydrogen phosphate.

All the pyrophosphates degrade to orthophosphates under certain conditions, although the rates of degradation vary. For most cleaning purposes, these reversion rates are so low as to be of no practical importance. Only when cleaning solutions are held at high temperature for an extended period must this factor be considered.

Sodium pyrophosphate, tripolyphosphate, and polymetaphosphate hydrolyze in aqueous solutions to orthophosphate, the rate of hydrolysis increasing with temperature. However, the presence of alkalis will reduce the rate of hydrolysis.

Generally, the polyphosphates are excellent as detergent ingredients, being:

Free-rinsing.
Good water softeners.
Good peptizing agents.
Good deflocculants.
Good dispersing agents.
Good suspending agents.
Good emulsifying agents.

Selection of optimum individual factors makes for development of a truly balanced detergent.

Acids

Acids are used to dissolve carbonate scales and certain mineral deposits. In many cases the disruptive action caused by effervescence with carbonate is sufficient to remove co-precipitated protein and fat deposits. The most widely used are:

Inorganic acids such as
- Nitric acid.
- Phosphoric acid.
- Sulphamic acid.

Organic acids such as
- Hydroxy-acetic acid.
- Gluconic acid.

These raw materials are used in formulaions designed for the removal of tenacious soil, such as milkstone, which is frequently encountered in sterilizers and evaporators.

These materials should be handled with care because they can cause severe burns on the skin. In addition they are corrosive to certain metals, and for this reason they may have to be used with corrosion inhibitors.

Sequestering agents

Prevention of water hardness precipitation may be achieved by using polyphosphates: however, ethylenediamine tetraacetic acid (EDTA and its salts) and gluconic acid (and its salts) have the advantage of being heat-stable and are also compatible with quaternary ammonium compounds (QAC's) thus permitting the formulation of combined detergent-sanitizer specialities.

Selection and conditions of use of the sequestering/chelating agents must be carefully considered as the specific activity depends upon the nature of the metals in solution. Nowadays the method of dealing with really difficult deposits of protein and calcium salts is to have present in the alkali a chelating agent for calcium. These compounds are able to 'hold' calcium ions in alkaline solution so that solution of the protein by alkali can proceed to completion, and the danger of re-precipitation of calcium salts such as phosphates and carbonates from alkaline solution is greatly reduced. There are three main classes of sequestering or chelating agents. The first is ethylenediamine tetraacetic acid (EDTA) which is also marketed as mono, di, tri, and tetra sodium salts (6).

The second class consists of sodium salts of gluconic and heptonic acids which are rather stronger chelating agents for calcium (and magnesium) than is EDTA. However, their optimum sequestering action for calcium and magnesium salts is developed in caustic soda solutions of 2 – 5% strength. This concentration is far above that normally used in most dairy applications (7).

The third class comprises the polyphosphates, such as sodium hexametaphosphate, sodium tripolyphosphate, and sodium pyrophosphate (8). These compounds have the disadvantage that they have insufficient long-term stability in alkaline solutions and slowly lose their chelating power.

Suspending agents
Suspending agents assist in keeping undissolved soil in suspension. Typical examples are starch and sodium carboxymethyl cellulose.

Inhibitors
Inhibitors are used to minimize the corrosive attack of acids and alkalis on metals. For example, sodium sulphite is used to protect tinned surfaces from attack by alkalis, and sodium silicates protect aluminium and its alloys from attack by mild alkalis.

Anti-foaming agents
Foam may be generated by pumping and jetting action during detergent recirculation. Sometimes crude soaps are formed by saponification of fats with caustic soda. Anti-foaming agents may be incorporated for special applications – a typical example is in bottle washing.

Surfactants (Surface-active agents)
To promote good liquid/soil/surface interfaces the surface tension of the aqueous medium must be reduced. Surfactants fulfil this requirement and contribute many other useful properties to detergent compounds, namely emulsification, dispersion, suspension, and improved rinsability. Some surfactants possess all these properties, whilst others contribute only one or two.

Surface-active agents are classified as anionic, non-ionic, or cationic depending upon how they dissociate in aqueous solution. A fourth category consists of amphoteric or ampholytic surface-active agents, which contain anionic and cationic groupings. These agents possess anionic properties in the alkaline range and cationic properties in the acidic range.

Anionic and cationic surface-active agents are mutually incompatible.

Anionic wetting agents
This is the most common group and consists of essentially neutral materials that can be adjusted for use in either acid or alkaline media. These compounds ionize with the negative anion as the active species. Chemically, the sulphated alcohols and the alkyl aryl sulphonates are the most common (9,10).

Non-ionic wetting agents
Many of these are liquids and, as they do not ionize, they are compatible with either anionic or cationic materials. Foaming characteristics vary from low to high. Typical members of this group are condensation products between ethylene oxide and an alkyl phenol (11).

Quaternary ammonium compounds
These are dealt with later, as their main use is as sterilizing agents.

Typical detergent formulations for various cleaning duties

Bottle-soaking detergent

Caustic soda	68%
Trisodium phosphate	4%
Soda ash	14%
Tetrasodium pyrophosphate	8%
Sodium metasilicate	6%
Total solids	100%

Acid-descaler-cleaner

Non-ionic surfactant	0.30%
Phosphoric acid	31.00%
Water	68.70%
	100%

CIP Heavy duty detergent

Caustic soda	95%
Sodium gluconate	5%
Total solids	100%

Pipeline cleaner

Surfactant	3%
Sodium tripolyphosphate	25%
Sodium metasilicate	10%
Sodium carbonate	30%
Sodium sulphate	32%
Total solids	100%

Manual cleaning detergent

Dodecylbenzene sodium sulphonate (LAS) 40% active	10%
Non-ionic surfactant	4%
Sodium tripolyphosphate	25%
Sodium metasilicate	10%
Filler: borax or sodium sulphate	51%
Total solids	100%

FUNDAMENTALS OF THE STERILIZING PROCESS

In the food industry the soil remaining on equipment after use is often contaminated with micro-organisms and is a good medium in which they can multiply. If improperly cleaned equipment is subjected to a sterilization process:

Micro-organisms present in the soil residues will be protected from contact with chemical sterilizers.

The strength of any chemical sterilizing solution, and hence its effectivemess, may be reduced by excessive quantities of soil.

Heat sterilization will render the residual soil more resistant to subsequent cleaning processes.

Micro-organisms surviving either heat or chemicals may multiply in moist soil residues and, if sufficient time elapses before use, the equipment may become seriously contaminated.

Build-up of soil as a result of continued inadequate cleaning will accentuate these effects.

It is essential that sterilizing agents are applied at the appropriate time, and that the construction and physical condition of equipment is well designed and maintained.

There are many types of sterilizing/sanitizing procedures which may be employed; they fall into two major categories – heat or chemicals.

Heat

The efficiency of processes using heat depends on the temperature reached, the humidity, and the time for which that temperature is maintained.

The required degree of microbiological destruction will be achieved, provided that the method of application and the design of the equipment permit adequate penetration of heat to all parts of the plant or equipment. Temperatures should be measured by means of thermometers of known accuracy, and always at the outlet pipe.

Steam

Where steam at atmospheric pressure is used the recommended time of application depends on the method. For example, for milk cans, steaming on a steaming stool for 1 – 2 minutes (depending on the capacity of the can) is recommended as adequate. For milking equipment or milk bottles in a steam chest, steaming should be continued for at least 10 minutes after the temperature in the chest reaches 96°C. For storage tanks and other large vessels, steam should be injected until the condensate issuing from the outlet of the tanks reaches 85°C, and should then be continued for at least 10 minutes. Steam at atmospheric pressure will not destroy all bacterial spores but is effective against vegetative bacteria, yeast and moulds if applied as recommended.

Hot or boiling water

This method is normally employed on processing equipment, such as plate heat exchangers.

Where the temporary (alkaline) hardness of the water supply exceeds 60 mg/l, water scale will be deposited on the surfaces of equipment unless the water is suitably softened. The temperature of the circulation water at its coolest point, usually the outlet, determines the time of treatment. Common time and temperature combinations for milk, milk products, and ice-cream processing plant are 85°C for 15 minutes or 80°C for 20 minutes. A higher temperature should be used if the time is to be reduced. Circulation of water at such temperatures is a convenient and effective method for treatment of plant after cleaning in place (CIP), and where destruction of bacterial spores is not required. The volume of water used and its flow rate will influence the time taken by the components to reach the required temperature.

Immersion in water which is then raised to boiling point may be used to sterilize small components. But pouring so-called 'boiling' water into buckets and similar utensils is not a reliable method of sterilization, because of the difficulty of ensuring that the utensils have been adequately heated.

Chemicals (including combined detergent/sanitizers)

The efficiency of all sterilizing agents is influenced by concentration, contact time, temperature, organic matter (soil), pH, water hardness, combination with detergents, and types of micro-organisms. All chemical sterilizing agents lack penetrative power, therefore micro-organisms in mineral soils and in crevices may survive prolonged treatment. The presence of less-resistant films of soil, such as air dried residues, will hinder immediate contact of the chemicals with micro-organisms.

As normally used, chemical sterilizing agents are not effective against bacterial spores, and should not be relied on to kill mould spores.

Chemical sterilizing agents may be formulated with detergents to provide balanced products which clean and sterilize in one operation. These may be preferred for applications where it is possible to achieve effective cleaning at moderate temperatures, for example below 60°C, and provided that the soil load is light.

At temperatures of 70°C and above, detergent solutions alone kill most spoilage and pathogenic bacteria, and the inclusion of a chemical sterilizing agent may thus be unnecessary at this stage. The use of detergent/sterilizers is therefore largely confined to manual washing-up operations and situations where the maintenance of high temperature cannot be ensured.

Chlorine

Sodium hypochlorite solutions and brands of chlorinated trisodium phosphate may be used as sterilizing agents alone. Hypochlorite may also be added to solutions of suitable detergents to provide combined detergent-sanitizers. Organic chlorine-release agents, for example dichlorodimethyl hydantoin and sodium dichloroisocyanurate, are most commonly formulated with detergents and marketed in powder form (12,13).

The available chlorine from hypochlorite and other chlorine-releasing chemicals reacts rapidly with, and is inactivated by, residual organic matter; but when used as recommended the volume of chlorine solution and its concentration are such that the quantity of residual soil present on equipment does not seriously impair the sterilizing efficiency of the solution. Storage of used solutions may, however, result in a marked decline in strength, and only freshly-prepared solutions should be used.

Hypochlorite solutions are corrosive to most metals including stainless steel. At low concentration in alkaline solutions, at low temperature and with short contact time, these corrosion hazards are minimized, and the sterilizing action remains effective.

The pH values of hypochlorite solutions diluted to contain 50 – 200 mg/l of available chlorine fall within the range 8.0 – 10.5, depending on the chemical composition of the water supply and the caustic alkalinity of the hypochlorite.

Where previously-cleaned equipment is to be sterilized with hypochlorite solutions the following precautions are necessary:

Equipment should be rinsed free of detergent residues.

If acid has been circulated to remove mineral salts, all traces of acid should be removed, and for this purpose circulation of an alkaline solution is advisable.

Sterilizing solutions containing chlorine should not be left in contact overnight with metal equipment.

Because of their materials of construction, stainless steel plate heat exchangers are particularly prone to corrosion by hypochlorite solutions, and the precautions mentioned above are essential to prevent damage to such equipment.

It is unnecessary, and it may be harmful to the equipment, to use solutions containing more than 200 mg/l of available chlorine at a temperature exceeding 40°C for longer than 10 minutes. For most purposes treatment with cold solutions containing 100 mg/l for 15 minutes is adequate.

Where possible, the available chlorine content of sterilizing solutions should be checked at the time of use.

Quaternary ammonium compounds (QACs)

Unlike hypochlorite, QAC sterilizing agents should not be added by the user to detergent solutions for combined cleaning and sterilizing, because the QAC may be seriously inactivated by certain detergent ingredients such as anionic wetting agents, and to a lesser or unpredictable extent by others. Formulations with compatible detergents may enhance the bactericidal activity of QACs, for example by increasing the alkalinity (14).

The more important properties of QACs influencing their performance as sterilizing agents and their uses are as follows:

In concentrated form they are highly stable and have a long shelf life.

Compared with undiluted hypochlorite they are much safer to handle, but they may cause skin irritation.

Being relatively non-corrosive to metals, if necessary they can be used on equipment at higher temperatures and for longer times than is acceptable with hypochlorite.

Their high surface activity may be disadvantageous; for example, if excessive foam is produced during circulation in pipeline systems it may hinder effective circulation and may be difficult to rinse away.

At low concentration (less than 50 mg/l) of QAC and low temperatures (less than 10°C) QACs are selective in their bactericidal activity being less effective against Gram-negative bacteria such as coliforms and psychrotrophs, than they are against Gram-positive bacteria such as staphyloccoci and streptococci. Hard water reduces the bacterial activity of QACs. Combination of such adverse conditions may encourage the development of QAC-resistant micro-flora on imperfectly cleaned equipment treated with QAC solutions. Selective bactericidal action is unusual at normal use concentrations (150 – 250 mg/l of QAC), above 40°C, and with a minimum contact time of 2 minutes.

QACs do not kill bacterial spores but may inhibit their growth. As with hypochlorites, the bactericidal effectiveness of QACs will be impaired by the presence of organic food matter.

Iodine (iodophors)

Elemental iodine is rendered water soluble by 'complexing' it with suitable non-ionic surface active agents such as nonylphenol-ethylene oxide condensates. Such complexes are known as iodophors. Acidic conditions enhance their bactericidal activity, and those approved for use are invariably modified, usually with phosphoric acid. The presence of surface-active agents and acids confers detergent properties on these iodophors, and all are classed as detergent-sterilizers.

Approved iodophors used at the recommended concentration usually provide 50 – 70 mg/l of free iodine and yield pH values of 3 or less in water of moderate alkaline hardness. Excessive dilution of iodophors with water having a high alkaline hardness may severely impair their efficiency because their acidity is neutralized.

In concentrated form, correctly formulated iodophors have a long shelf life, but solutions may lose iodine by vaporization, and the loss can be rapid above 50°C. Some plastic materials absorb iodine and are stained brown. The rubber gaskets of heat exchangers may also absorb iodine, and if for example hot milk comes in contact with the affected rubber, the milk may acquire an iodine or 'antiseptic' taint.

Iodine stains most organic and mineral soil yellow, thus indicating clearly where equipment has been inadequately cleaned. As iodophor solutions are acidic they will, if used regularly, help to prevent accumulation of minerals, but they should not be expected to remove those existing.

The amber colour of iodophor solutions provides visible evidence of the presence of the sterilizing agent, but the depth of colour is not a reliable guide to the concentration of iodine.

Organic matter such as milk inactivates the iodine in iodophor solutions, and the amber fades. Unless excessive organic residues are present on equipment, the loss of iodine from solutions is slight but may increase if used solutions are stored. If they are to be re-used, iodiphor solutions should be checked and made up to the correct strength.

Amphoteric (ampholytic) surface active agents
These compounds have detergent properties and some have bactericidal properties. The high foaming characteristics of products of this type make them unsuitable for CIP.

Acid sterilizing agents
These are formulations containing surface active agents and inorganic acids, usually phosphoric acid. They may be used either as detergent/sterilizers or as sterilizing agents.

Sodium hydroxide (caustic soda)
This chemical because of its high alkalinity has good bactericidal properties ; a 1.5 – 2.0% m/v solution at 45°C is effective in 2 mins against most spore-forming bacteria.
Sodium hydroxide is included in bottle-washing detergents and, at the caustic alkalinities and temperatures normally recommended, these detergent solutions are highly bactericidal and may kill a proportion of bacterial spores.

Formaldehyde
This chemical is mainly used to disinfect rooms for example, as a fungicide in cheese rooms.

Selection of sterilizing agents
Steam at atmospheric pressure, water circulated at temperatures of 80°C and above, or chemicals, are used for sterilizing equipment and utensils in the food industry. The choice of a suitable sterilizing agent is influenced by:

The type and the materials of construction of the equipment to be sterilized.
The method of application of the sterilizing agent. (manual, spray, circulation).
The process or product for which the equipment is used.
The effectiveness, cost, and convenience of the sterilizing agent.

The following items of equipment, all from the dairy industry, illustrate the philosophy of sterilization/sanitization techniques.

i) Refrigerated farm bulk tanks should not be treated with steam or boiling water, because of the difficulty of raising the temperature of the surface in contact with chilled water and the wastage of the ice bank. There would be a risk of buckling or distorting the metal walls and damaging thermostats and thermometers if steam was used.

ii) Milking equipment is rarely steam-sterilized because of the high capital cost of steam-raising equipment and steam chests on a farm. It is common practice to use acidified boiling water on this type of equipment.
iii) Milk cans and lids washed in mechanical washers are sterilized (sanitized) by injection of steam, which ensures that the cans are hot enough to be dried quickly.
iv) Silo tanks are not sterilized by steam because of the length of time that would be required for the tank surfaces to reach a sterilizing temperature. These tanks are equipped with spray devices, and sterilization is accomplished by spraying solutions of chemical sterilizing agents.
v) Where smaller storage tanks or transport tankers are similarly equipped, chemical sterilization is alsoappropriate, but where tanks are cleaned manually, steam sterilization is to be preferred, because of the difficulty of ensuring adequate coverage of surfaces when chemical sterilizing solutions are applied manually.
vi) Plant cleaned in place (CIP) is best sterilized (sanitized) in place either by recirculating water at a suitable temperature or by circulating a chemical sterilizing solution. Steam sterilization would require the injection of steam at various points in the circuit, and provision for drainage of condensate to to ensure adequate penetration of steam. There is also a greater risk of damage to the equipment and injury to personnel with steam hoses.
vii) Ultra-high temperature (UHT) milk processing plant is required to be free of all micro-organisms including the most heat-resistant bacterial spores. On no account should chemical sterilization be attempted on this equipment. To achieve the high temperatures required for sterilization, pressurised water at 140/150°C is used. The water hardness should not exceed 60 ppm when expressed as calcium carbonate.

MICRO-ORGANISMS ON SURFACES AND THE EFFECT OF STERILIZING AGENTS

A wide variety of micro-organisms may be present on equipment and plant after use. Taking the dairy industry as an example, some appropriate main groups are listed below, and an indication is given of their resistance to sterilizing agents. Situations where some groups may be of particular importance are noted.

It is emphasized that the list is not exhaustive and that there may be specific organisms within the groups which do not necessarily conform to the heat resistance limits.

Non-thermoduric micro-organisms

These are killed by pasteurization at 72°C for 15 seconds.

Milk-souring bacteria, such as lactic acid streptococci.

Staphylococci and other gram-positive micro-cocci.

Coli-aerogenes bacteria and other gram-negative rods.
Psychrotrophic bacteria.
Yeasts.
Moulds (some are heat-resistant).

Hot water, steam, and all chemical sterilizing agents used as recommended are effective against all these types.

Thermoduric micro-organisms

These survive 72°C for 15 seconds but are killed at 80°C for 10 minutes.
Thermoduric micro-cocci and coryneform bacteria.
Some mould spores.
Phages attacking starter cultures (some may survive 80°C for 10 minutes).

Sterilizing procedures employing hot or boiling water, steam, or approved sterilizing agents are effective against these types. The more heat-resistant of the thermoduric coryneform bacteria sometimes present in milking machines may survive the boiling water treatment usually used for this type of equipment.

Micro-organisms surviving 80°C for 10 minutes

Bacterial spores.
Some phages.

Neither prolonged steaming at 100°C nor special treatment with chemical sterilizing agents, such as prolonged soaking (using non-corrosive types) can be relied on to be effective against all bacterial spores, but some types may be reduced in numbers. If contamination by bacterial spores becomes a problem, treatment to remove minerals or dismantling and thorough cleaning may assist by physical removal of the spores.

CLEANING-TEMPERATURE–CONCENTRATION–FLOWRATE–TIME RELATIONSHIPS

CIP procedures aim to provide sufficient energy to a system to change soil adhering to a surface into a suspended or dissolved state. Within the context of CIP, energy forms may be visualized as follows:

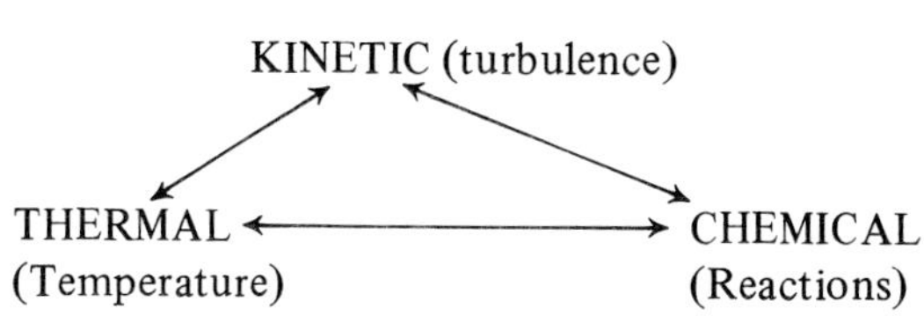

The mechanisms of soil adhesion are complex. Soil is held to surfaces by occlusion in surface irregularities, by electrostatic forces between surface and soil, and by the attraction of soil fractions such as minerals and protein to each other. The sum total of all these forces may be expressed as the energy of soil adhesion.

From the visualization of energy forms given above, it can be seen that a deficiency of one component can be compensated for by increasing one or both of the others. For example, if thermal limitations are applied to a cleaning process, increasing the flowrate and chemical concentrations may compensate for the reduction in temperature, but may well adversely affect the cost of the operation.

It has been shown that the change from laminar flow to turbulent flow condition occurs in pipelines at certain critical flowrates, and this is dependent upon pipe diameters and temperature conditions. Successful cleaning is usually obtained only when turbulent flow is achieved (that is, in pipes, Reynolds number > 3000).

At constant temperature, the Reynolds number increases with increasing flowrate. At constant flowrate, the Reynolds number increases with increasing temperature (assuming that the increase of temperature results in a decrease in viscosity).

Graphs have been prepared to enable flow velocities, flowrates, and pump requirements to be calculated so that a CIP system can provide maximum turbulence at all times.

For some years the criterion of 1.5 m/sec (5 ft/second) has been adopted as the required flowrate in pipelines, irrespective of pipe diameter and solution temperature. It follows that larger pipelines carrying high-temperature solutions would require unrealistic flowrates if this velocity requirement were rigidly applied.

The application of heat to the cleaning solution changes the physical state of the soil (it melts fats), accelerates chemical reactions and alters the turbulence of the cleaning solution.

As a generalization, increasing the solution temperature by 10°C increases the rate of chemical reaction by a factor of 1.5 – 2.0.

Complex relationships exist between soil loads, choice of detergent, time available etc., and it is only possible to make broad generalizations in this text. As an example, the interrelationship between time to clean, flow velocity, and temperature at a fixed detergent concentration for a heat-denatured milk soil is illustrated in Fig. 11.6.

Similarly, optimization for cost-effective cleaning is equally complex and is a subject demanding detailed in-plant study.

In Fig. 11.7 the same detergent concentration has been employed as in Fig. 11.6, but the individual costs of detergent, temperature, and flow velocity components have been illustrated in bar chart form.

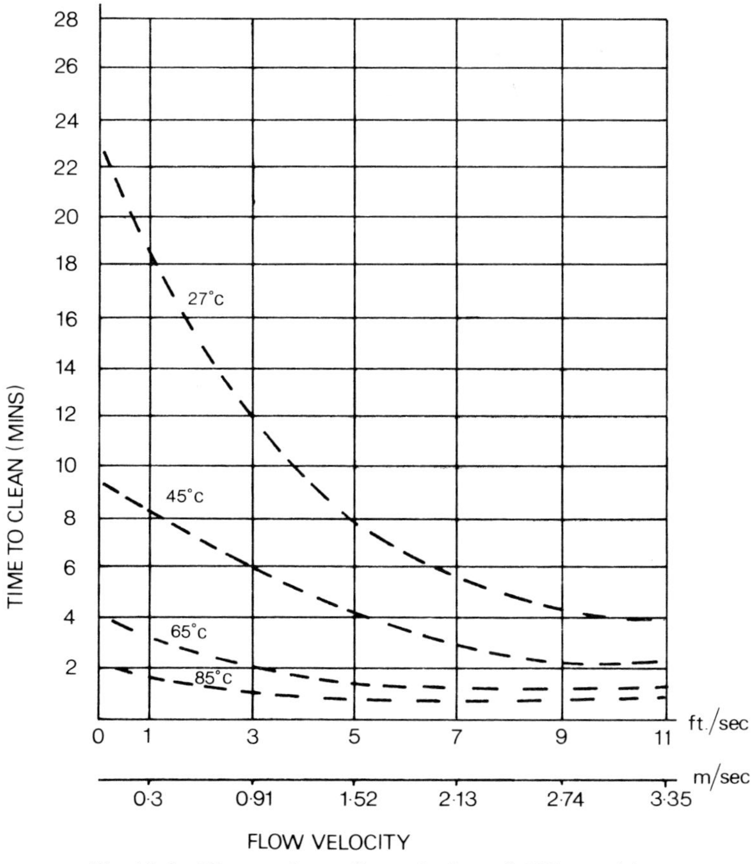

Fig. 11.6 – Time to clean v flow velocity at 0.35% causticity.

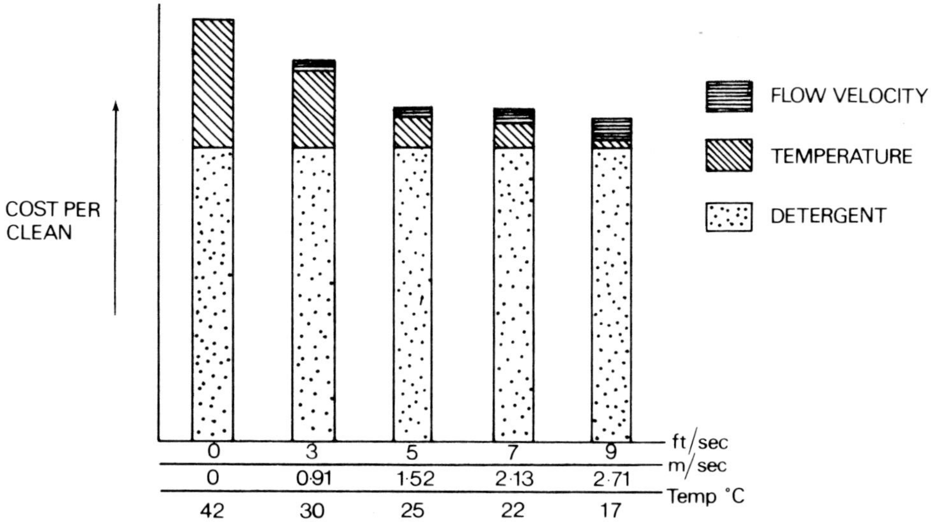

Fig. 11.7 – Typical CIP costs: 10-minute clean at 0.35% NaOH.

REFERENCES & ACKNOWLEDGEMENTS

In the course of preparation of this text, reference has been made to, and extracts obtained from, the following publications.

B.S. 2756: *Recommendations for the use of detergents in the dairying industry.*

B.S. 5305: *Recommendations for the sterilization of plant and equipment used in the dairying industry.*

In place cleaning of dairy equipment (1959), *Society of Dairy Technology.*

Australian Standard Code of Practice AS 1162 – 1973: *Cleaning and Sanitizing Dairy Factory Equipment.*

Hygienic Design of Food Plant (1967) – Joint Technical Committee of the Food Manufacturers' Federation and the Food Machinery Association (reproduced in the present book).

In addition, modified extracts of the as yet unpublished work of IDF document 70 – 1978 'Automatic cleaning and disinfection of Milk Storage and Processing Plants' have been adapted for inclusion in this paper. The extracts are reproduced by courtesy of the IDF. The extracts from British Standards are reproduced by kind permission of the Institution.

APPENDIX 1.

DEFINITIONS AND ESSENTIAL TERMINOLOGY

The following definitions obtained from various sources have been used in this text. The list is by no means complete but is intended as a guide to preferred terminology in relation to dairy detergency and sterilization:-

Bactericidal power
The characteristic which gives additional protection if for some reason the cleaning is not 100% effective. It is important to note that an effective bactericide will not cover up for the inadequacies of poor physical cleaning.

Bactericide
A chemical agent which under defined conditions is capable of killing bacteria but not necessarily bacterial spores.

Bacteriostasis
A state in which multiplication of bacterial populations is inhibited.

Bacteriostat
A chemical agent which under defined conditions induces bacteriostasis.

Buffering action
Stabilizing the pH value of a solution under cleaning conditions. A state in which the hydrogen ion concentration, and hence the acidity and alkalinity, is practically unchanged by dilution, and there is a resistance to change of pH on addition of acid or alkaki.

Chelating power
The property which enables a cleaning solution to redissolve precipitated calcium or magnesium salts.

Cleaning/cleansing
The cleaning process as distinct from sterilization/sanitization. The term 'cleansing' is construed, as in various milk and dairies legislation, as applying to a combination of cleaning and sterilization.

Corrosion inhibitors
Substances capable in specific instances of minimizing the corrosion of certain metals.

Detergents
Substances capable of assisting cleaning when added to water. They include soaps, organic surface-active agents (such as synthetic detergents), alkaline materials, and acids in certain instances.

Dispersing and suspending power
The ability to bring into and keep in suspension undissolved soiling matter. Once this has been achieved soiling matter must be kept in suspension so that particles do not re-deposit and foul the clean surface.

Emulsifying power
The ability to bring into and keep in dispersed form residual oils and fats.

Fungicide
A chemical agent which under defined conditions is capable of killing fungi including their spores.

Organic dissolving power
The ability to solubilise proteins and fats.

Rinsing power
The property which ensures that the deposits and solutions can be rinsed from the plant.

Sanitizing
A process which reduces the number of micro-organisms in plant and on utensils to a level consistent with acceptable quality control and hygiene standards. After sanitizing, the surface shall not give a significant increase in bacteriological contamination to the product coming in contact with it.

Sanitizing agent
A substance that is capable of reducing the number of viable micro-organisms to an acceptable level on the product contact surfaces.

Sequestering agents
A class of chemicals which combine with calcium and magnesium salts, such as those occurring in hard water, to form water-soluble compounds, generally enhancing the detergent operation.

Soiling matter (soil)
The food residue, scale, and other deposits which have to be removed from plant and containers during the cleaning process.

Sterilization
This is the broadest of all the terms and demands the destruction of every form of life, be it plant or animal, visible or invisible under the microscope, harmful or innocuous.

Sterilizing agent
A substance capable of destroying any form of life.

Surface-active agents
Substances capable of modifying the physical forces existing at surfaces, such as between liquids and solids, permitting more intimate contact and facilitating mixing.

Suspending power
See Dispersing

Wetting power
The property which enables the components to reduce the surface tension of the solutions and thus promote penetration of the soils.

APPENDIX 2

CHEMICAL FORMULAE AND EQUATIONS

Where possible, chemical formulae and equations have been extracted from the text and incorporated in this Appendix.

$$CO_2 + H_2O \longrightarrow H_2CO_3 \quad (1)$$

$$CaCO_3 + H_2CO_3 \longrightarrow Ca(HCO_3)_2 \quad (2)$$

$$^{*}Ca(HCO_3)_2 + \Delta\,\text{heat} \longrightarrow CaCO_3 \downarrow + H_2O + CO_2 \quad (3)$$

$$^{*}CaSO_4 + Na_2CO_3 \longrightarrow CaCO_3 \downarrow + Na_2SO_4 \quad (4)$$

$$^{*}CaSO_4 + \Delta\,\text{heat} \longrightarrow \text{No reaction} \quad (5)$$

* For simplicity, only the calcium components of water hardness have been selected for illustration.

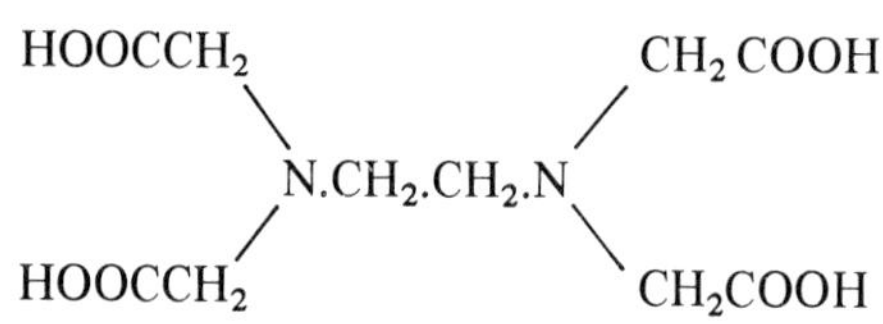

(6)

Ethylene diamine tetra acetic acid

$$CH_2OH\,(CH.OH)_4\,COOH \quad (7)$$

Gluconic acid

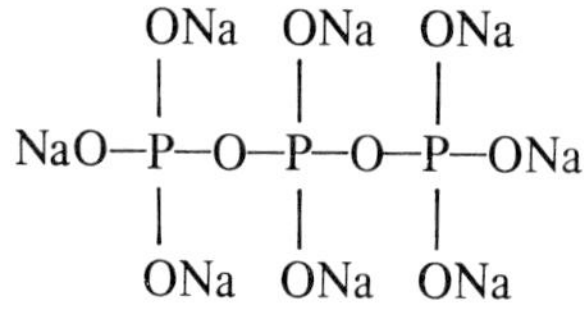

(8)

A sodium polyphosphate

$$C_{12}H_{25}{-}(OC_2H_4)_n{-}O{-}SO_3^{-} \quad Na^{+} \quad (9)$$

Sodium lauryl ethoxylate sulphate - n = 7 - 10
(A sulphated fatty alcohol ethoxylate)

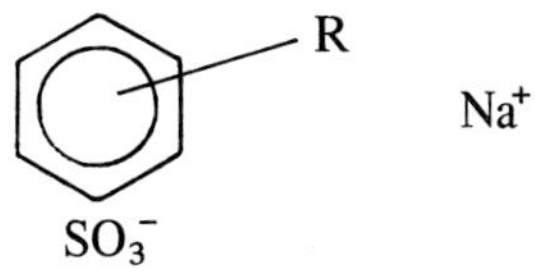

R≡ alkyl (10)

A sodium alkyl benzene sulphonate

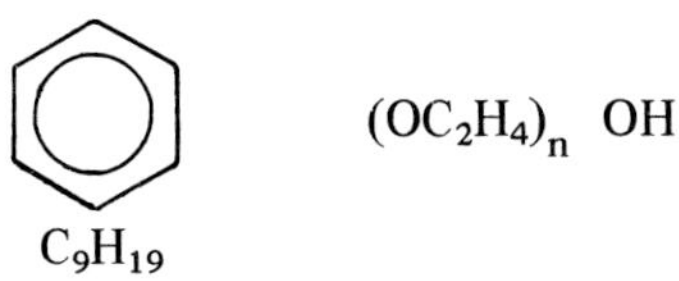

(11)

Nonyl phenol ethoxylate (n = 8 — 10)

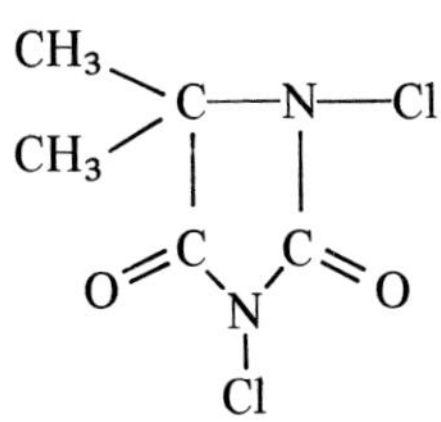

(12)

Dichlorodimethyl hydantoin

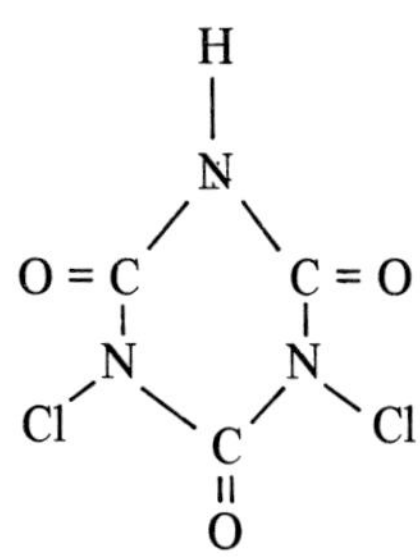

(13)

Dichloro isocyanuric acid

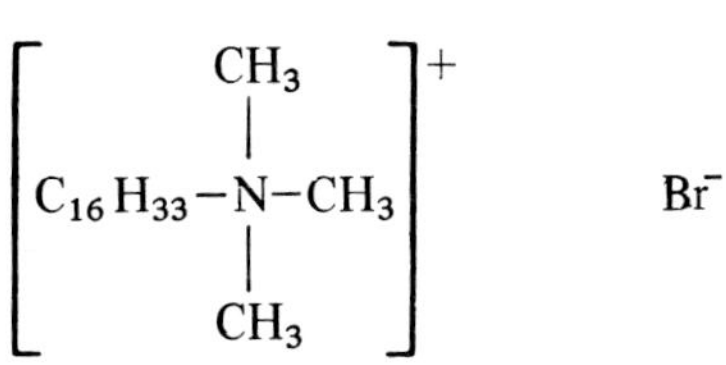

(14)

Cetyl trimethyl ammonium bromide

APPENDIX 3.

MANAGEMENT OF CLEANING AND STERILIZING OPERATIONS

Cleaning and sterilizing operations are an integral part of the production line, therefore successful management implies both close attention to the training of operatives in the use of detergents, detergent/sterilizers, and sterilizing agents, and continual supervision to ensure that there is no deterioration in standards of hygiene.

When solutions are being prepared the quantities of water and chemicals should be carefully measured.

Thermometers of known accuracy should be used for checking the temperatures of solutions and, in particular, checking temperatures at strategic points during heat sterilizing procedures. Carelessness can result in waste of chemicals, ineffective cleaning and sterilization, or damage to plant and personnel.

Solid detergent/sterilizers should be stored in covered containers in a cool dry place; liquids should be stored in original containers which should be kept closed. Solutions of sodium hypochlorite should be stored in a cool place protected from light; it is advisable not to carry large stocks in warm weather. Strict stock control of all chemicals should be exercised to avoid deterioration and waste and to ensure stock rotation.

DISCUSSION

Mr S. Sordy (Pedigree Petfoods): Does the use of hard water clog the spray balls?

Mr Tamplin: If one is using a cleansing solution based on, say, caustic soda with adequate sequestration – EDTA, gluconate or glucoheptonate or boroheptonate or similar – there would be no problem at all. You can demonstrate this in the laboratory with caustic soda and hard water. As you pour in the caustic soda, down comes a great precipitate. If one then adds some EDTA in accurate quantities, the solution becomes clear again, and obviously such formulated solutions are used routinely in detergency. If deposition is likely to occur from hard water and you don't want to go to the expense of EDTA, then separate recirculation of, say, nitric or phosphoric acid will remove hard water scale, and there are CIP systems available which include this operation for every CIP cycle. There is first a caustic recirculation, perhaps with hypochlorite, and then at the end of this comes the circulation of acid just to brighten the process.

Mr R. Jowitt: Is it, in general, cheaper today to use sequestering agents than softened hard water?

Mr Tamplin: EDTA is a most expensive component. Sequestrants are the most expensive components of all the detergents, and I would think that in a new plant certainly one would be advised to adopt water softening.

Mr J. Milledge: Would you say more about fail-safe systems to prevent contamination of product with detergent/sanitizers in CIP systems?
Mr Tamplin: Can I refer to a slide that I didn't use in my lecture? (Fig. 11.8). It is becoming more and more important these days that companies guarantee absolutely the requirement that there shall be no intermixing. It is no good having a system where a CIP solution is adjacent to the same valve as the product, because leakage is then a major risk. It is not even good enough these days to say that the pressure is higher on the product side than the CIP solution side, and argue therefore that any leakage is bound to occur that way. This claim is no longer valid. In the simplest systems you can solve this with two valves and an additional leak to atmosphere. Any leakage that occurs will then drain out through the drain between them.

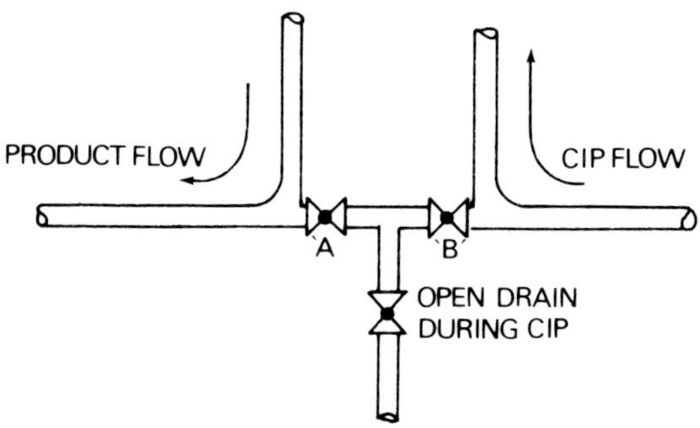

Fig. 11.8 – Fail-safe system: leakage via valves A or B during CIP means that fluids discharge to drain.

The other technique which is readily available is to use a 'keypiece' system referred to earlier (Fig. 11.5), where before one can undertake cleaning, a particular component has to be removed and replaced in a different way or with a different component, so that when it is correctly assembled the appropriate CIP route is established and legitimate CIP routines can commence.

CHAPTER 12

Operators - Personal Aspects of Hygiene

G. A. **Steel**, H. J. Heinz Co. Ltd.

In spite of following all the procedures for plant hygiene described in the previous papers at this symposium, a manager of a food processing plant could still be faced with the situation where product from his plant has been implicated in a food poisoning outbreak. This is a very stressful situation, and I will describe it in some detail.

The local health authority will have been informed, indeed they may have already been informed from other sources, and the manager gets his first information from them, which is in itself a stress situation. Environmental health officers will have visited the plant, asking a lot of very personal questions and taking a lot of very personal samples. The press will soon be aware of the situation and are likely to be probing and hostile. The plant operators will be scared and, because they are scared, they will be on the defensive. Because they are on the defensive, they may be uncooperative. It is very likely that production will be stopped and shipping may be stopped. The Sales Manager may well make this an excuse for any errors or weaknesses in his department in the past. Above, the Board of Directors will be baying for a human sacrifice, and the manager knows that he is top of the list. Faced with the threat of this situation, a manager, if he is going to sleep at night, is going to know about food poisoning over and above the incidental knowledge he will have acquired as part of his working knowledge of plant hygiene, and he is also going to train his operators with care.

This paper is concerned with food poisoning, the attitudes of plant operators to personal hygiene, and the training aids available.

The personal aspects of hygiene of operators are a factor in the prevention of food poisoning, The consumer has a legal right to expect that food is produced under hygienic conditions. The consumer has also the right to expect that food is produced in an aesthetically acceptable way, and this implies cleanliness.

This paper is based on experience as an occupational health physician for the past twenty years in two food manufacturing units with about 4000 employees, not all of whom, of course, are food handlers, but all of whom have to conform to the factory rules of hygiene. However, if one considers food hygiene in a historical context or in a global context, scientific medicine and health supervision apply to only a small minority of food handlers. Until the middle of the 19th century, hygiene, as applied to food handling, was largely a matter of taboos and tradition. Food taboos are prehistoric, but some have been on record for more than 2000 years and are still sound. For example, in the Old Testament – Deuteronomy, Chapter 14, verse 21, 'Ye shall not eat of anything that dieth of itself,' – a very important basic rule, because the very earliest civilization had recognized that meat from an animal which had died from disease was harmful. However, the advice goes on 'Thou shalt give it unto the stranger that is within thy gates that he may eat it.' In other words, 'fit for hotel and restaurant trade', and finally, 'Or thou may sell it unto an alien.' In other words, 'fit for export.' So you can conclude that the conflicts between commercial expediency and hygiene are very old. It is an interesting concept of lateral thinking to consider that the present strictness of export licence requirements for some Nordic countries may be traced to the Reformation and the subsequent dissemination of biblical advice in the common tongue. Not all taboos are logical. An old farmer was told by his wife that there would be tongue for tea. He reacted strongly and said, 'I will eat nothing that has been in the mouth of a cow,' so she fried him a couple of eggs. Now if you consider the anatomical details of egg production, that was not very logical from the food hygiene point of view. We are on surer ground when we consider rules for personal hygiene, based on culture patterns. Even before the work of Pasteur in the middle of the last century gave the explanation of the bacterial origin of food poisoning, the culture pattern associating cleanliness and freedom from disease was established by the writings of Chadwick and Florence Nightingale. Florence Nightingale's life extended to this century, and to her death she did not believe in bacteria but achieved a revolution in the standard of patient care and prevention of infection, based on cleanliness and removal of the source of bad smells. In terms of culture pattern, the basic rule, that having been to the lavatory you wash your hands, is of very recent origin in this country. My parents had a late Victorian childhood. My mother would certainly wash her hands before preparing food – that was part of the general philosophy of cleanliness; but they were never taught to wash their hands after going to the lavatory, and they never taught me. Perhaps you believe that the rule would have been taught at my school. It certainly wasn't. The lavatory was at the farthest end of the school playground, a dark insanitary hole without any possibility of washing your hands as it was without light and water supply. There may have been a wash-hand basin in the school itself, but if you were caught using that, you would be punished for splashing water around. You may well believe that it would be different when my children went to school – well, they went to a rural school, and the sanitary facilities had not changed in 25 years. Nowadays, when my grandchildren go to school, it will be different – yes of course, it is different. Every school has good toilet facilities and hand-washing facilities. These are frequently vandalized and the basins kicked in. So the practice of hygiene, as part of a culture pattern in schools, is still inadequate for food handling.

Finally, to bring up to date the significance of a culture pattern of cleanliness in food hygiene, here is a quotation from Schumacher's book *Small is Beautiful*.

> 'Most of us try to keep ourselves reasonably clean. Why? Simply for hygienic reasons? No, the hygiene aspect is secondary; we recognize cleanliness as a value in itself. We do not calculate its value; the economic calculus simply does not come in. It could be argued that to wash is uneconomic: it costs time and money and produces nothing – except cleanliness'.

To sum up:

1. You need rules for personal hygiene in food handlers.
2. If the rules are to be followed, they have to be explained and understood. This involves a training programme.
3. The rules will be more meaningful and are more likely to be followed if they are linked with a culture pattern of cleanliness, and cleanliness in food preparation in particular.

Now let us deal with the significance of the food handler and personal hygiene as a cause of food poisoning. We are at present, in Britain and in Western Europe in general, involved in a fundamental reappraisal of the relative importance of human-origin and animal-origin food-transmitted disease. In 1977-1978, the information and recommendations on which policy is based have shown important changes. I will try to draw together four separate threads. Firstly, a Parliamentary question on the 1 February this year (1978).

Food Poisoning.

Mr Patrick Jenkin asked the Secretary of State for Social Services what plans he has to tackle the growing problem of food poisoning; and if he will make a statement.

Mr Ennals, pursuant to his reply, (Official Report, 27 January 1978. Vol. 942, C 822), gave the following information.

I am glad to say that, while final figures are not yet available, the indications are that the number of food poisoning incidents in England, notified for 1977, will be lower than that for 1976. Nevertheless, the Government attach great importance to all possible measures being taken to reduce the incidence of food poisoning.

What is required is, in our view, not so much the adoption of fresh measures as the strengthening of efforts along existing lines; in particular there is need to impress on all those engaged in handling food the importance of maintaining good hygiene and food safety. Within the limits of available resources, officers of local authority environmental health departments give advice and guidance to this end in the course of their food inspection duties and as part of wider education measures. In addition, my Department publishes a variety of material stressing the importance of this subject and giving appropriate advice. My right hon. Friend the Minister of Agriculture, Fisheries and Food also accepts the importance of taking steps to reduce the incidence of infection in live animals and feeding stuffs.

Now of course, a Parliamentary Question and Answer is never as simple as it appears in print – in fact you probably all know the definition of the ideal Parliamentary answer which is 'short, accurate, and adds nothing to what is already known'. In this particular case, the Government department concerned has produced an excellent discussion document – a draft memorandum on the investigation and control of a food poisoning outbreak. This is still a draft document, but I have extracted (with the author's permission) some of the information relevant to this subject.

Chance contamination of food by a few organisms is probably not harmful to the healthy individual, as the ingestion of large numbers of organisms is needed to cause disease, but if the lightly-contaminated food is allowed to stand at room temperature for a few hours, multiplication of the organisms will take place. The majority of outbreaks are due to contaminated meat and poultry, although other raw food or ingredients of food are sometimes responsible.

Animal reservoirs of salmonella organisms include chicken, turkeys, and ducks (providing poultry and eggs and egg products), cattle (providing meat, offal, and milk), pigs (providing meat and offal), horses (providing meat for pets and humans).

In nearly all cases of human salmonellosis the infection derives directly or indirectly from farm livestock or poultry. The investigation of outbreaks has frequently shown that the responsible organisms can be isolated from the local abbatoir or farm of origin. Surveys have demonstrated that 30% of poultry, between 2% and 10% of bucher's meat, and 11% of knacker's meat sold for pet food may be contaminated with salmonella.

Although outbreaks are sometimes caused by contamination of food by a transient human excretor, infected food-handlers are more often the victims rather than the source of an outbreak.

Some salmonella infections are not food-borne and can be acquired in a number of ways, including transmission from pets (such as *S. java* infection from terrapins) or by person-to-person spread, particularly in hospitals and nurseries.

The significance of animal origin, compared to human origin, is apparent.

Thirdly, you will remember that the Ministerial reply refers to the incidence of infection in live animals and feeding stuffs. Let us just consider the chain of events. We import feeding stuffs, particularly fish meal and cereals from countries where the raw materials are very likely to be contaminated with indigenous bacteria or are contaminated during processing. These raw materials are compounded into animal feed in large units in this country, ensuring a thorough mix and distribution at the compounding plant. Again, the distribution system within the country is such that we get country-wide distribution to the wholesale and retail agricultural suppliers. Increasingly, beef cattle and poultry are reared in large units from prepared feeds with the maximum opportunity of cross-infection. Abattoirs and poultry processing plants are large, needing high throughput for economic production, leading to further cross-infection. Post-slaughter processing is again concentrated in large units for final distribution of the product to predominantly large units, prepacked for the retail sale. Now if you were a foreign exporter with a product that could be used by every man, woman, and child in the country, and you wanted a distribution system that would reach say 90% of the households in the country, I put it to you that you would be hard pressed to devise a more effective system. But worse is already happening and worse is to come. Offal and excreta are rich in available nitrogen as a source of further protein. It is a relatively cheap source and freely available. It follows that much potentially infected material is recycled into animal feed. The ultimate is the recycling of the animal's own excreta into its food. In eating habits and food processing habits we tend to follow the United States. In the *Farmers' Weekly* of the 5 January 1978 there was a technical article about an American farm where silage, made from hay and an equal quantity of slurry solids and a little grain, was fed direct to beef cows. To be fair, there is lactic fermentation in the silo which will destroy pathogens but, even so, the risk of cross-contamination is a very real one.

Fourthly, on the 21 March 1978 a report by a study group of the British Association for the Advancement of Science was published with the title of 'Salmonella – the Food Poisoner.' This is an excellent publication, written in non-technical language, again drawing attention to the need for action to reduce the disease in animals as a source of disease in man. I quote from its postscript.

> In dealing with this most complicated problem, much could be achieved in the short term by the further education of the public in matters of food hygiene.
>
> Economics are not the only factors of importance. People matter, and some people become ill from salmonellosis and some die.

Here I would emphasize that the specific responsibilities in a food-manufacturing plant will be apparent to you all, and that hygiene saves lives.

All this information has been very much the concern of medical officers working in the food industry who meet together from time to time and are, of course, particularly concerned with the health supervision of food handlers.

Recently, they have discussed the question of routine stool examination of food handlers. This is a current requirement for some categories of food handlers in the EEC countries and Sweden, but is not a requirement in Britain. There now seems a good chance that the British point of view will carry the day in the discussion with the other EEC countries, and we will not be required to introduce this procedure in Britain. In my view, the examination of a stool specimen for pathogens has a place firstly, in the diagnosis and response to treatment of an individual patient and also in subsequent fitness for work if the patient happens to be a food handler. It also has a vital function in the investigation of an outbreak of food poisoning and, in particular, if that food poisoning outbreak involves a food manufacturing unit. I do not consider there is any place for routine stool examination, pre-employment, for the generality of food handlers, though there can be exceptions to this. For example, if we are considering a sensitive product such as meat or semi-processed meat products handled by a vulnerable group of food handlers who have spent a substantial time on the Indian sub-continent. It is still a matter for further discussion, and we are still at variance with a number of EEC directives and codes of practice, but I believe responsible opinion is swinging towards Britain's point of view. One routine test with a negative result is only of value for that point in time, and unless very strict procedures are followed, it is not even of value for that individual because stool samples can be bought or changed.

I have mentioned the importance of training for food handlers. Is there a qualification for food handlers? The answer to that is 'Yes'. The Royal Society of Health run courses on food hygiene with an examination leading to a certificate, and the Royal Institute of Public Health & Hygiene run similar courses. These are held at various centres throughout the country. More recently, St John Ambulance, who for many years have granted certificates in food hygiene, in particular, have re-launched a short course in food hygiene, run in conjunction with the Environmental Health Officers' Association.† It is particularly appropriate for the catering and retail food trade, but the principles of the course apply to all food handlers. In-plant training of food handlers should start with an induction programme, and many industrial organizations have produced their own training films or other training aids.††

It is not sufficient to display the Food Hygiene Regulations. They must be explained to all food handlers.

I began with a quotation from the Old Testament. I would like to end with a reference to classical mythology. Zeus had two daughters. The elder was called Panacea. Much of our civilization today worships Panacea. However, the younger, and to my mind more beautiful, daughter was called Hygiea. Anyone connected with the food industry will be doing themselves and others a service if they pay their tribute to Hygiea.

† The Royal Society of Health, 13, Grosvenor Place, London, S.W.1.
The Royal Institute of Public Health & Hygiene, 28, Portland Place, London,W1N 4DE.
St John Ambulance, H.Q. St John Ambulance, 1, Grosvenor Crescent, London, SW1X 7EF.
†† *Training Films.*
'The Clean Way': H. J. Heinz Company Ltd. 'The Key to Cleanliness': J. Lyons & Co. Ltd.

DISCUSSION

Dr J. G. Davis (Reading): Have you come across an incurable salmonella carrier like Typhoid Mary in your experience?

Dr Steele: Typhoid Mary is a classic. We have moved away from the large pool of typhoid infection in this country over 60 years because we have had a good water supply. That case occurred in the States at a time when their water supply was not as well-controlled and there was a lot of typhoid in the States, so the simple answer to your question is 'No'. There are legal constraints about such people working in food at all. I have known, through the literature of two cases in recent history, by that I mean the last 10 or 15 years, where that constraint has had to be applied, but we haven't had anything like Typhoid Mary in this cointry.

Dr Davis: There have been two cases which could not be cleared up?

Dr Steele: I agree, they are in the literature, and they had to have legal constraints (permanently).

Dr Davis: That is extremely rare?

Dr Steele: Yes.

Chairman: How well-known is Typhoid Mary to the majority of the audience? Do you all know about Typhoid Mary? No, so perhaps Dr. Steele had better explain very briefly the significance of the expression.

Dr Steele: In the *New Yorker* some years ago there was a fascinating article in lay terms about Typhoid Mary. She was the public health bane of their existence in the States for a period of ten years or more. They'd have a typhoid outbreak, they'd do a lot of work and trace it back to this person – low intellect, always engaged in the lowest catering/cleaning type of work in a food establishment, moved around the country, lost supervision – it was easy to lose supervision then in the States – and Typhoid Mary as she became to be known was responsible for dozens of separate typhoid outbreaks in the United States about 40 years ago.

Mr Barnes (Marks and Spencer): Could I ask Dr Steele to expand his views a little more on the use of pre-employment stool tests for people working with highly perishable foods – sliced meats and so on?

Dr Steele: I work in a good industry in the sense that canning is a safe process, and we are not concerned about that test. One of my friends, a doctor in industry, is at that side of the spectrum; his population contains many immigrants, his products are the ones we described, and he says 'Whatever the generality of opinion is, I believe that in my particular situation it is right that we require pre-employment stool examinations for workers on certain parts of the process, and that is done'.

Mr J. Bennet (Mars Ltd.): Are there good reasons for food handlers to wear gloves?

Dr Steele: We did some work on this, and although it was a long time ago it is still valid, but I can't give you the reference. Gloves were worn by handlers of a sensitive product; in our particular case they were stripping chicken meat off bones. It was found that there was a higher bacterial count on the gloves after the same length of time than there was on bare hands washed regularly, so that in this particular process (and we are very glad that we don't do it any more) the answer to the question is that we may well end up less satisfactory than with regular hand washing. Wearing gloves is *not* a solution.

CHAPTER 13

General Discussion

R. Jowitt, Chairman

Mr R. E. Welborn: Glass-fibre reinforced plastics vessels are being used increasingly for storage. Has anyone any experience of their cleanability or of any product taint problems?

Mr Tamplin: Many people are using GR plastics for the storage of water and also for the storage of wine. They seem to be very well made indeed, but one has to be careful. If you start using chlorine-based products and there have been phenols in the resins, you can get chlorophenols which will give you particular taint problems associated with ‘antiseptics’. On general cleanability they seem to have a very good track record. One could itemize certain instances of problems on poorly produced surfaces where there might have been air bubbles which will behave like little caves, and inside the caves micro-organisms can give rise to problems, but in the main they are very valuable.

Dr von Brockelmann: Perhaps I could add on the cleanability of plastics that in my experience it is very important in manual cleaning to be careful in the choice of the brushes or other aids so that they are not harder than the plastic. If they are harder they will damage the surface and cause increasing problems from day to day. There is one more point with plastics cleaning; one has to be extremely careful in choosing detergents because some of the wetting agents used in composite detergents will react with the plastic components, and after some time there is a risk that the surfactant has invaded the plastic and it will turn black and cause off-flavours in the product. Even if it could not be a health risk it could endanger the food quality, but I agree with the last speaker: they are quite useful, plastic vessels, but one has to know how to handle them.

Dr J. G. Davis: Some years ago I made an investigation of the cleanability of various materials commonly used in the food industry. Our results showed that glass was the most hygienic material, closely followed by stainless steel and vitreous enamel. The next best, but definitely not so good, was aluminium, then after this came various plastics which varied considerably in their behaviour from the point of view of ease of removal of soil and bacteria by orthodox sanitizing methods. The plastics tended to give anomalous results, possibly because of the presence of plasticizers in them which exerted an inhibitory effect on bacterial growth. Much worse than these were painted surfaces, and very much worse than any of these was wood.

Chairman: I have often wondered just how far the use of metals – and that's about the only thing left other than plastics and glass – can give rise to metallic flavours. We are all familiar with metallic flavours in canned foods which have perhaps not been stored under ideal conditions. Would any of the conferees care to comment on any evidence that the use of even stainless steel can give rise to metallic taints in the flavours of food? I think it's well known the distilling industry will use nothing but copper. This, I think, is a negative taint situation. There seems to be some evidence, but we don't know by any means all that would be helpful to know about this question of metallic taint. Would anyone like to take this one up?

Dr von Brockelmann: I know of only one situation, and that is an indirect case where you have milk in stainless steel and copper in contact with the stainless steel. If you had copper coils in the hot water boiler on the farm and stainless steel piping in the pipeline connecting system, you may get copper together with the hot water, and that will eventually adhere to the stainless steel surfaces during the cleaning procedure. After cleaning, during the next milking copper will be transferred to the milk and give a metallic off-flavour.

We have had many cases of that, and we have solved them by introducing a rinse with citric acid after alkaline cleaning. It so happens that a citric acid rinse will remove the copper residues and so remove the risk of a metallic flavour: but that is only for milk.

Chairman: Would Dr Burton like to add anything to the comments of Dr von Bockelmann about milk taint?

Dr H. Burton (National Institute for Research in Dairying): I can't make much additional comment on this, I'm afraid. The effect of copper specifically in the case of milk and presumably other fats is well known in catalyzing oxidation. The only other experimental work that we have done was with aluminium foils and aluminium foils alloyed with various other metals to give improved mechanical characteristics. This was for the capping of milk in glass bottles, and with none of these foils, either ones commonly used or the ones with additional alloying agents, was any influence in the flavour of the milk detectable.

If I can just revert to GRP tanks, 15 to 20 years ago we did try GRP tanks for milk storage. At least we were asked to try them by other people, and the results were absolutely catastrophic. Whether they are any better now than they were then, I would not know.

Chairman: I do not know if it is still the custom in any part of the world to add tin salts to pale canned fruits which are 'canned' in tin-less containers such as plastic pouches, but I think it is fairly well known that the leaching of tin salts into light-coloured canned fruits has been responsible for the retention of the pale colour. This is something rather different, and I wonder if anybody would like to comment on the hygienic or health aspects of this phenomenon which is established by practice, if not by *good* practice.

Dr Steele: I have no experience of that, but going back to public health and food poisoning there are cases where antimony in the glaze on enamelware in contact with acid products has produced food poisoning.

Chairman: Mr Thorpe, would you like to comment on that?

Mr Thorpe: I think the only thing I would say is that it is not permitted legally. The only instance I can think of where it is legally permitted is in the United States, and that is to add tin salts to glass-packed asparagus.

Chairman: Would anyone like to discuss any aspect of yesterday's proceedings on hygienic *design* of food plant?

Mr D. H. Halliday (Unilever): Although it was mentioned in the papers, the question of building materials was not discussed very much. It is becoming increasingly important in view of the EEC regulations to get the right materials for walls, floors, ceilings, etc. In another symposium of this nature it would be useful to concentrate a bit more on this aspect.

Dr Lawson (Unilever): I would add to Mr Halliday's comment and say that with increasing requirements upon engineers to take into account environmental aspects in the design of new factories (and this is another aspect of the point Mr Halliday has just been making), we are going to find ourselves – from the hygienic design point of view – in somewhat of a compromise situation. I am thinking, for example, of a mezzanine floor which might, with food machinery mounted on it, give rise to noise and vibration, but which is relatively easily kept clean. Now if requirements or even legislation make us use sound-deadening material on the underside, then certainly the sound-deadening materials that are available at present would be very dangerous harbourers of contaminants, and certainly at the moment they are impossible to clean. I'd like to hear if any members of the symposium have, within their factories, any examples that they could quote and of any progress that they might be making in this area.

Chairman: The Food Engineering Panel recently held a half-day symposium on the problem of noise in food factories and, other than recognizing the point Dr Lawson has made, of which everyone was very much aware, namely the incompatibility of sound-absorbing materials and hygienic finish, no solutions were offered. Perhaps it does emphasize the need to reduce the sound generation at source. That seems to be where most of the effort in the food industry is being directed.

Mr Whitman (Leatherhead Food RA): I think the problem is a very serious one. Sound reduction at source – yes; it's often possible to make some improvement on current practice, but there are many machines where one would have to do a radical re-engineering of the whole process in order to alleviate the problem. This simply is not practical. We have been very conscious of this lack of a hygienic building material for sound reduction purposes for a very long time. I have discussed it with various people with no success at all. I really think here that we have something that ought to be interesting to people in the universities, our basic physicists, to go back and see whether there isn't some way almost round the laws of physics, because on talking with people from the National Physical Laboratory the answer was 'No, it couldn't be done, it's against the laws of Physics. You can't do this sort of thing'. But there must be a solution somewhere if only we can turn the right sort of brains on to it.

Mr J. Harms: In relation to hygienic operation, not much comment has been made on the role of top management. The speakers from Marks and Spencer showed some horrific examples, and I wonder if they have any comments to make on these bad examples where top management really wasn't interested in hygienic operation.

Mr Robson (Marks and Spencer): I am sorry that this point didn't come out clearly enough in presenting our paper. It is mentioned in the last section in which we make the point that management has a specific responsibility, firstly to ensure that operators are properly trained and educated in these matters as Dr Steele has pointed out so graphically, but, secondly, to set an example themselves. I tried to make the point that if you are wandering around your factory on a daily inspection to see what is going on and you ignore even the slightest transgression of the hygiene rules and you overlook it and pass it by, this will be seen and observed and taken as an indication that it is not important: management are not interested in it, and therefore no one will ever take any notice of it again. This is the sort of responsibility we believe that management have. You really have to go out of your way and make a fuss about it so that people make sure they are not there the next time you come round. You achieve this standard of hygiene only if the people at the top are determined to make it work. There is no doubt about this at all. We often say in our stores that if a store manager is determined to have a clean store he will have a clean store. It doesn't matter what his staff problems are; it entirely stems from the top.

Mr Harms: One other point might be of interest in relation to the removal of copper from stainless steel. Way back before stainless steel became such a common material, citric acid used to be processed in monel metal containers, and I think I am right in saying that it is quite common to find the copper being dissolved out of the monel metal by the citric acid.

Chairman: Now the last item on the programme is Chairman's summing up. It is not my intention to try to sum up the proceedings, but I would like to make a few comments on the extent to which our intentions have been achieved or indeed what our intentions were.

I think it has emerged, if it hasn't already been explicitly stated, that in a sense this symposium itself is almost incidental – but let me hasten to say that I think it was one of the best accidents that came out of the general feeling that the *Hygienic design of food plants – a Guide to good practice* booklet should be updated after ten years. It was felt that as we couldn't get down to updating it and expanding it to include both operation and design, we ought to get together in a symposium, the proceedings of which might form an updating of this booklet. So in a sense this is just an excuse to get a book, but I think it's been much more. I feel personally, and I think the organizing committee would also feel, that the symposium has been well worthwhile in its own right. It has shown the interrelation between subjects which have been the topics of the individual papers. It has left a number of questions unanswered. It has shown that, owing either to external pressures or to an increasing desire to improve the hygienic standard of the food in this country and of our export customers in the face of evidence that food poisoning is increasing, things are being done; that an awareness exists of the need to do even better in terms of design and of operation; and that these two things which need to be looked at separately for various good reasons are really the opposite sides of the same coin and so inextricably interconnected.

One thing which hasn't emerged to the extent that it might have done, and which is literally the $64 question, is the economics of the interaction of hygienic design and hygienic operation. Some years ago in relation to work we did here at the College, it became quite clear that *any* surface is cleanable if you are prepared to spend the time and the money in cleaning it, and that certain surfaces are literally unsoilable provided you are prepared to pay the cost of them. Between those two extremes, neither of which is very practical, there is a whole spectrum of combinations of more or less expensive surfaces and more or less expensive schemes of cleaning available to the food engineer and the food processor. It would be useful if some facts and figures could be published on these alternatives to help those who have to make the choice.

One of the outcomes of the symposium and the published proceedings will be evident to a reader who might sit down and read it from cover to cover; that is, the fact that certain solutions to certain problems in certain papers exist in other papers.

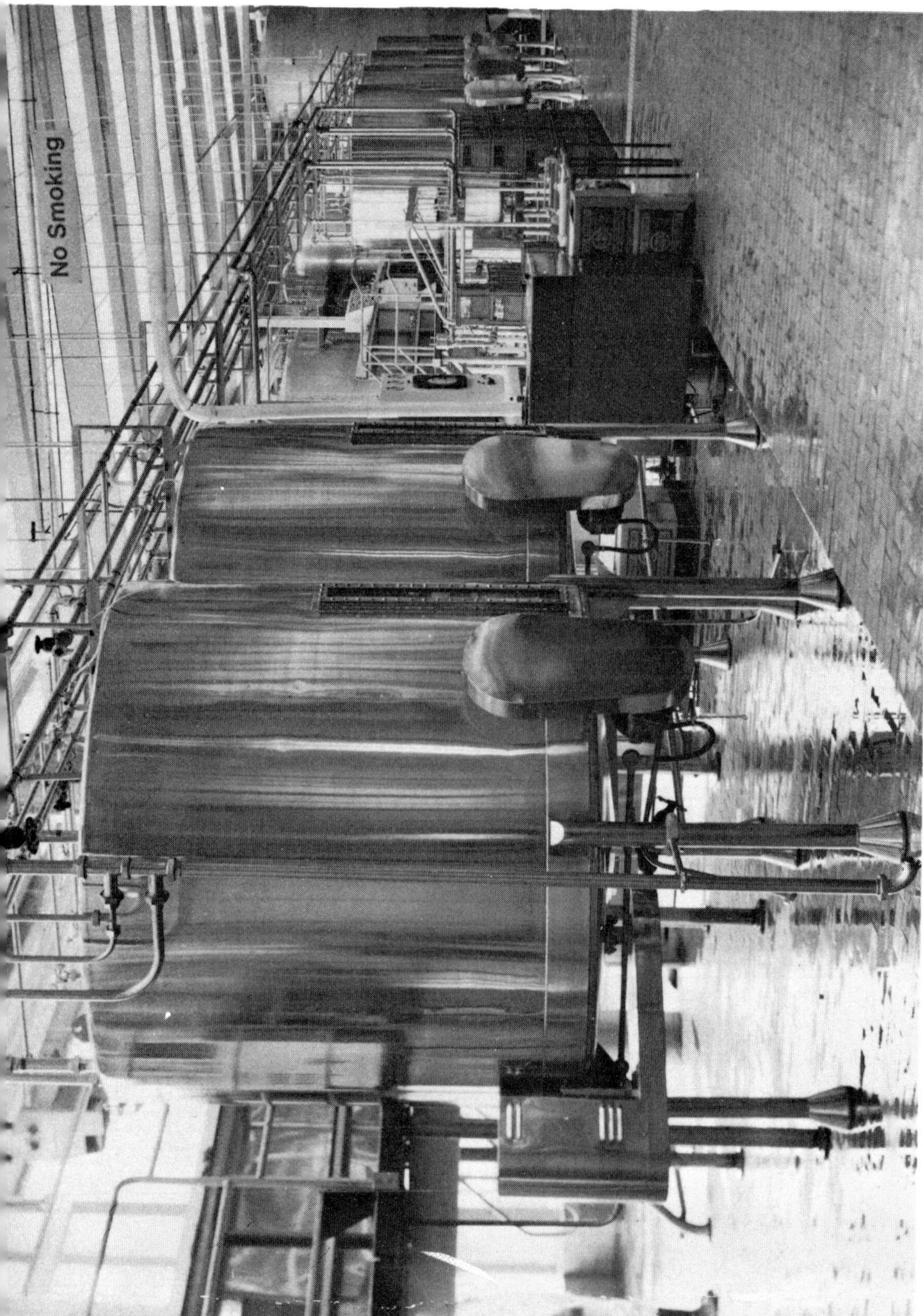

An example of well-designed hygienic plant and layout.

APPENDIX

Hygienic Design of Food Plant (1967)

Joint Technical Committee, FMF/FMA

INTRODUCTION

The detailed preparation of this publication was carried out by a Working Party appointed by the Joint Technical Committee of the Food Manufacturers' Federation and the Food Machinery Association in October 1966.

The composition of the Working Party was as follows:

Mr D. T. Shore, M.Sc.(Eng.), A.C.G.I., C.Eng., F.I.Mech.E., A.M.I.Chem.E.
—Food Machinery Association
Mr S. Brightwell, M.Sc.
—Food Manufacturers' Federation
Mr G. A. Lea, B.Sc., A.R.I.C., M.R.S.H., F.I.F.S.T.
—British Food Manufacturing Industries Research Association
Mr R. Jowitt, B.Sc.(Eng.), D.L.C., Dip.Chem.Eng.(U.C.L.), C.Eng., M.I.Chem.E., M.I.Mech.E.
—National College of Food Technology
Mr G. G. Popham, B.Sc., C.Eng., M.I.Mech.E.
—Food Manufacturers' Federation
Mr F. de Saulles
—Food Machinery Association
assisted by:
Mr J. B. Wells, B.Com.
Mr K. Rowe
—Food Manufacturers' Federation
Mr S. C. M. Salter, B.Sc.(Tech.), A.M.C.T., C.Eng., A.M.I.Chem.E.
—Food Machinery Association
Mr P. Lloyd-Jones
Mr G. M. Wootton, C.Eng., M.I.Mech.E.,

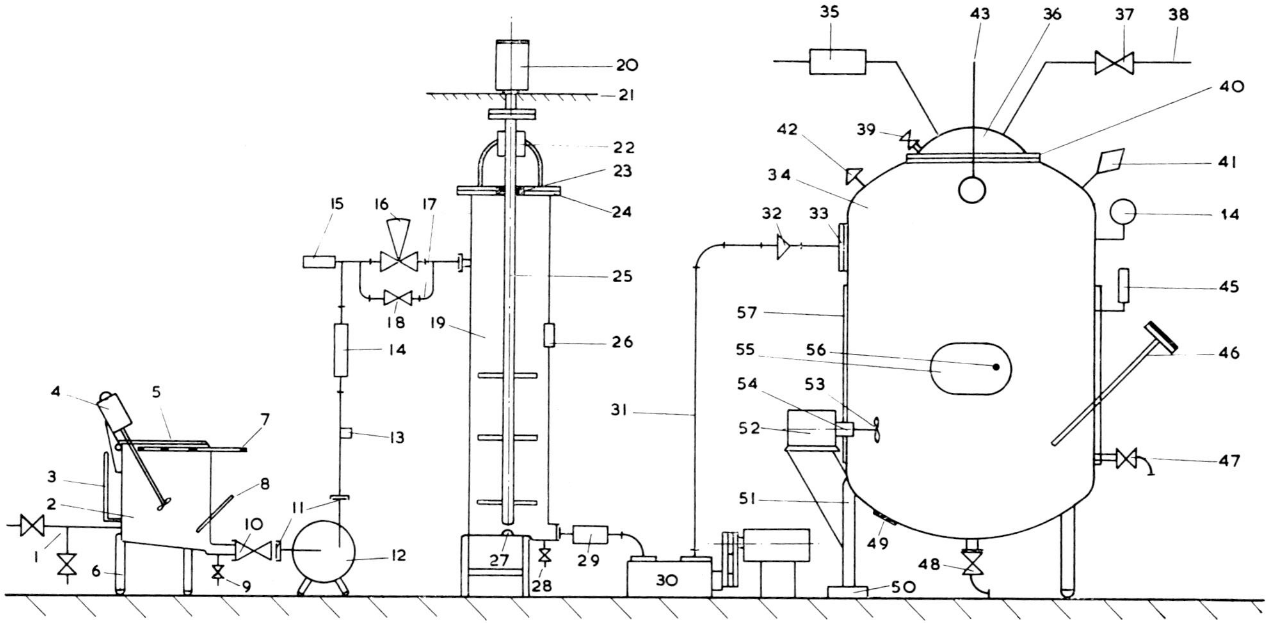

KEY TO FIG. 1

1. Product/water inlet
2. Vessel open to atmosphere
3. Level gauge
4. Protable agitator
5. Cover
6. Feet
7. Spray tube
8. Steam lance
9. Drain
10. Cock
11. Pipe fittings
12. Centrifugal pump
13. Pressure switch
14. Flow meter
15. Temperature probe
16. Control valve
17. By-pass
18. Valve
19. Sealed vessel
20. Drive and coupling
21. Drive support
22. Bearing
23. Seal
24. Joint
25. Agitator
26. Sight glass
27. Bottom bearing
28. Drain
29. Pipe line filter
30. Positive pump
31. Welded pipe line
32. Non-return valve
33. Flanged connection
34. Pressure vessel
35. Air filter
36. Top manway
37. Steam valve
38. Steam line
39. Vent
40. Manway joint
41. Pressure relief valve
42. Anti-vacuum valve
43. In-place cleaning
44. Pressure gauge
45. Thermometer
46. Thermometer pocket
47. Sample valve
48. Outlet valve
49. Differential pressure element
50. Load cell
51. Legs
52. Drive
53. Agitator
54. Gland
55. Side manway
56. Sample point
57. Jacket

Fig. 1 – Items requiring attention to hygienic design.

Background

The Joint Technical Committee had felt that, whilst there had been great improvement in the hygienic design of much food processing equipment in recent years, there was a lack of standards and general guidance in this important field. The Working Party was accordingly instructed to consider what codes of practice or design standards were at present in use by groups or individual companies both in the UK and elsewhere and to prepare an authoritative guide to good practice which would be helpful to a wide range of suppliers and users of food processing equipment and so to raise the overall standard of hygiene.

It was soon obvious that the range of products, processes and equipment involved was both large and diverse. It was therefore agreed to limit this publication to what may be regarded as a pilot exercise dealing with tanks, pumps and interconnecting pipework primarily concerned with the handling of liquids, although it is believed that much of the material contained should be of general interest and value.

Initial search revealed there to be no official standards relating specifically to hygienic design in the UK, although a few standards issued or in preparation by the British Standards Institution for specific items of dairy equipment contained references to certain hygienic design features. (The relevant standards issued are referred to in the appropriate sections of the text.) The Working Party also noted the provisions of Part II Section 6 of the Food Hygiene (General) Regulations 1960.

Investigation of the position on the Continent, revealed that no standards or codes of practice relating to hygienic design existed there either.

Consideration was given to information from America made available by the 3A Sanitary Standards Committee, the US Baking Industry Sanitation Standards Committee and the National Canners Association of USA and to the publication 'Sanitary Design of Food Processing Equipment' issued by the journal, 'Food Processing', and based largely on recommendations of the aforementioned bodies.

In order to produce a practical document in a short space of time it was necessary for the Working Party to proceed without formal contact with other bodies. Hence, as stated in the title, this publication is to be regarded as a guide to good practice and not as a formal statement of standard requirements.

Scope

This guide deals with the hygienic design aspects of tanks, pumps and pipework.

The individual features which may be present and require consideration are indicated in Fig. 1. Tanks may be of open or closed design, pressurised or subjected to vacuum operation. Pumps may be of a wide variety with direct or indirect coupled drives, while circuit pipework may contain fittings such as pressure gauges, thermometers, etc., necessary for the operation of the process. Similarly, the vessels may contain agitators, mixers, etc.; product sampling points and devices for in-place cleaning may also be required.

To assist in the specification of equipment which must be manufactured and supplied for hygienic operation, the guide deals first with hygienic design principles and with criteria for materials of construction applicable to any items of equipment, then considers the requirements of particular items under the following broad heads:

Tanks, open and closed
Pumps
Valves
Product Piping (including fittings)
Motors and drives

The sections contain drawings illustrating particular features of design appropriate to the particular sections. In addition a number of photographs are grouped in a final section, each illustrating a number of hygienic features of some interest.

HYGIENIC DESIGN PRINCIPLES

The Committee agrees with the seven basic principles for hygienic design outlined in the American document 'Sanitary Design'* as follows:

'1. All surfaces in contact with food must be inert to the food under the conditions of use and must not migrate to or be absorbed by the food.

2. All surfaces in contact with food must be smooth and nonporous so that tiny particles of food, bacteria, or insect eggs are not caught in microscopic surface crevices and become difficult to dislodge, thus becoming a potential source of contamination.

3. All surfaces in contact with the food must be visible for inspection, or the equipment must be readily disassembled for inspection, or it must be demonstrated that routine cleaning procedures eliminate possibility of contamination from bacteria or insects.

* Reprinted from 'Food Processing', October 1964 and April 1965 and 'Food Processing Catalog 1964/5'.

4. All surfaces in contact with food must be readily accessible for manual cleaning, or if not readily accessible, then readily disassembled for manual cleaning, or if clean-in-place techniques are used, it must be demonstrated that the results achieved without disassembly are the equivalent of those obtained with disassembly and manual cleaning.
5. All interior surfaces in contact with food must be so arranged that the equipment is self emptying or self draining.
6. Equipment must be so designed as to protect the contents from external contamination.
7. The exterior or non-product contact surfaces should be arranged to prevent harboring of soils, bacteria or pests in and on the equipment itself as well as in its contact with other equipment, floors, walls or hanging supports.'

There is no substitute for common sense, and no specification can be complete enough to ensure an hygienic design. Good design requires much attention to detail. It is seldom that a single plant item can be considered in isolation; one must consider the process itself, the environment in which the equipment is placed and, of course, the maintenance which will be provided throughout the life of the equipment. The compatibility of the equipment with the product, the environment and also the cleaning fluids are of vital importance.

It must be recognised that there are degrees of hygienic design generally related to the permitted tolerance of microbial infection in the final product. This document is not primarily concerned with process plant design for completely aseptic operation, but rather with the maintenance of a general standard of hygiene throughout the process equipment. Designs must allow for easy dismantling of components for rapid cleaning or in-place cleaning methods must be incorporated as part of the basic design. It is suggested that the latter will give more reliable microbiological results, particularly on large installations and where an automated cleaning cycle is justified.

The frequency of cleaning will be determined by the nature of the product and process but must not permit significant contamination of the product by residues which may have undesirable microbial growth. In this connection it should be noted that combinations of product and process are not uncommon which necessitate that the plant be cleaned after operating periods as short as 4 hours.

In applying the principles indicated in this section the object must be to design food plant which will either remain clean during its normal operation or be such that cleaning will enable the equipment to be restored to the desired degree of cleanliness.

MATERIALS OF CONSTRUCTION
(including Coatings, Finish and Jointing Materials)

1. Design criteria

a. Inertness

All surfaces in contact with food should be inert to the food under the conditions of use, and must not migrate to or be absorbed by the food. Surfaces should also be inert to such cleaning materials as may reasonably be employed and to approved methods of sterilising. Inertness includes freedom from corrosion (whether stress, crevice, electrolytic, shielding, weld decay, or other type) and from catalytic activity. Of itself, staining may not be harmful, but is objectionable psychologically, and may decrease the visibility of soil.

b. Mechanical stability

Materials used should show resistance to major deformation, denting, chipping, flaking, and delamination.

c. Surface finish

All surfaces in contact with food should be smooth and non-porous, and free from pits and crevices. The aim in all cases must be to provide a surface from all parts of which food residue can readily be removed during appropriate cleaning procedures, thereby leaving no material which can serve as a medium for bacterial growth. A high surface polish is valuable in helping to make soiling visible. The relationship between cleanability and surface finish is by no means clear at the present time. Recent work at the National College of Food Technology, directed towards clarifying the subject, is summarised on page 273.

d. Surface stability

Materials used should be such that the original surface finish is maintained under all conditions of use for which designed, and under all reasonable cleaning and sterilising conditions. No development of porosity should occur.

e. Permanent joints

Where permanent joints are required in contact with food, these should be made by welding or brazing. If material other than the parent metal is used for this purpose, this should be chosen with due regard to the possibility of dissimilar metal corrosion under the conditions of use.

f. Coatings and linings

Coatings, linings, or plating over a constructional base material may be employed where appropriate, in order to provide a surface with desirable characteristics in contact with food. The criteria set out in the preceding paragraphs should apply to any lining material. In addition particular attention should be paid to the avoidance of crazing, cracking, or chipping due to either mechanical action or temperature changes. The base material should be such that, in the event of its exposure to foodstuffs following failure of the lining, no hazard from toxicity will arise, nor any marked chemical activity occur.

g. Jointing materials

Jointing materials may be of natural or synthetic rubber or of other suitable material, of approved food quality. They should be inert to the food and no migration into the food should occur. In particular, they should not impart to the food any toxic substance, colour, odour or flavour. They should be suitable for cleaning and sterilising by the normal procedures. Joints should be free from patches, blisters, porosity, embedded foreign materials, and physical defects. They should be mechanically stable, in so far as this is compatible with the necessary resilience.

h. Non-contact surfaces

Non-contact surfaces (*i.e.* surfaces not normally in contact with food materials) should be mechanically stable, smoothly finished, and easily cleanable. Coatings generally recognised as being of a toxic nature should not be used.

i. Materials identification

The nature of the material(s) of construction should be indicated on the exterior of a tank, together with any temperature limitations which may be appropriate.

2. Pointers to the suitability of specific classes of materials

The preferred material in most cases is austenitic stainless steel, and grades such as 321 S12* (En 58B) or 304 S16* (En 58E) are frequently satisfactory. Pitting attack may be troublesome where acidic liquors are to be handled in the presence of salt, and in such cases, better resistance to this form of corrosion may be obtained by the use of a molybdenum-bearing stainless steel such as 316 S16† (En 58 J). In severe conditions, where high temperatures are also encountered, it may be necessary to use a steel containing greater proportions of nickel, chromium and molybdenum.

For tanks, other materials which are used are aluminium; glass-lined steel; steel lined with other materials (*e.g.* epoxy resins); high density polyethylene, polypropylene, acrylonitrile–butadiene-styrene copolymer, chloroprene, polytetrafluoroethylene and polyester resins reinforced with glass fibre.

* See B.S. 1449: Part 4: 1967.
† See B.S. 1449: Part 2: 1967.

Pipelines are generally of stainless steel of appropriate grade, but in some cases glass is used. For flexible pipes, where these cannot be avoided, food quality rubber (natural, synthetic or silicone) or plastic materials such as polyethylene, polypropylene and nylon are suitable.

Pump parts in contact with food may be entirely of stainless steel, or may incorporate non-metallic materials such as food quality rubber (natural or synthetic) and nylon for seals and bushes. Stainless steel castings find extensive application in pumps and particularly as pipeline fittings. They are produced in several corrosion-resisting grades and may be welded without undue difficulty.

For gaskets, food quality rubber is used. This may be natural or synthetic (*e.g.* chloroprene, butadiene/styrene, butadiene/acrylonitrile or silicone) according to the particular duty. Canvas reinforcements should not be exposed to the product.

With certain notable exceptions (*viz.* in brewing, distilling and manufacture of sugar confectionery) copper is generally unsatisfactory for food equipment. It should be specifically avoided in contact with meat, fats and fruit and with vegetables, especially when brine is present.

Tinned surfaces, while generally satisfactory in contact with foodstuffs, carry the hazard of exposure of the base metal if perforation, damage or excessive wear occurs.

Nickel, nickel alloys, silver and titanium are useful materials in some circumstances.

Materials to be avoided include zinc (except for galvanised steel pipes carrying water of pH greater than 7); lead (except as a constituent of solder, in which it should not exceed 5%); cadmium and antimony; plastic materials containing free phenol, formaldehyde or plasticisers; wood.

OPEN OR CLOSED TANKS

1. General comments

In order to encourage the cleaning of equipment, reduction of the time involved and ease of access are important considerations.

The design, materials, construction and installation should be such as to facilitate in-place chemical cleaning. The units of equipment should contain the minimum number of parts so that, when dismantling for cleaning is necessary, subsequent reassembly may be effected readily by unskilled labour. The equipment should be placed so as to permit easy access for hygienic, as well as mechanical, maintenance.

The notes and comments, which follow, are generally compatible with extracts from the following British Standards:—

BS 3719	Stationary Milk Tanks
BS 3441	Milk Tankers
BS 1515: part 2	Fusion Welded Pressure Vessels for use in the Chemical, Petroleum and Allied Industries. Austenitic Stainless Steel
CP 3003	Lining of Vessels and Equipment for Chemical Processes.

2. Design and construction

(a) All surfaces in contact with food should be readily accessible for cleaning and visual inspection.

Where conditions render this impossible provision should be made to remove or expose hidden parts for inspection and cleaning.

(b) Outlets should be finished flush inside the tank. Exposed threads should not be used.

(c) Equipment should be arranged to be self-emptying or self-draining and pockets or depressions are to be avoided.

(d) The equipment should be designed to protect the contents from external contamination.

(e) Demountable type hinges should be fitted and, wherever possible, consist of the simple hook-on type without bolts. It is essential that lids, when opened, do not cause drainage into the tank. Lid joints should be easily removable for cleaning.

(f) The exterior or non-product contact surfaces should be readily cleanable and should be arranged to prevent harbouring of dirt, bacteria or pests. When cleaning is taking place no material from the exterior should be allowed to contaminate the inside of the tank.

(g) If the tank legs are of hollow stock they should be completely sealed. Ties and braces should be minimal and where used should avoid acute angles, crevices and other dirt-harbouring surfaces.

(h) All external nuts should be captive with a minimum showing of threads.

(k) Shaft seals, glands and bearings (mechanical) should be easily removable for inspection, maintenance and cleaning. Design of shaft seals, glands and bearings for mechanical agitators should be hygienic, *e.g.* mechanical rotary seals rather than packed glands.

(l) All welding should be designed so that the completed weld can be adequately ground.

(m) Where it is necessary to have stiffening bars on the top of a tank, they should be of the stand-off type or continuously welded.

(n) Where clean-in-place (CIP) is not used, the diameter of horizontal tanks or height of vertical tanks should be such as to allow manual cleaning of the tank.

(o) Attention should be directed to the possibility of internal fittings masking tank surfaces, or themselves having masked surfaces, where CIP is used.

(p) Stainless steel ball feet are preferred, but where flanged feet are necessary for any reason, these feet should be fixed to the floor on adhesive pads.

(q) Manways should be in accordance with BS 3719. Manway covers should be of a design which will not produce interior pockets.

(r) Design of the vessel should be such as to prevent flexing under load conditions and thus creating hollows or pockets.

(s) Agitators wherever possible should be of the top entry type. The shaft hole in the tank top should be shielded to prevent the ingress of oil or foreign matter into the contents of the tank. Where side or bottom entry agitators must be used special attention should be paid to the design of glands.

3. Fabrication

(a) All internal corners should be radiused and, where possible, have minimum radii of 2″.

(b) Care should be taken to avoid all possible sources of surface contamination during fabrication. Where flame cutting is used, the surface should be removed by grinding to prevent slag inclusion.

(c) All stainless steel welds should be argon arc and should be continuous. (See BS 3719, para. 2(f).)

(d) All joints should be butt welded where possible. If fillet welds are used they should be given generous radii. Filler wires should be of similar composition to the parent metal.

(e) Where it is necessary to use mild steel brackets or supports, these should not be welded directly to a stainless steel tank. In all cases stainless steel backing plates should be used. Damage to the tank by external welding must be avoided.

4. Location

(a) Tanks should be installed at a height sufficient to provide adequate access for cleaning and inspection and preferably not less than 8 inches off the ground, or should be installed completely sealed to the floor or plinth.

(b) All parts of equipment should be installed at a sufficient distance from wall and ceiling areas to provide access for cleaning and inspection.

(c) All ancillary items and services related to the vessel should be located either on the vessel, or sufficiently clear of the vessel, in such a way as to allow proper maintenance and cleaning.

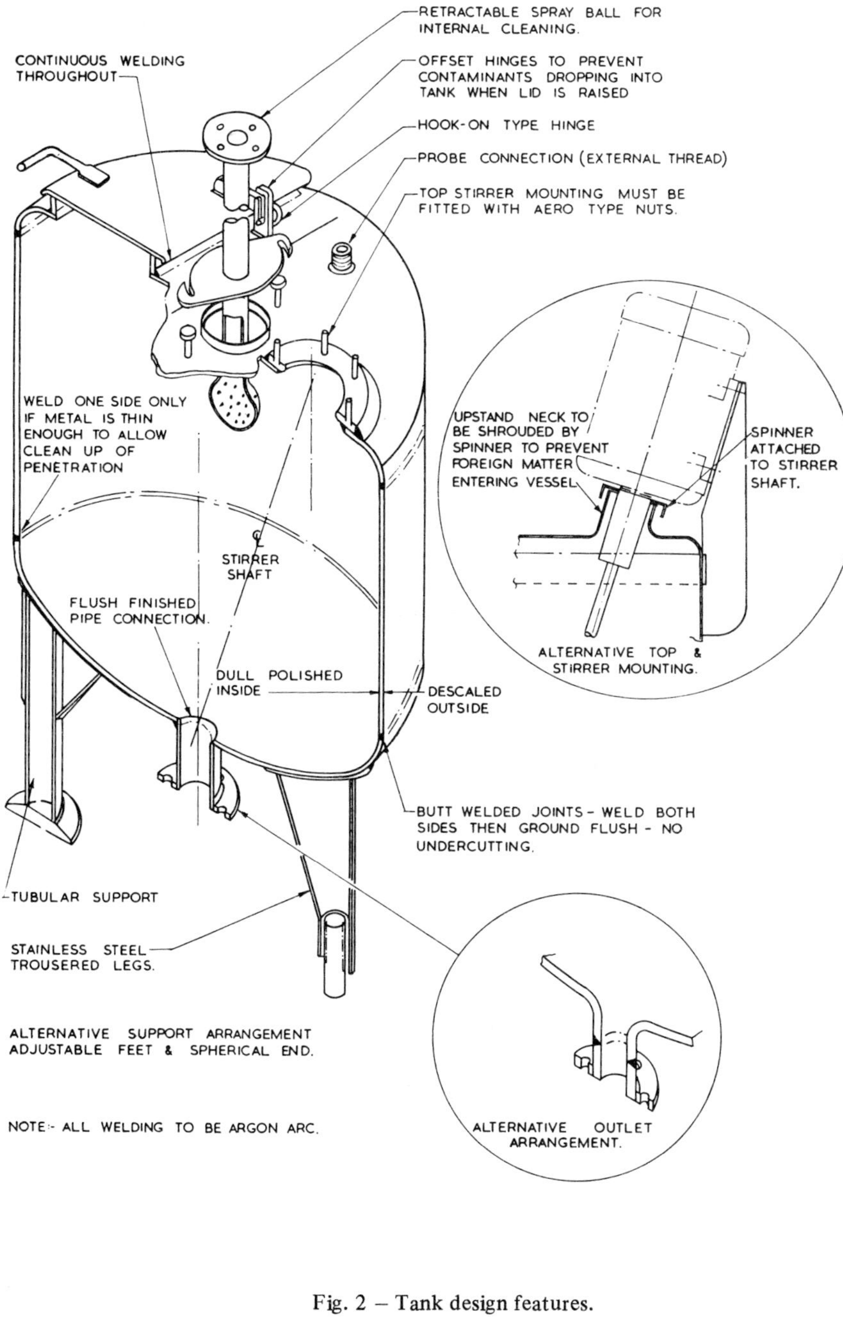

Fig. 2 – Tank design features.

PUMPS

1. Pump types

Some types of pump are inherently more hygienic than others. As a general guide the various types are listed below in approximate order of decreasing inherent hygiene:

- Peristaltic
- Fluid diaphragm
- Diaphragm
- Air-lift
- Ejector:
  - Steam-operated
  - Air-operated
- Open impeller kinetic:
  - Propeller (axial flow)
  - Centrifugal
- Closed impeller kinetic:
  - Centrifugal
  - Screw (axial flow)
- Rotary positive displacement:
  - Single rotor flexible lobe
  - Screw in flexible stator
  - Double rotor lobe
- Various gear types:
  - Sliding vane
  - Worm and wheel
- Reciprocating:
  - Single plunger (external valves)
  - Multi-plunger (external valves)
  - Single plunger (internal valves)
  - Multi-plunger (internal valves)
  - Single acting piston (external valves)
  - Double-acting piston (external valves)
  - Single-acting piston (internal valves)
  - Double-acting piston (internal valves)

In practice hygienic design has to be reconciled with functional requirements. A pump of good inherent hygienic design may not be suitable for a particular pumping duty.

Further, in considering the list it should be borne in mind that different makes of a particular type may be more or less hygienic in design. Where care has been paid to details of design and construction some pumps which might generally be classified as of relatively low inherent hygienic design may be pre-eminently suitable for certain food pumping duties.

Design or adaptation for food use should include consideration of the following requirements:

2. Design

(a) Passage shapes should be smooth, sharp changes in cross-section should be avoided and dead spaces or turbulence-promoting features minimised.

(b) When cleaning-in-place (CIP) is intended this will be facilitated by meeting the above criteria. Otherwise ease of dismantling is essential to allow access for cleaning all surfaces which contact food material. The number of parts should be a minimum.

(c) Parts requiring periodic replacement should be easily replaceable and designed so that they cannot be wrongly assembled. Joints and seals should be so designed that leak-proof assembly is most easily achieved with the correct components without recourse to sealing compounds.

(d) Screw-threads in contact with food material should be avoided, *e.g.* by retaining impellers with cap nut and gasket. Where unavoidable, threads should be male, coarse and shallow, preferably not less than 60° nor more than 8 tpi.

(e) Location of moving components should be by flats rather than by keyways or splines.

(f) Clamp rings or bayonet couplings of smooth, 'clean' shape are preferable to bolts as fastenings for pump bodies.

(g) Pumps should be so designed as to be readily emptied of product. In the case of non-positive pumps adequate clearances and appropriate arrangement of branches, internal ports and components should permit self-draining.

(h) Positive pumps should be either similarly self-draining or capable of being operated so as to be self-emptying. This usually implies suitability for operation empty for short periods.

(i) Pump overload prevention should not involve venting to atmosphere or recirculation of process material at the pump.* Where this is unavoidable careful consideration of the design with reference to the foregoing requirements is advisable.

(j) Bearings should be located outside the product zone and be of sealed or self-lubricating type.

(k) Wherever possible shaft seals should be of the mechanical type and accessible for inspection, adjustment and maintenance.

(l) Any leakage which might occur should be readily visible and should be to the open (*i.e.* not into closed spaces such as motor casings).

(m) All external parts should be easily cleanable and capable of withstanding frequent hosing or such other cleaning down procedures as are commonly used in the intended location.

* Possible alternatives include electrical overload protection, excess-pressure-switched relays, mechanical overload protection (slipping clutches, shear pins) or ring-main re-circulation provisions.

3. Location and ancillaries

(a) In general, pump location should be such as to facilitate cleaning of pump, drive, motor, adjacent equipment and floor, and to avoid dirt-traps.

(b) Ancillaries mounted on or with the pump should meet the relevant design requirements in section 2 above and should be located in accordance with 3(a) above.

(c) Portable pumps (*i.e.* pumps intended to be used for short periods only in any one location and small enough to be carried from place to place) and non-portable pumps should preferably be mounted on legs. Legs should be smooth with rounded ends, and free of exposed screw threads.

(d) Mobile pumps (*i.e.* pumps intended to be used for short periods only in any one location but not suitable for carrying from place to place) should be provided with wheels designed in accordance with the appropriate hygienic requirements in this and in other relevant sections. Wheels and chassis should in particular comply with 2(m) above.

(e) Fixed pumps supported other than on legs should have their base plates and plinths separate from those for their motors. Base plates and plinths should be free from ribs, flanges or crevices and have smooth surfaces. Upward-facing surfaces should be given an outward fall to ensure drainage. Intersections between plinth and floor should be concavely radiused.

(f) Supporting framework and legs should be constructed from tubular stock rather than rolled steel sections. Hollow stock should be sealed.

(g) When supports are not sealed to the floor, *e.g.* by plinths, a minimum ground clearance of 4″ should be provided for cleaning access.

(h) Piping and valves should be supported independently of pumps, which should be levelled to enable hygienic connections to be made without strain on pump, piping or joints.

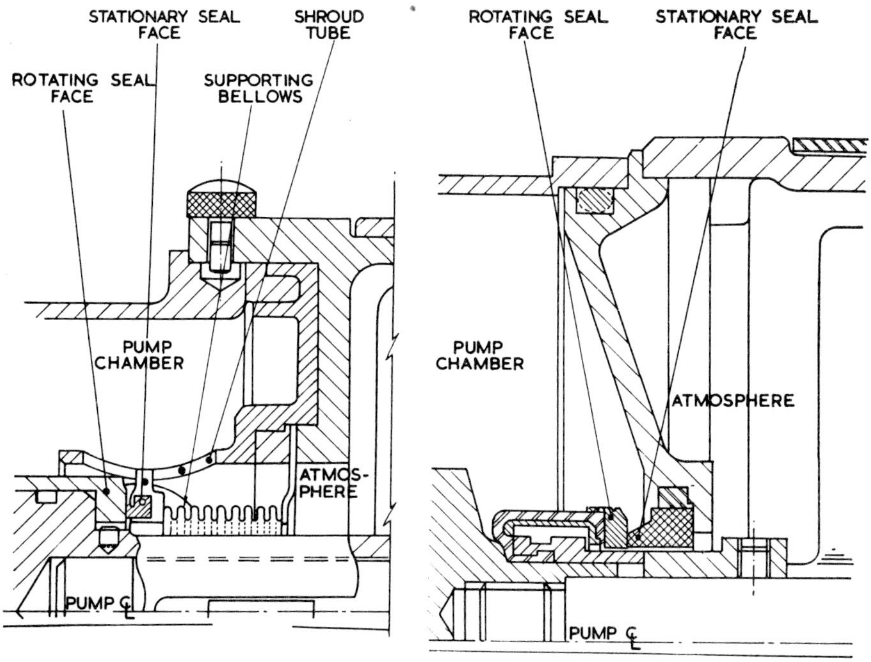

a) OLD SEAL DESIGN
Metal bellows supporting stationary seal face and shroud tube tend to obstruct free flow of fluid and to trap particles.

b) IMPROVED SEAL DESIGN
Flow obstructions and particle traps eradicated.

Fig. 3 – Mechanical seal in food pump at entry of driving shaft through wall of pump chamber.

a.) Initial design.

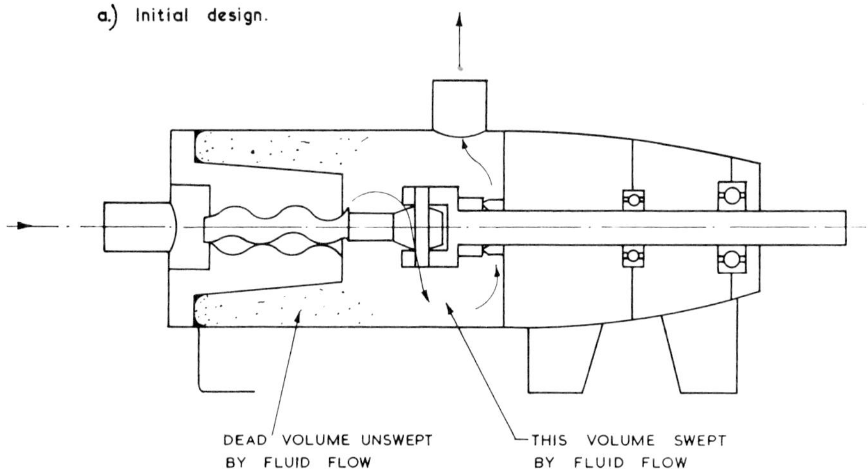

b.) Modified design.

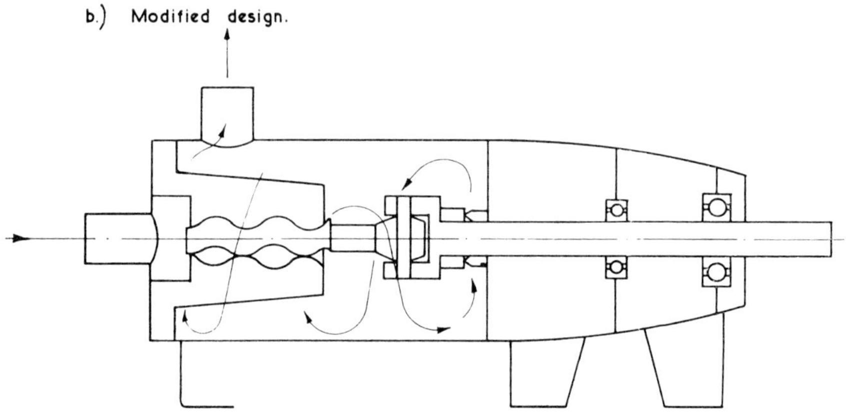

FULL VOLUME SWEPT BY FLUID FLOW.

Fig. 4 – Hygienic design of pump improved by repositioning outlet branch.

VALVES

1. General classification

The types of valve available may be generally classified in approximate order of decreasing suitability from the point of view of hygiene as follows:

1. Glandless valves
   a) Pinch cock (mechanically or fluid operated)
   b) Diaphragm
   c) Diaphragm sealed (between the product and activating mechanism)
2. Butterfly valves
3. Plug cocks, including ball type
4. Standard globe, needle and gate valves, etc.

It is not possible to state any absolute order of hygienic suitability (although some valves, *e.g.* plug type, are obviously more hygienic than others, *e.g.* gate) since other factors are of importance, in particular the method of sealing the valve mechanism. These methods, in usual order of hygienic suitability are:

a) Diaphragm
b) Lip seal
c) 'O' ring
d) Packed gland.

2. Stop and regulating valves

(*a*) *Glandless valves* (Figs. 5 a–d)

The most hygienic valve will be without joints or crevices in which food particles can lodge and remain during normal product flow and normal in-place cleaning. The only valves which can meet this standard are the pinch type or diaphragm valves. These valves can be supplied with normal hygienic end connections, and the flow of the product through the fully-open valve is completely uninterrupted. The tube or diaphragm of the valve makes a complete seal in the closed position and the operating mechanism is simple and situated entirely outside the bore of the valve.

Its limitations in use are due to the flexible diaphragm which can distort after extensive service and may, in fact, rupture. The diaphragm material also limits its temperature and pressure of operation and where in-place cleaning is involved care has to be taken in selecting the temperature and composition of the cleaning fluids.

This valve is especially suitable for automatic operation.

b. Butterfly valve (Figs. 5 e and f)

This type of valve incorporates many of the features required for good hygienic design and, being of all-metal construction with the exception of the glands, it is not subject to the same limitations of temperature and pressure as is the pinch type.

However, insofar as this type of valve must be fitted with a stem with a moving part in the valve body, there is a possibility that the product may seep back into the valve stem.

c. Plug cocks (Figs. 5 g and h)

The plug cock is widely used in the food industry and has the advantage of being easily dismantled and reassembled. When the valve is open there is no interruption to the product flow and as such the valve is completely hygienic. However, as the valve relies on the entire cock turning in the valve body it is possible for product to remain between the plug and the valve body, and this necessitates a dismantling of the valve for cleaning.

Glass plug cocks are sometimes used, mainly in conjunction with glass pipelines. In addition to the general comments on plug cocks listed above these have the normal advantages and disadvantages of glass as a material of construction and further are subject to severe limitation when using in-place cleaning with hot alkaline detergents.

The ball cock is an adaptation of the plug cock principle in which the plug is replaced by a spherical ball, the prime reason being to reduce the frictional resistance to turning the cock. However, as compared with the plug cock there are undesirable dead pockets, and more parts to dismantle for cleaning.

d. Globe, needle and gate valves

These valves as a class present two problems of hygienic design. Firstly the actuation requires a spindle moving through a gland between the body and atmosphere. Secondly, sealing requires a complicated flow chamber to receive the globe head, needle or gate, resulting in serious interruption to smooth flow or in dead pockets.

Valves with packed glands are generally unsatisfactory since it is impossible to clean this area without dismantling the packing.

In-place cleaning techniques may, however, be adequate for cleaning the body of valves in this class particularly when the design and construction or the physical orientation of the valve in the production line permits a thorough scavenging of the contact surface.

These valves are, in general, not suited to the handling of food products but examples of this type, in which a spindle moves through the product and in which attention has been given to hygienic design, are given in Figs. i and j.

3. Pressure relief safety and diversion valves

Examples of hygienic designs of these types of valves are given in Figs. k and l. Fig. k is superior in design to Fig. l as the former is moulded integrally with a section of the product flowline and provision is made for diversion of the product under high pressure conditions to a tank or other vessel. The valve shown in Fig. m is mounted in a 'T' which is in itself unhygienic and no provision is made for containing the vented product.

4. Design criteria

(a) Within the limits of each valve type, the flow passage should be smooth with no abrupt changes in cross-section.

(b) The finish of metal parts should be smooth and free from defects (see reference to 'Surface finish' in section on 'Materials of construction'). Other materials should have at least an equivalent finish. Outside surfaces should have smooth contours and a finish which is easily cleaned.

(c) The design should allow for easy dismantling for maintenance and cleaning and should be inherently self-draining.

(d) The design should ensure that any leakage is immediately evident and the source easily detected.

(e) Gaskets and joints should be installed to give an effective seal and be flush with adjacent surfaces. They should be positively retained so that they do not distort or move from their position when under pressure or vacuum.

(f) There should be complete isolation of the product from the valve mechanism and from external contamination.

(g) Seatings should be designed so as to make an effective seal where shut off is required and should not hinder self-draining. Seatings should give a smooth contour to the bore. Where soft seatings are used, they should be so retained that they are not easily displaced when either pressure or vacuum is applied. In particular, seatings should be designed to resist wear and to allow regular maintenance since wear or distortion will affect hygienic character.

(h) The direction of opening and closing and the open or closed 'state' of the valve should be readily apparent. This is desirable to avoid process problems due to operation faults. For in-place cleaning evidence of valve state is a safety requirement.

(i) Connections should be by hygienic fittings and of the same type throughout the installation. Fittings should preferably be integrally cast or otherwise rigidly secured to valve or cock by welding.

(See also 'Pipe connections' in the section 'Product Piping'.)

(j) Valve and cock sizes should normally be designated by the bore dimensions of the pipeline or fittings for which their end connections are made.

(k) Exposed threads must, and screw or bolt heads or nuts should, be eliminated from the product area.

(l) Where diaphragms are used in contact with the product they should be well secured and capable of withstanding the temperatures and pressures required during product flow, sterilisation and cleaning.

(m) Where lubricants are required the design must be such that edible or other approved grades will be suitable.

(n) Where part of the valve mechanism is unavoidably within the product area, for example the spring of a relief valve, it should be capable of being easily dismantled for frequent cleaning.

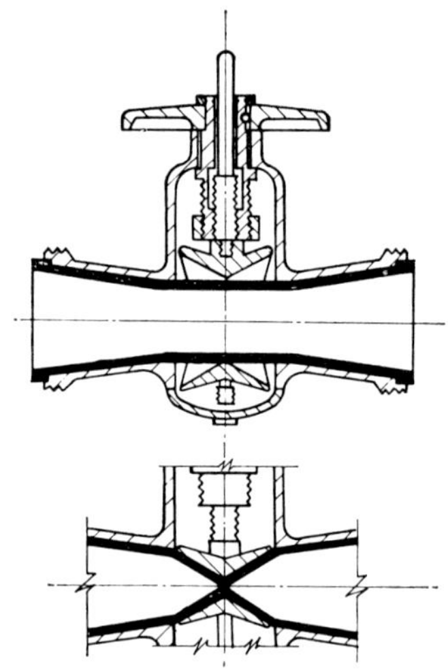

Fig. 5a – Mechanically-operated pinch cock.

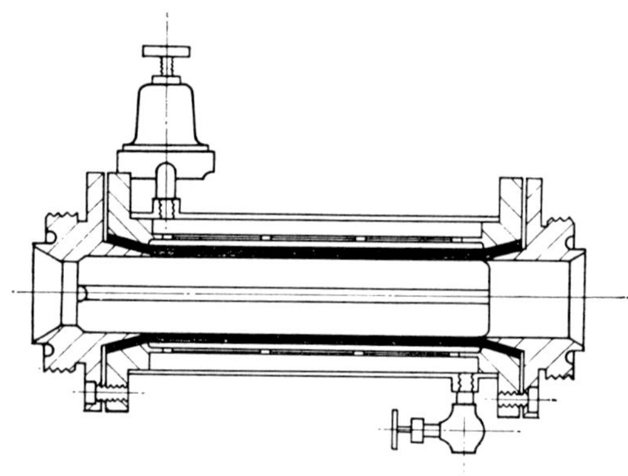

Fig. 5b – Pneumatic valve air-operated pinch cock.

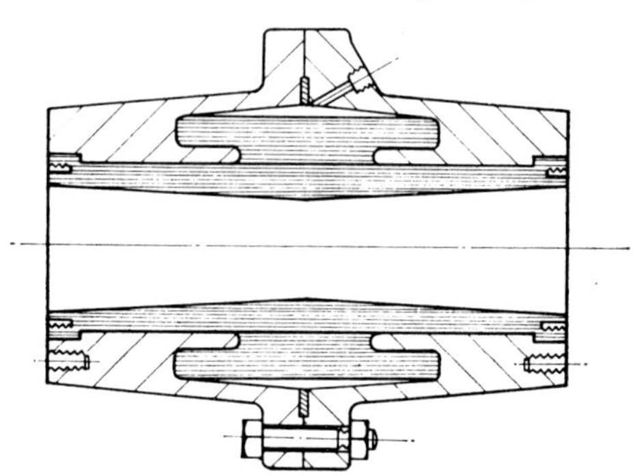

Fig. 5c – Fluid-operated pinch cock.

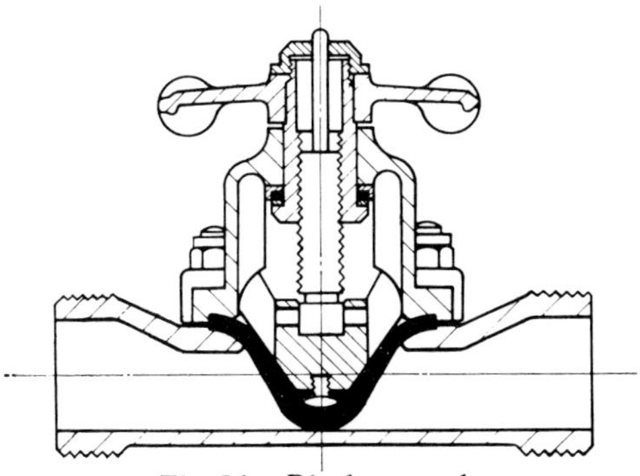

Fig. 5d – Diaphragm valve.

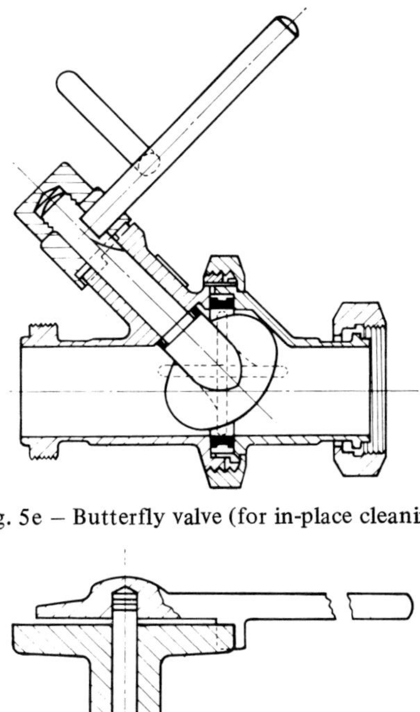

Fig. 5e – Butterfly valve (for in-place cleaning).

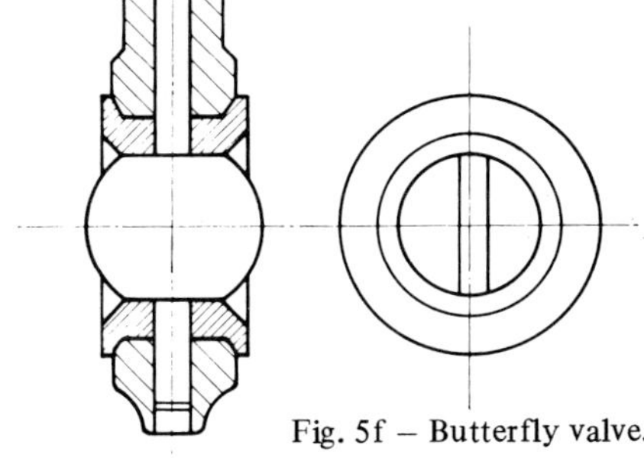

Fig. 5f – Butterfly valve.

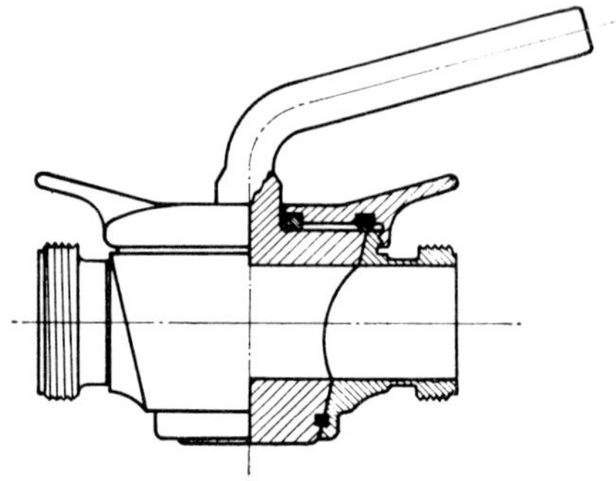

Fig. 5g – Plug cock with smooth bore.

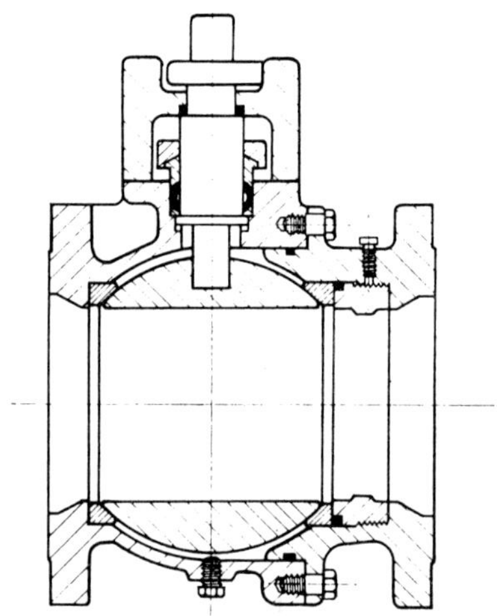

Fig. 5h – Ball cock.

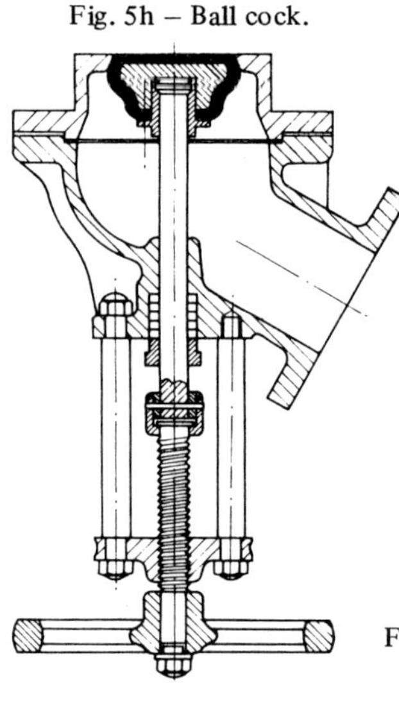

Fig. 5i – Tank outlet valve.

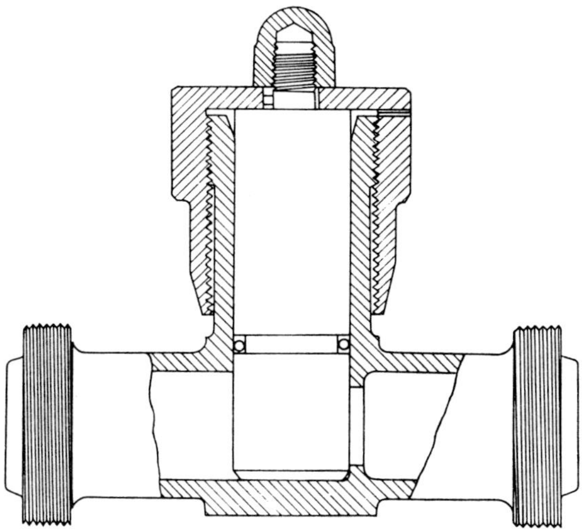

Fig. 5j – Graduated flow control valve.

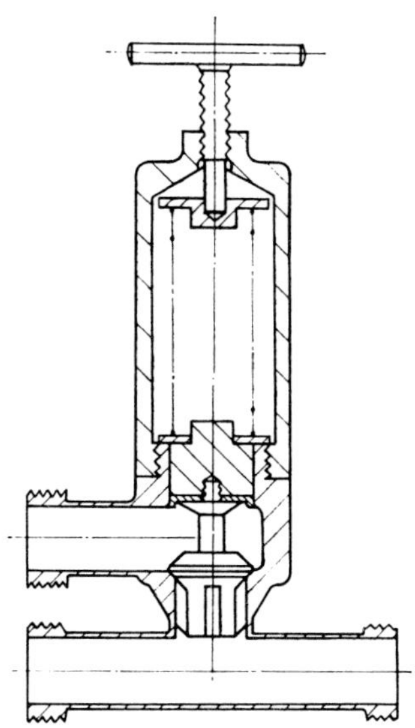

Fig. 5k – Relief valve spring-loaded.

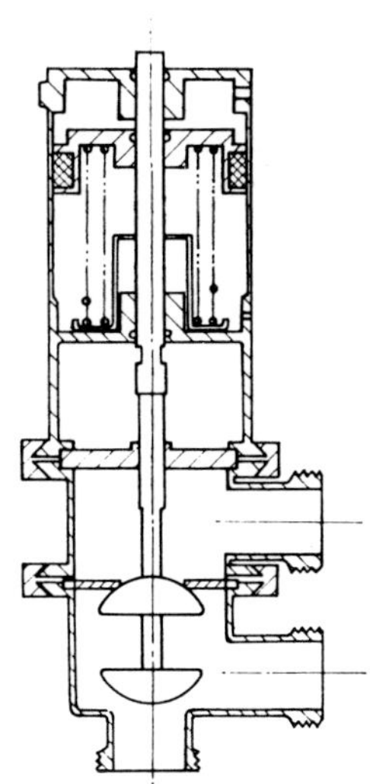

Fig. 5l – Air-operated diversion valve spring assisted.

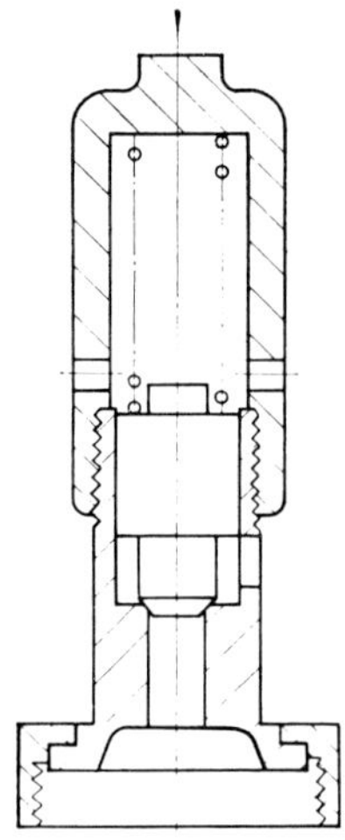

Fig. 5m – Relief valve spring-loaded.

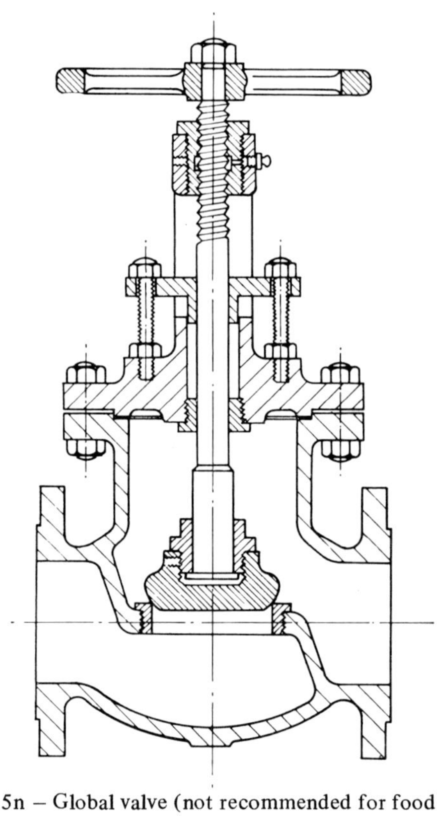

Fig. 5n – Global valve (not recommended for food use).

PRODUCT PIPING

1. Pipe connections

Pipe lengths may be joined by butt welding or by the use of hygienic fittings.

(a) Butt welding should provide a smooth and crevice-free inside bore with a weld bead not exceeding 1/32″ in depth.

(b) Fittings of stainless steel should be in accordance with one of the following standards:

BS 1864	Stainless steel milk pipes and fittings. Recessed ring joint type (RJT)
BS 3581	Stainless steel cone joint pipe fittings. (American 3A sanitary standard)
IDF 14*	Milk pipe fittings (ISS)
DIN 11851	Stainless steel pipe fittings.

Various designs of hygienic pipe connections are shown in the diagrams (Fig. 6) at the end of the section.

Fittings of stainless steel must be rigidly secured to the pipe by welding or by an expanding method suitable for the process conditions.

Attachment by 'expanding' is only satisfactory where the design of fitting prevents access by product to the expanded joint.

2. Gaskets and joints

Gaskets and joints should be installed to give an effective seal, being concentric and smooth with the inside bore. They should be retained so that they are not distorted from position when either pressure or vacuum is applied.

3. Connections to tanks

These should normally be made by fittings of the same type as used for pipe length connections. (It is suggested that fittings are preferable to welded joints in order to facilitate inspection of product surfaces.)

4. Fastenings

Exposed threads, screw or bolt heads, nuts, etc., should be eliminated from the product areas.

5. Bends

Bends should be dimensioned to include a centre line radius not less than the pipe outside diameter. End connections should be the same type as those used for pipe length connections. Where fittings are welded on to the ends of a bend the weld should be made on a straight length and be accessible for polishing and grinding.

* IDF 14 is at the time of publication under revision within the International Dairy Federation and is under consideration as basis for an ISO (International Standards Organisation) Recommendation to cover hygienic fittings for the food industries generally.

6. Tee pieces

At the junction of a tee piece, the pipe should be necked out, the side branch weld being on a straight length and accessible for polishing and grinding. End connections should be the same type as those used for pipe length connections.

7. Reducing pieces

Change of cross-sectional area should be effected by a smooth taper without abrupt changes or sharp edges. They should be self-draining in either the vertical or horizontal position and have end connections of the type as used for piping.

8. Installation

Piping should be installed so that pipes are in good alignment and well supported to prevent sagging. All installations should be suitable for either manual or in-place-cleaning and sterilising. Piping should be self-draining with a recommended fall of 1 in. in 10 ft, a minimum being 1 in. in 20 ft for in-place cleaning with the fall towards the CIP return line.

9. Jackets and insulation

Jackets and insulation round the outside of the piping should be free of sharp edges and leave a clear space on each side of pipe connections for inspection and servicing.

10. Layout

The layout should be designed so that as far as practicable all product surfaces may be made visible for inspection.

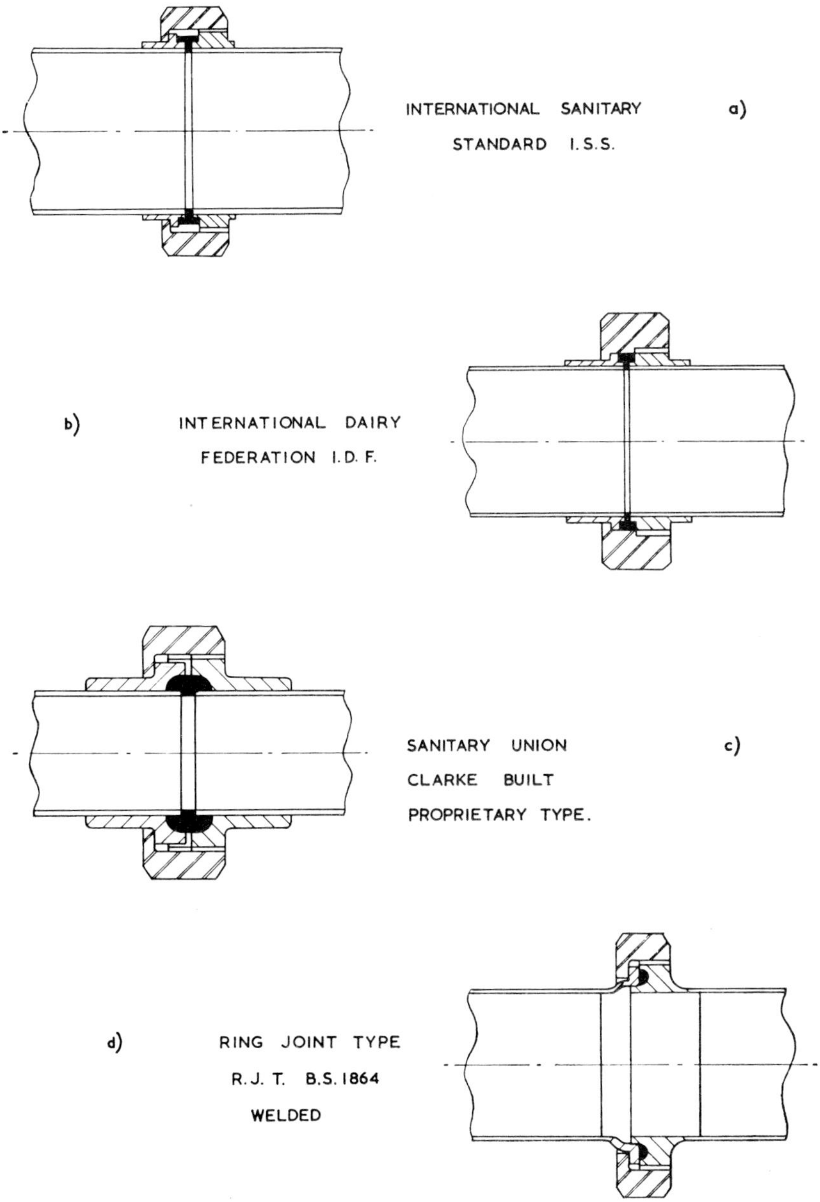

Fig. 6 – Pipe connections.

e) RING JOINT TYPE
R.J.T. B.S. 1864
EXPANDED

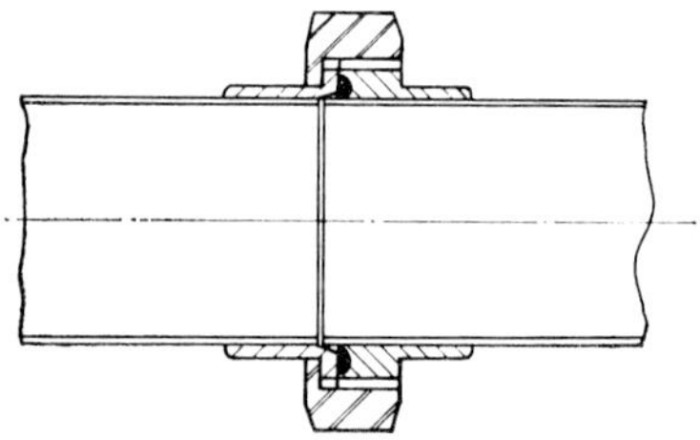

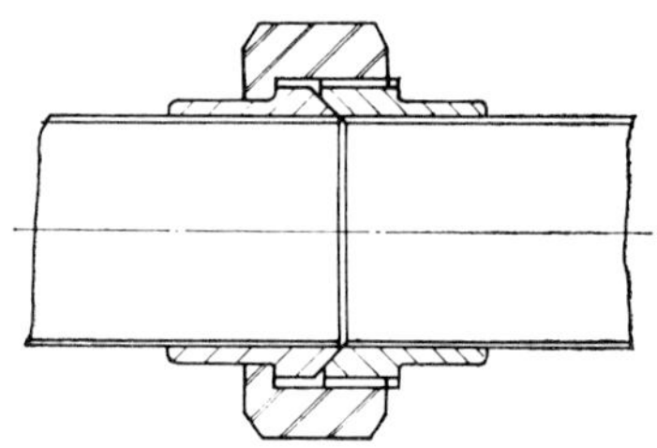

f) AMERICAN 3A CONE JOINT
GROUND SEAT B.S. 3581

g) AMERICAN 3A
GASKET SEAT

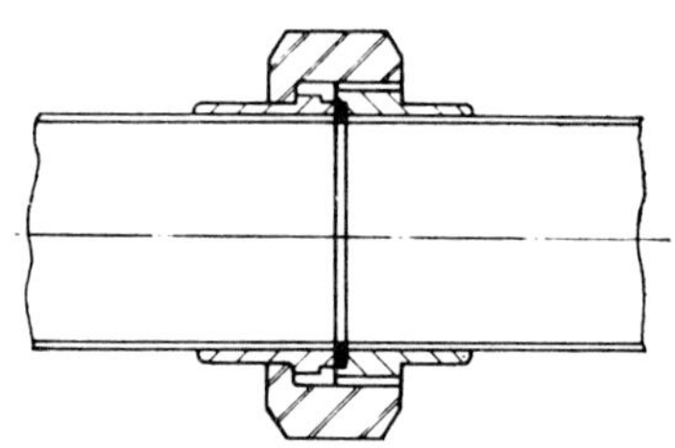

h)

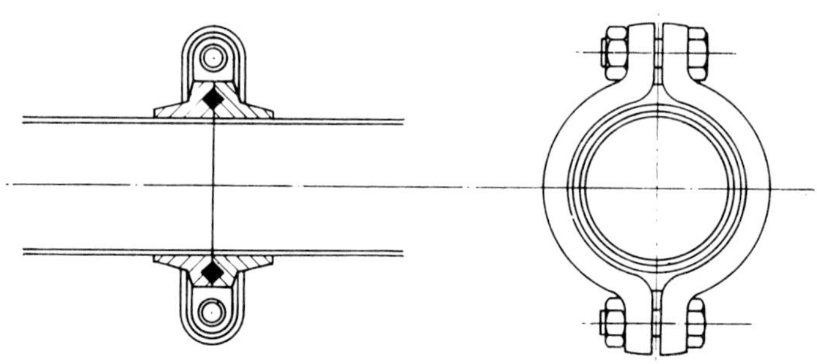

SWEDISH DESIGN CLAMP — SANDVIK PROPRIETARY TYPE

Fig. 6 – Pipe connections (continued).

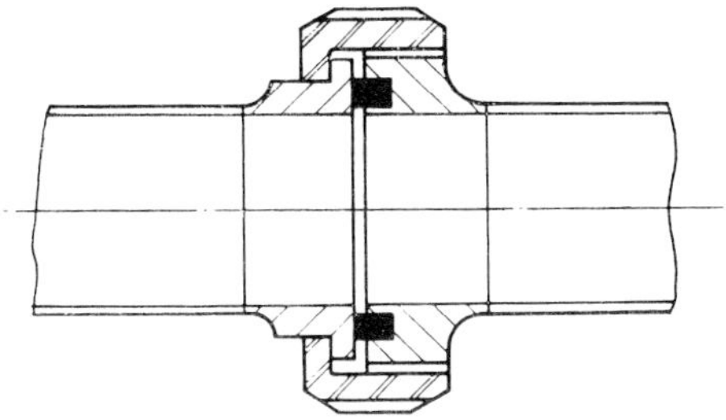

i.) D I N STANDARD
WELDED

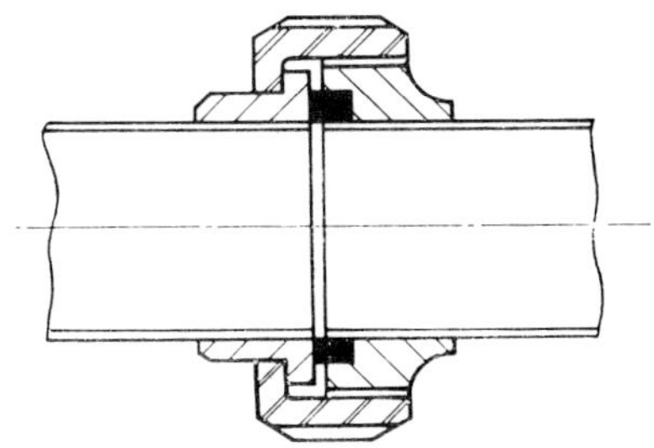

j.) D I N STANDARD
EXPANDED

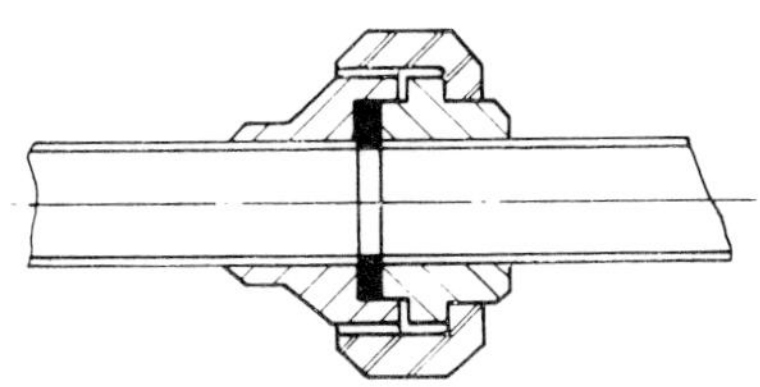

k.) UNION FOR SMALL BORE PIPE
REALM ENGINEERING
PROPRIETARY TYPE

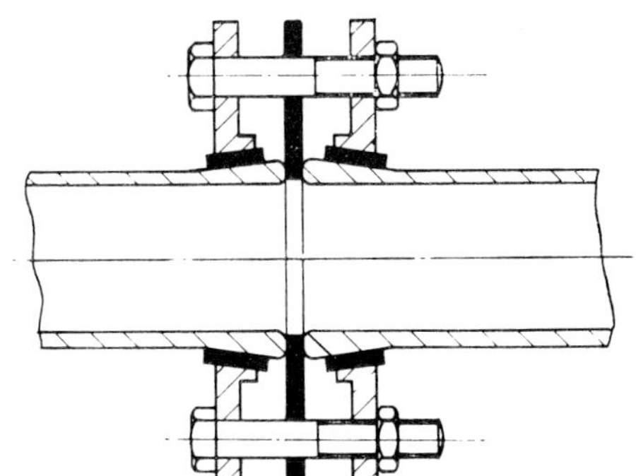

l.) FLANGED UNION FOR
GLASS PIPELINES
Q V F PROPRIETARY TYPE

Fig. 6 – Pipe connections (continued).

a) to B.S. 1864

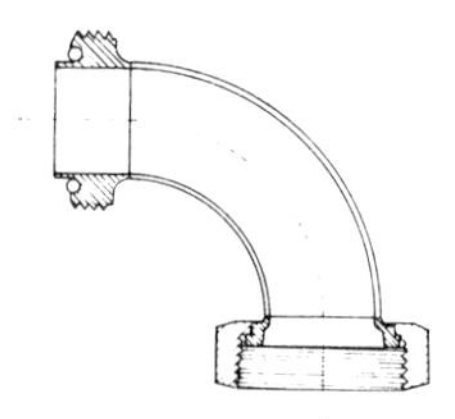

90° BEND - ENDS MALE AND NUT

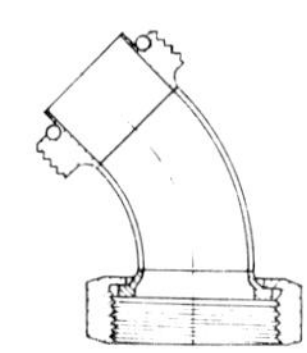

45° BENDS - ENDS MALE AND NUT

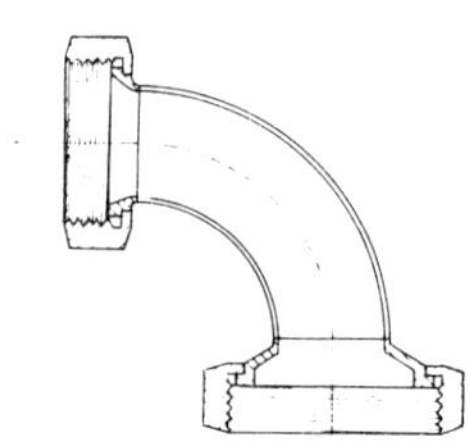

REDUCING BEND - BOTH ENDS NUT

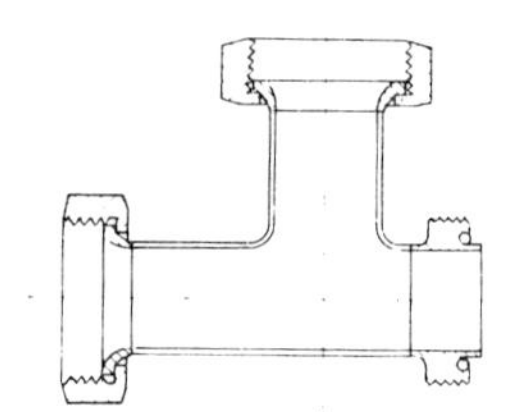

TEE - ENDS MALE AND NUT, BRANCH NUT

Fig. 7 – Typical fittings.

b.) I.S.S. Type.

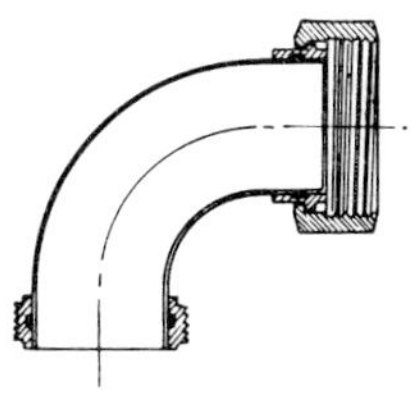

90° BEND - ENDS MALE AND NUT.

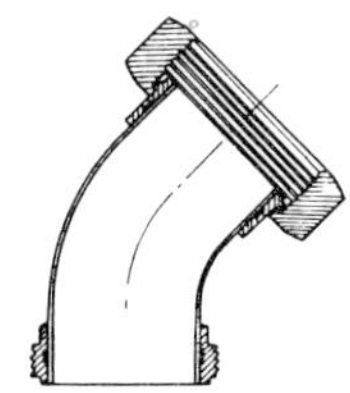

45° BEND - ENDS MALE AND NUT.

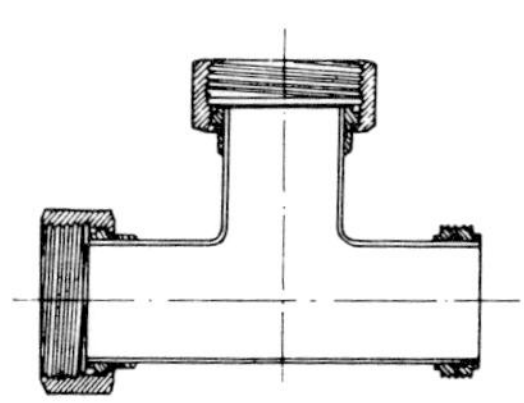

TEE - ENDS MALE AND NUT, BRANCH NUT.

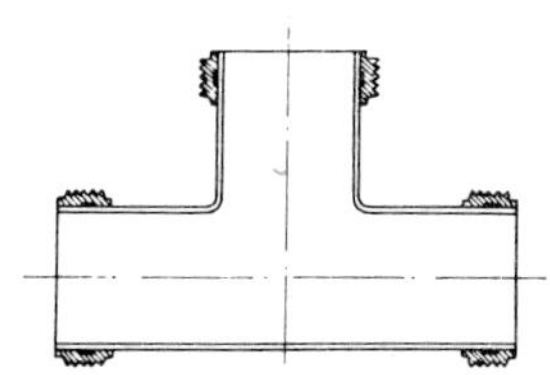

TEE - ALL ENDS MALE.

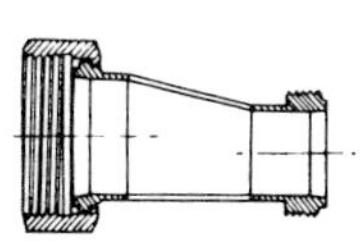

REDUCER - ENDS MALE AND NUT.

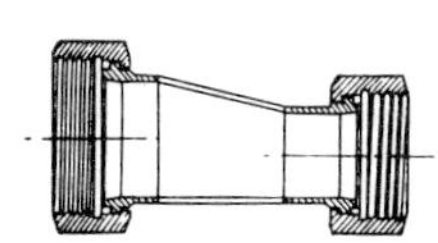

REDUCER - BOTH ENDS NUT.

Fig. 7 – Typical fittings (continued).

MOTORS AND DRIVES

The hygienic design of *driven* plant is dealt with elsewhere in the appropriate sections. This section is concerned with the hygienic design considerations of the *driving* of such plant. This involves two principal aspects:

1) The driving motor
2) The inter-connecting mechanism whereby the drive is transmitted.

1. Motors

In general, the characteristics which give rise to the wide choice of motors available may have little bearing on the hygienic character of the motor provided the motor is *effectively enclosed* (from the hygienic point of view). This may or may not involve 'total enclosure' in the normal sense of the words. The interior of the motor can then be disregarded and the hygienic suitability of the motor assessed on its external features.

From the point of view of hygiene, requirements are few and confined to:

a) a smooth, inert crevice-free and easily-cleaned exterior;
b) adequate clearance for cleaning between the motor body and plinth or floor *or* adequate sealing to the floor to exclude product from this region;
c) lubrication arrangements which either prevent leaking of lubricant from the motor or ensure that leaking lubricant is both immediately visible and safely contained;
d) Suitability of the motor externals in both design and material for the general cleaning processes used in the area (*e.g.* hosing down).

Control gear, if local to the motor, should be housed integrally with the motor in accordance with the above hygienic design considerations or else mounted remote from the motor at a high level on an adjacent structure.

2. Drives

The simplest inter-connection is the direct drive which passes between the seals respectively on the driving motor and the driven plant. The intervening length of shaft is either exposed or, particularly in the case of 'monobloc' type construction, enclosed by the outer casing of the composite unit.

In both cases provision should be made for preventing contamination of the motor internals by leaking product and contamination of the product by leaking lubricant from the motor. In many cases simple thrower rings and housings on the shaft between the driver and the driven casings are sufficient, but when the shaft at this point is enclosed provision should be made for easy inspection by removal of a section of casing or otherwise.

More elaborate forms of drive are common and include V-belt drive, gear train, chain and sprocket, hydraulic transmission. Whenever possible these should be totally enclosed so as to prevent ingress of product or egress of lubricant. In the case of gear, chain and hydraulic drives this is essential, hygienic and functional requirements serving mutual ends. Where cost or other factors preclude complete enclosure the drive is unlikely itself to be designed to meet specific hygienic requirements and should, therefore, be able to withstand frequent hosing down, steam-detergent or other effective cleaning procedure, at appropriate intervals.

NOTE

Effect of surface finish on 'cleanability'

Because of the limited and somewhat contradictory literature on this subject a project was initiated at the National College of Food Technology (a) to survey the literature and (b) to clarify, if possible, any relationship between cleanability and the surface finishes commonly used in British food plant. Since stainless steel is the predominant contact material, work was confined to this.

The scope of the work was naturally limited and considerable extension to alternative soiling and cleaning systems is required but the indications may be summarised as follows:

(a) The nature of soil adherence is as yet little understood.

(b) Relative ease of cleaning can only be determined by strict control of

i) the 'standard' soiling procedure
ii) the 'standard' cleaning procedure
iii) statistical evaluation of a large number of replicate tests.

(c) 'Surface finish' may be expressed in several different ways which do not all measure the same thing and hence would not all result in the same relationship to another variable such as cleanability.

(d) High degrees of surface finish by traditional grinding and buffing do not necessarily result in more easily cleaned surfaces when compared to apparently less polished surfaces such as pickled or descaled surfaces.

(e) Remaining surface irregularities need not be *small* but probably need to be *rounded*, not *jagged*.

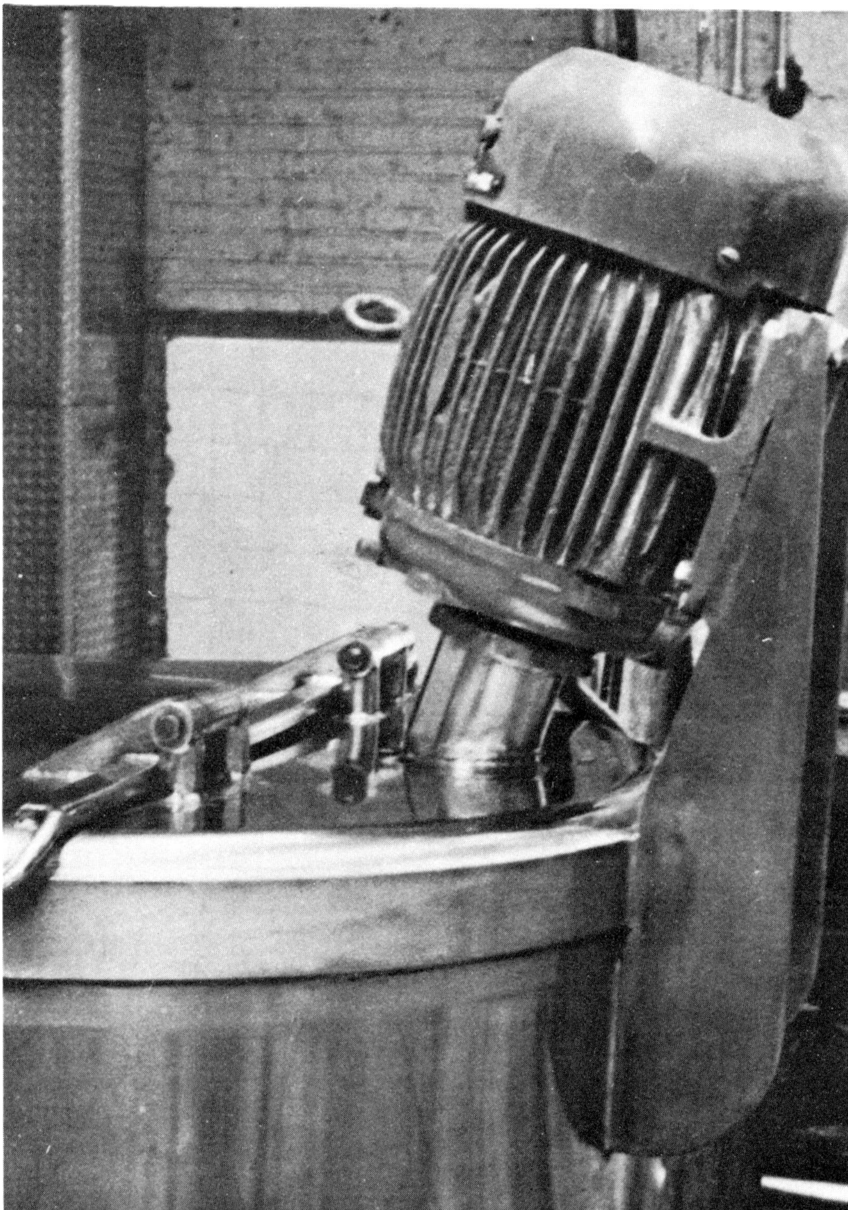

A
Well-designed entry of stirrer drive into vessel. Curved edges to top of vessel. Note hygienic hazards of conventional ribbed motor casing.

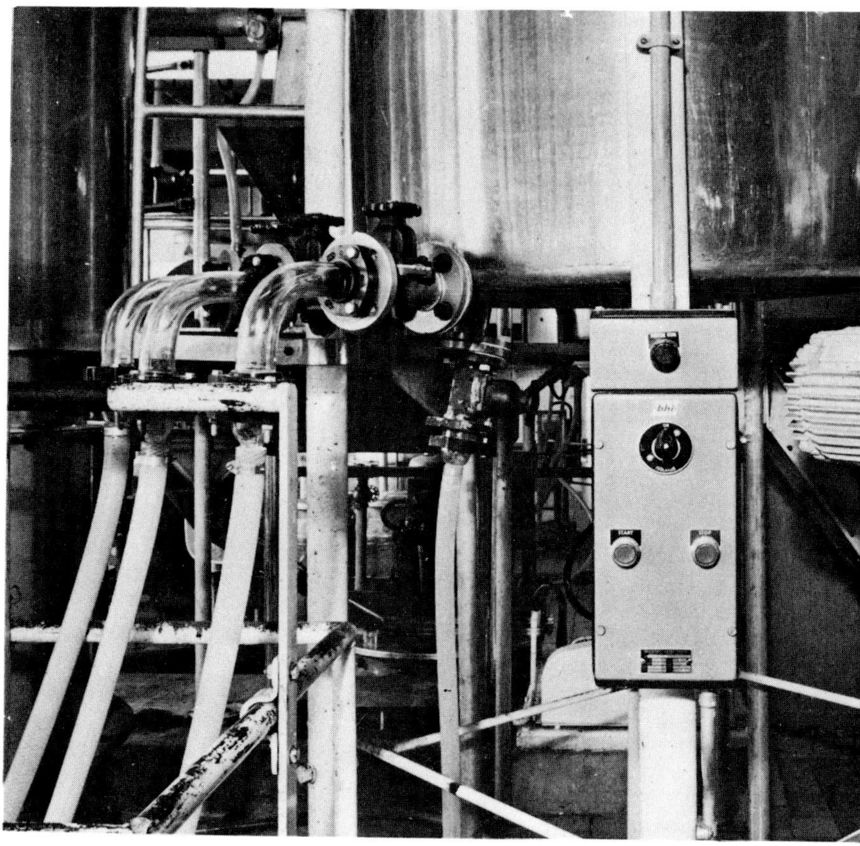

B
Side outlets from dished tank, making it impossible to drain completely.

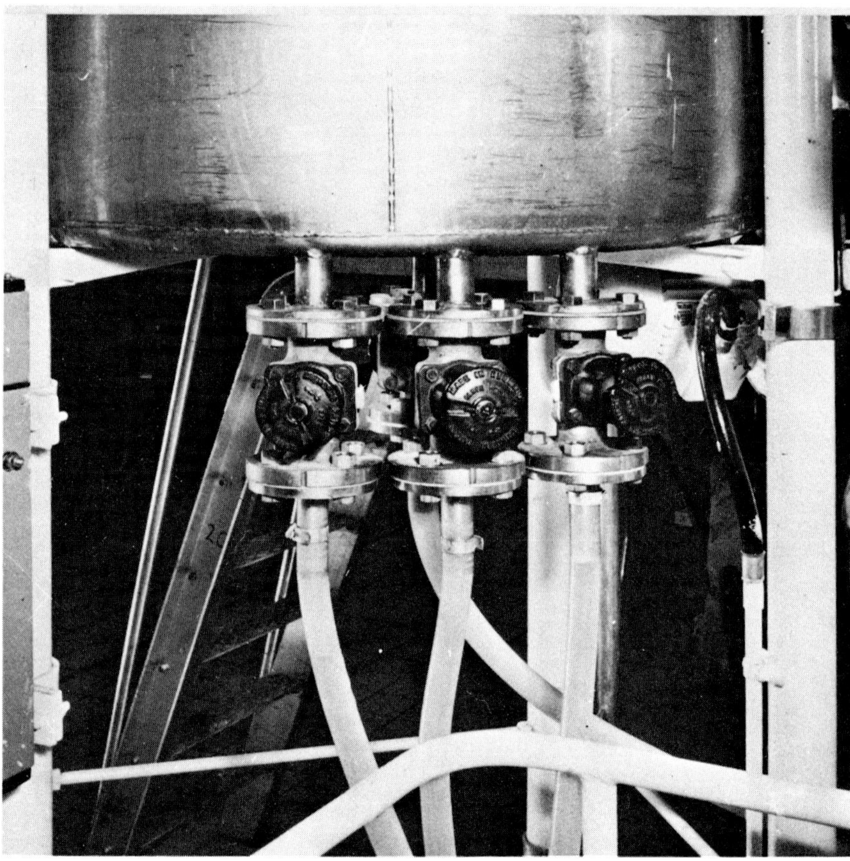

C
Correctly placed outlets from or sloping bottomed vessel.

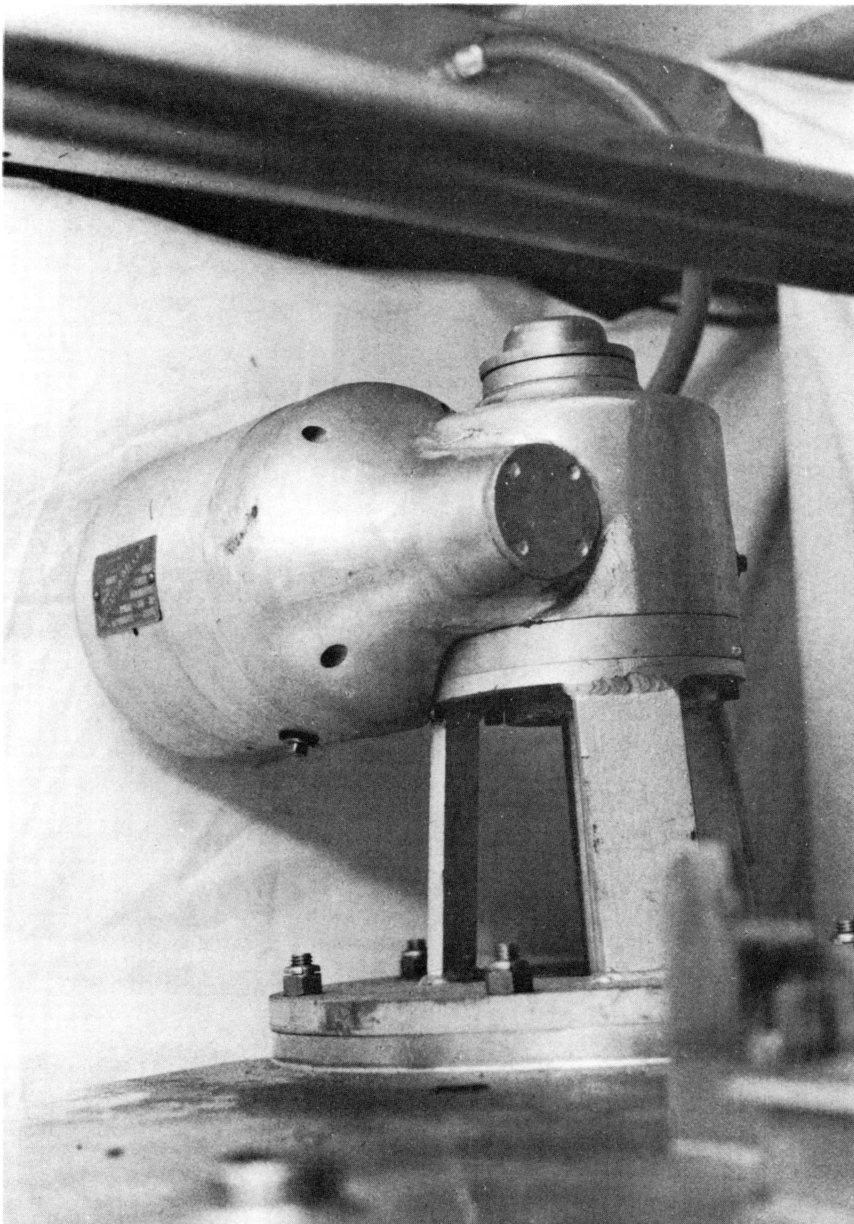

D
Top agitator design with integral motor and gearbox. Note that exposed threads should have been covered with cap nuts.

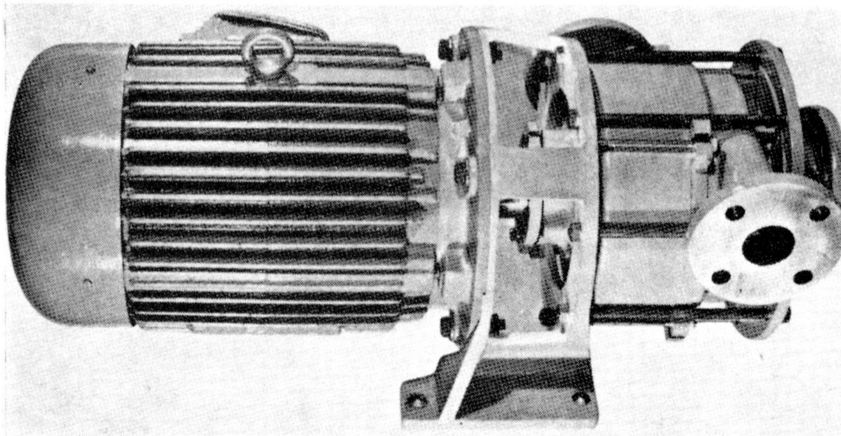

E1
Silicon-iron centrifugal pump, specially designed for the chemical industry, would never be used for foodstuffs but makes an interesting contrast to . . .

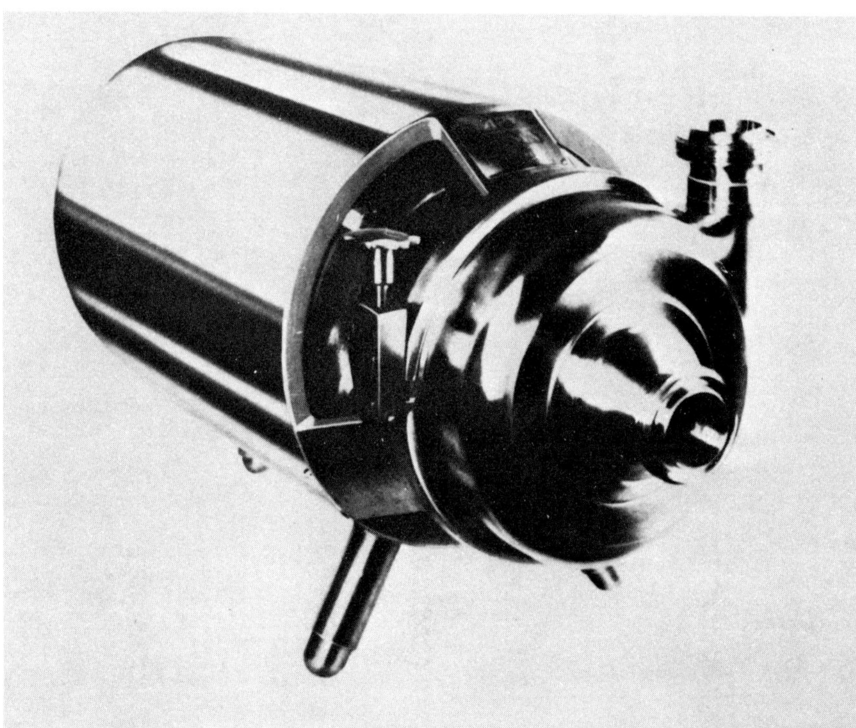

E2
. . the above which is a centrifugal pump specially designed for foodstuffs.

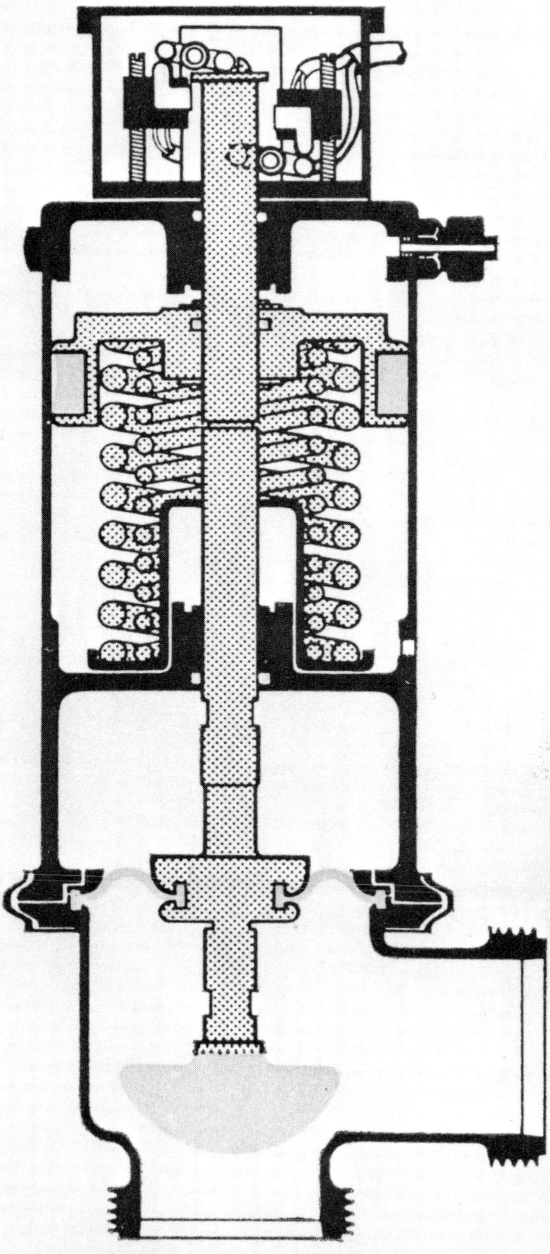

F
Section through diaphragm-sealed hygienic valve.

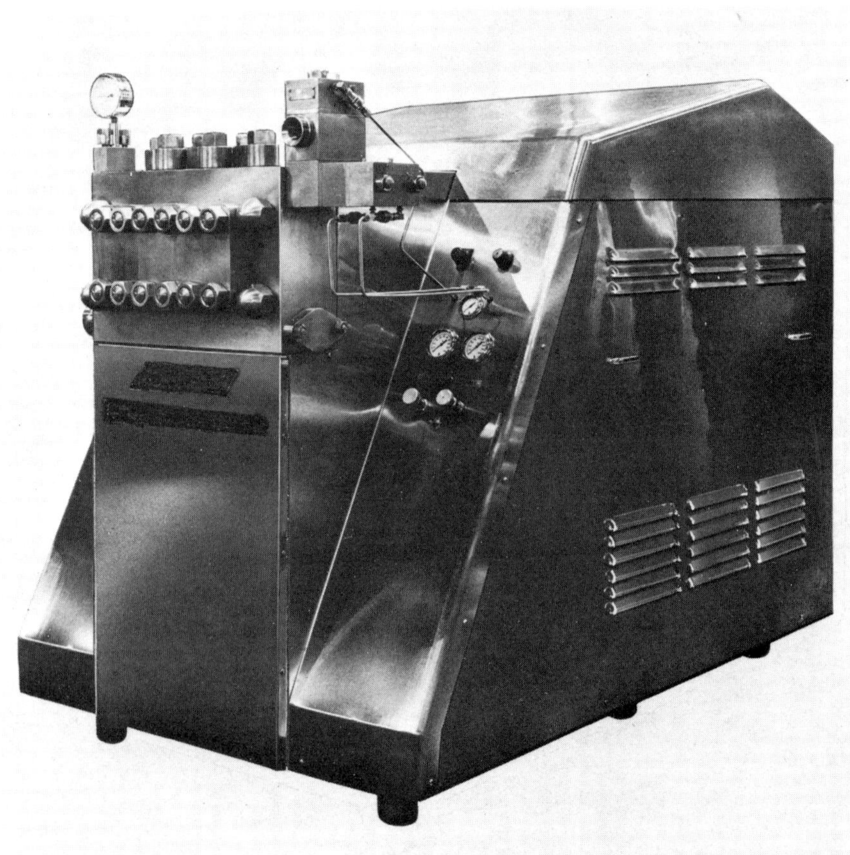

G
Hygienic casing for motor and drive of 100 h.p. homogenizer.

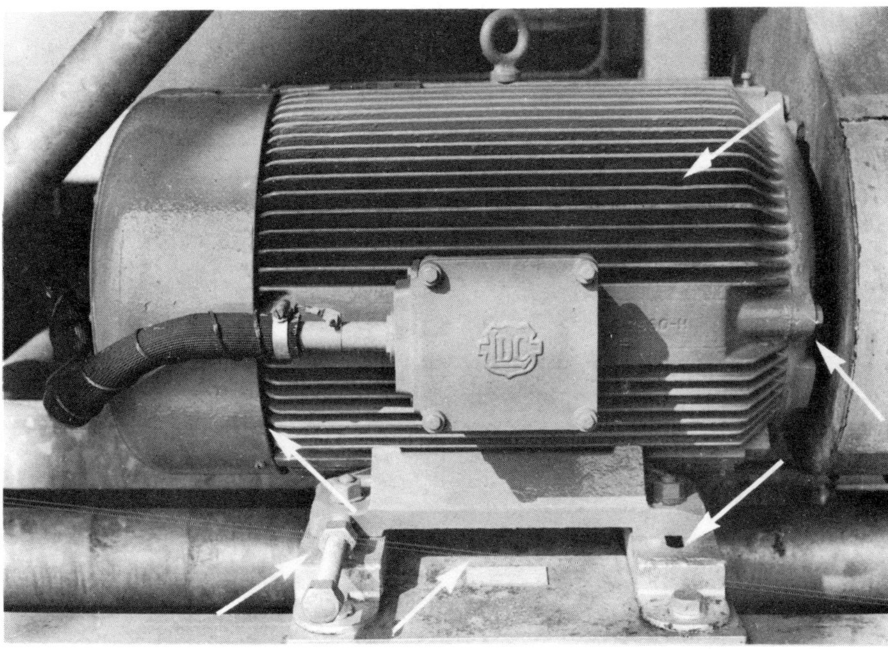

H
Arrows indicate crevices, all of which should be avoided.

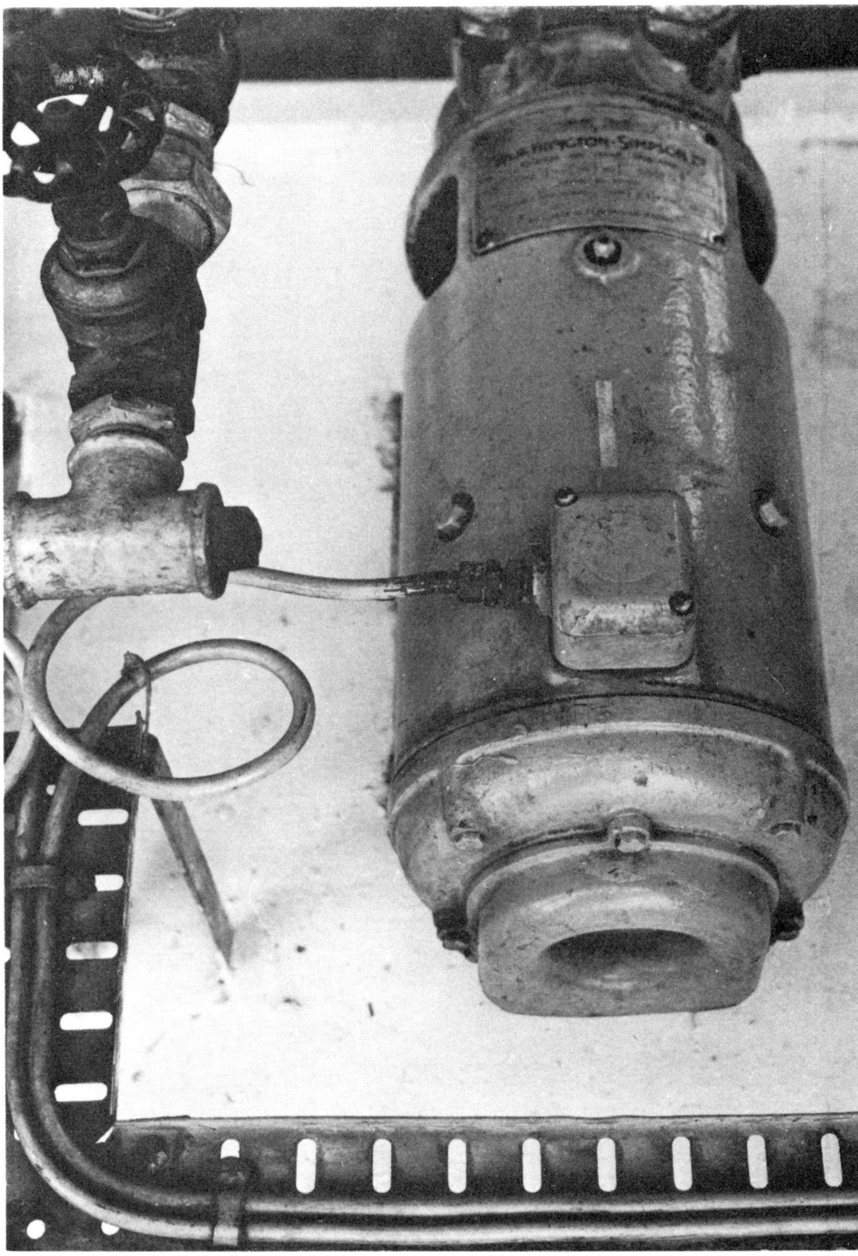

I
Unsatisfactory cable connection to motor and unhygienic support.

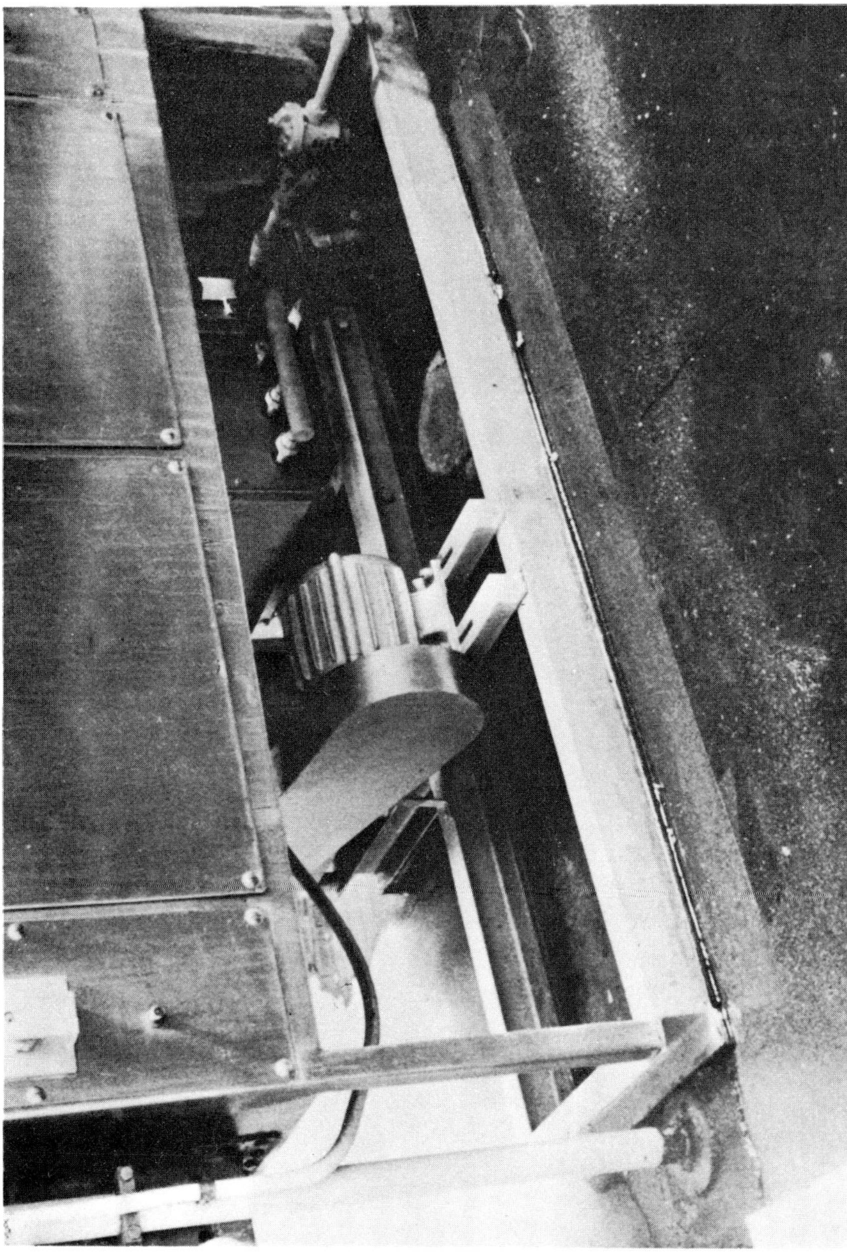

J

Stringers direct on floor, making it impossible to clean inside base.

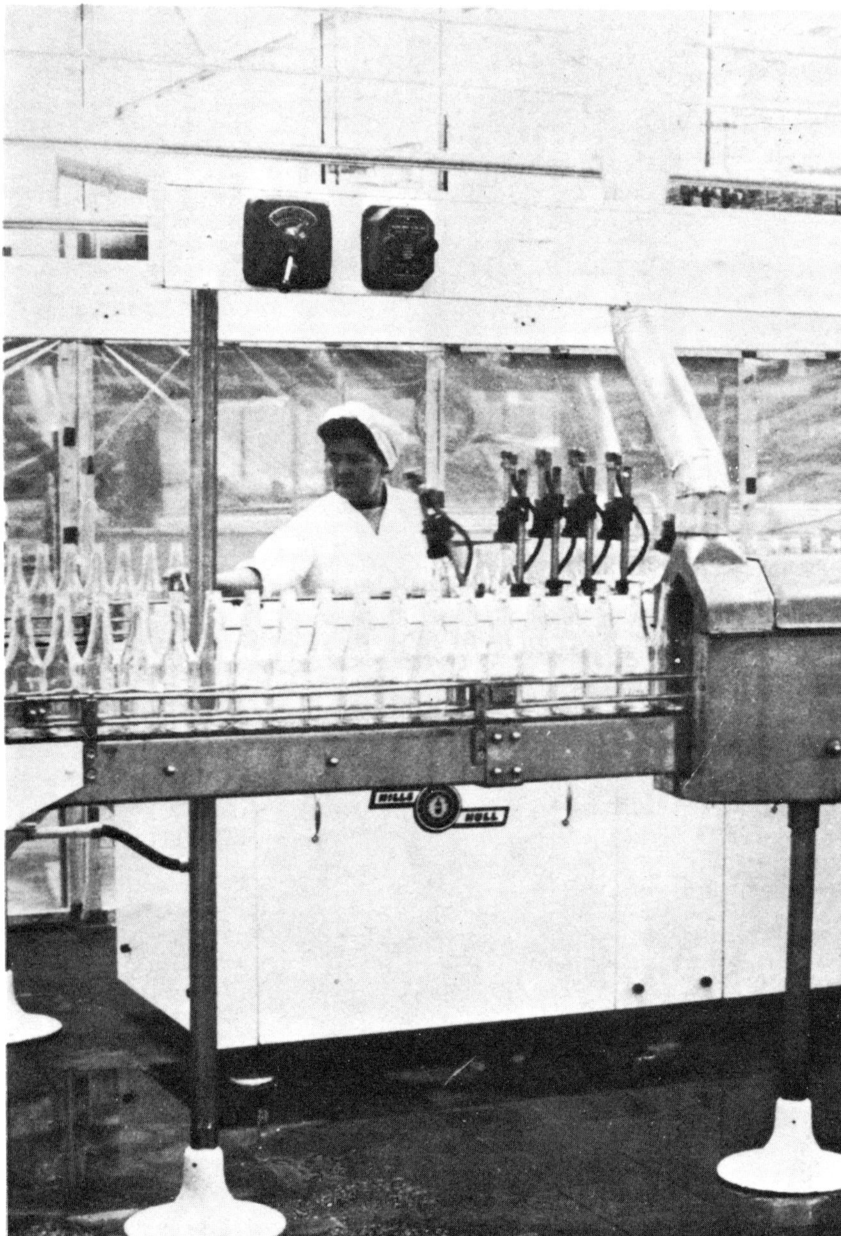

K
Well-designed machine supports. Electrical switchgear mounted well away from floor and plant.

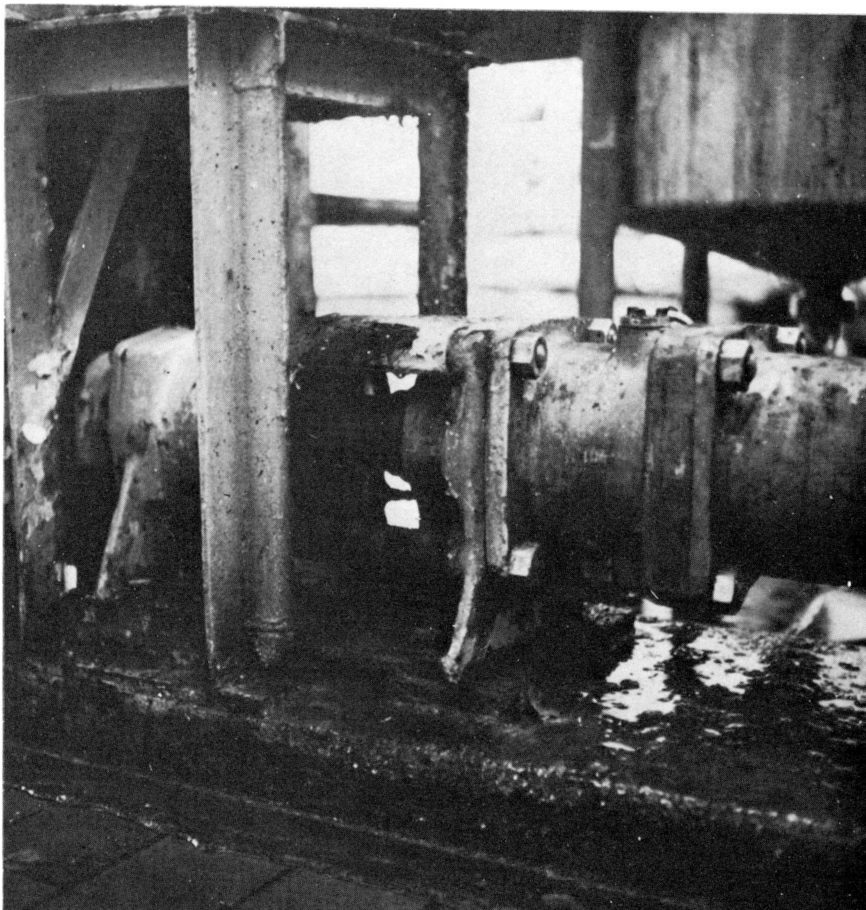

L
An unlimited number of undesirable crevices and corners.

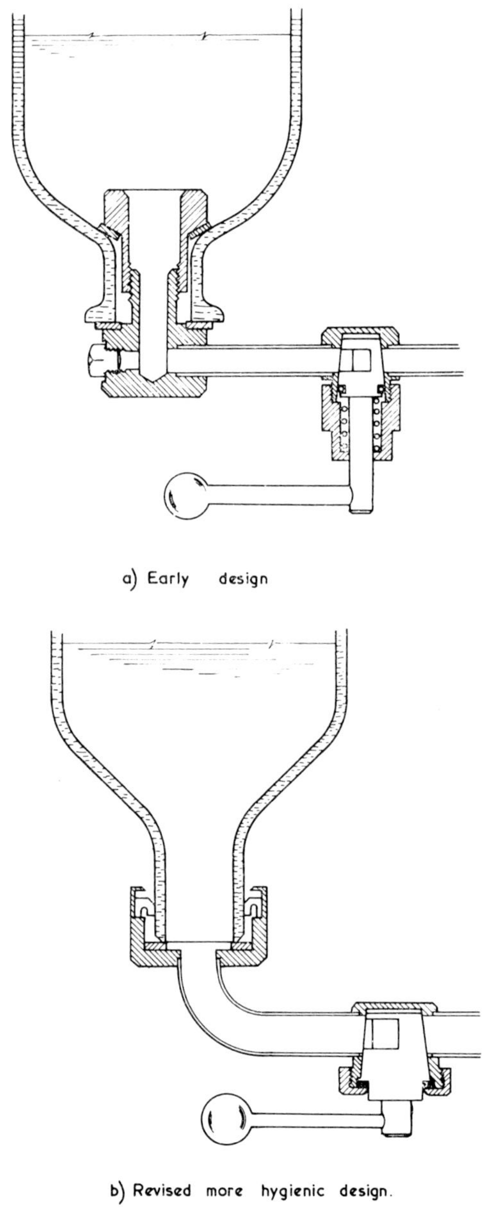

Fig. 8 – Outlet from ultrasonic homogenizer.

Author Index

Subject Index